Clinical Microbiology

Clinical Microbiology

An Introduction for Healthcare Professionals

Jennie Wilson BSc RGN

Surveillance Co-ordinator, Nosocomial Infection Surveillance Unit,
Public Health Laboratory Service, London, UK

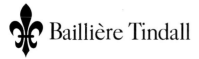 Baillière Tindall

EDINBURGH LONDON NEW YORK OXFORD PHILADELPHIA ST LOUIS SYDNEY
TORONTO 2000

BAILLIÈRE TINDALL
An imprint of Elsevier Limited

First published 1959 (as Bacteriology for Nurses)
Fifth edition 1978 (as Microbiology for Nurses)
Sixth edition 1982
Seventh edition 1993
Eighth edition 2000
    Reprinted 2001, 2003, 2004, 2005 (twice), 2007 (twice)

ISBN-13: 978 0 7020 2316 3
ISBN-10: 0 7020 2316 7

British Library Cataloguing in Publication Data
A catalogue record for this book is available from the British Library

Library of Congress Cataloguing in Publication Data
A catalogue record for this book is available from the Library of Congress

Note
Medical knowledge is constantly changing. As new information becomes available, changes in treatment, procedures, equipment and the use of drugs become necessary. The editors, contributor and the publishers have taken care to ensure that the information given in this text is accurate and up to date. However, readers are strongly advised to confirm that the information, especially with regard to drug usage, complies with the latest legislation and standards of practice.

The Publisher

your source for books,
journals and multimedia
in the health sciences
www.elsevierhealth.com

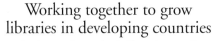

Working together to grow
libraries in developing countries

www.elsevier.com | www.bookaid.org | www.sabre.org

ELSEVIER   BOOK AID International   Sabre Foundation

The publisher's policy is to use paper manufactured from sustainable forests

Printed in China

Contents

Acknowledgements

My thanks go to Dr Dinah Barrie for spending so many hours reading the text for me and providing invaluable advice on the content.

JW, 2000

This book is a new edition of *Microbiology for Nurses* by Vivien Stucke. The publishers wish to acknowledge the work of Vivien Stucke and to thank her for her continuing contribution.

1

The history of microbiology

PLAGUES, PESTILENCE AND CONTROL MEASURES

Microbiology, as a science concerned with the study of organisms not visible to the naked eye, dates from the invention of the microscope. However, measures to protect people from communicable disease, even though the causes were not understood, have been used for thousands of years. The Egyptians believed that plagues and illnesses were punishments from angry gods, but were also the first to record the theory that vapours released from decomposing flesh would cause disease. In the time of the Babylonian empire, 600 years BC, dead bodies were removed from among the living to protect others from infection (Coleman, 1985). In Biblical times, leprosy was recognised to be a communicable disease and lepers were segregated and ostracised. Unfortunately, the diagnosis was frequently inaccurate and in many cases their deformities were due to illnesses other than leprosy.

The ancient Greeks, who had a close association with the Egyptians, were the first to introduce the concept that events were not the result of supernatural influences, rather that there were natural laws that governed them. Hippocrates, and later Aristotle, promoted the use of logic and empirical evidence to demonstrate facts and explain events. Nonetheless, some influential figures of the time, including Galen, a Greek physician, continued to support vague concepts such as the miasmal theory, which associated vapours that fouled the air with the spread of diseases. The belief in miasmas as the cause of disease continued well into the 20th century.

1

The Romans were great proponents of public health. Their towns were planned with wide streets, sewerage systems for waste disposal, aqueducts supplying fresh drinking water, and in some places latrines flushed by running water. Unfortunately, after the collapse of the Roman empire, the influence of the church increased in the West, bringing with it a belief in the supernatural origin of disease and a lack of interest in hygiene. In the East – in Arabia and India, for example – an appreciation of science continued and progress in understanding diseases such as smallpox was made in these parts of the world.

During the Middle Ages in Europe, infection was a common cause of death, although records were poor and different diseases were not clearly defined. Leprosy was imported by travellers from the East and bubonic plague was thought to be introduced in the 13th century by Tartars who catapulted their dead into a city they were besieging. The rats that were the natural host of the plague bacterium, *Yersinia pestis*, flourished in the overcrowded and unhygienic conditions found in many cities and were the source of infection for many poor people. The bacterium could also be transmitted directly from person to person, and by human fleas, which were common during that time. Efforts were made to isolate affected people in an attempt to prevent spread. The Venetians introduced the concept of quarantine by requiring incoming ships to wait for 40 days on an island before being allowed to enter the city. The first epidemic, 'the Great Pestilence' (commonly known as the Black Death), was probably responsible for the deaths of a third of the population of Britain in the 30 years after 1348. The disease then became endemic in Britain, periodically causing outbreaks, when thousands of people died, for the next 300 years. Syphilis was also a common infection, and a major pandemic occurred in Europe towards the end of the 15th century.

Plague declined after the end of the 17th century but was replaced by other infections. Smallpox became the most widespread fatal disease in the 18th century and typhus, spread by the human body louse and associated with poor hygiene and overcrowding, caused major epidemics in the 1740s and 1750s. Children commonly died of throat infections such as diphtheria and scarlet fever, and tuberculosis was a constant threat.

In the 1800s the problems were compounded by an increase in population, together with the industrial revolution. This saw the development of new industrial towns, built with minimal planning and with no form of drainage for sewage or supplies of fresh water. The resulting communities were crowded and squalid. Excreta were discarded in the streets and carcasses and other waste material left to rot in the open. Infections spread by contaminated water, such as typhoid and infantile diarrhoea, became widespread under these conditions. In 1831 cholera, until then not seen in Britain, was introduced from India via traders from Russia. It spread rapidly through the country, causing the deaths of 60 000 people, especially those living in poor and overcrowded conditions.

THE FIRST VACCINE

The concept of vaccination was known in India and China, where the inoculation of fluid from a smallpox vesicle on to a scratch on a child's skin was used to induce a mild illness and subsequent immunity from the infection. When knowledge of smallpox inoculation spread from the East into the Western world in the 18th century, this practice was used by some in an attempt to prevent infection. However, it was Edward Jenner, in 1796, who introduced a much safer practice that was eventually to be given the name 'vaccination' by Louis Pasteur. Jenner noticed that dairy-maids who had developed cowpox lesions on their hands were protected against smallpox. He proposed that the fluid from a cowpox lesion could be used to protect against smallpox if it was inoculated into the skin and duly carried out the procedure successfully on an 8-year-old boy (Figure 1.1). Since cowpox was not a serious infection this form of vaccination was quite safe and enabled the spread of smallpox to be gradually controlled. However, it was not until the work of Pasteur in the mid-19th century that vaccines against other infections began to be made.

PUBLIC HEALTH REFORMS

The cholera outbreak finally forced the authorities to take action. The Poor Law was reviewed in 1832 and Poor Law Commissioners were appointed to oversee the changes required in local government. Edwin Chadwick became the secretary to the Commissioners. In 1942 he produced a detailed report analysing the living conditions of the poor and highlighting inadequate sewage disposal and contaminated water supplies as major sources of disease. This work was tremendously influential, resulting in the Factory

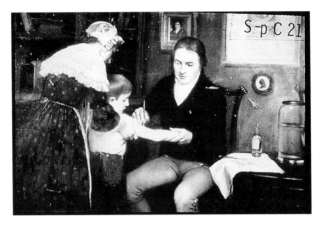

Figure 1.1 The first vaccination: Edward Jenner, 1796. Source: Wellcome Institute Library, London.

Act, passed in 1847 to regulate the working hours and conditions of work for women and children, and the Act for Promoting Public Health, passed in 1848. This act resulted in the establishment of sewage drainage systems and piped supplies of fresh water. It also established the role of the medical officer responsible for initiating the improvements and inspectors to monitor their implementation.

In 1836, the Births and Deaths Registration Act was passed and Dr William Farr was appointed to administer it. He was able to compile accurate records and make data available on which public health decisions could be made. These dramatic improvements were all made while the theory of miasmas as the cause of disease still predominated and was believed even by Chadwick. Clear evidence that such vapours from filth were not responsible was finally provided by a protégé of Chadwick's, Dr John Snow. Using Farr's data he studied the occurrence of cholera in London and realised that there was a concentration of cases around a public water pump in Broad Street, Soho. Once the pump was inactivated, the epidemic stopped. In a further analysis he demonstrated that the incidence of the infection was much lower in those areas with cleaner water supplies and the significance of clean water finally began to be appreciated (Figure 1.2).

Other doctors were also beginning to demonstrate that diseases were not spread by miasmas. Dr William Budd studied the epidemiology of typhoid in a village near Bristol and concluded that

MISTAKING CAUSE FOR EFFECT.

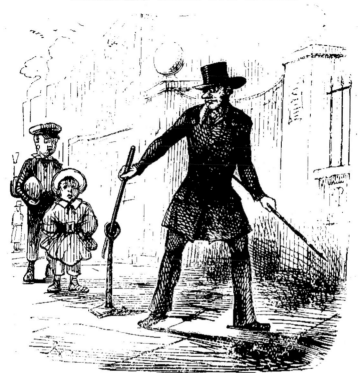

Boy. "I SAY, TOMMY, I'M BLOW'D IF THERE ISN'T A MAN A TURNING ON THE CHOLERA."

Figure 1.2   Cartoon from *Punch*, 1849.

the infection was spread by drinking water contaminated by excreta from the sick. He also proposed that tuberculosis was spread by germs in the sputum of those affected.

When Gladstone became Prime Minister in 1868 he began the creation of a national Public Health Service that encompassed food hygiene, disease control, child welfare and maternity and sexually transmitted disease clinics, as well as sewage and water supplies, and also had responsibility for municipal hospitals. This system continued until the National Health Service was formed in 1948.

THE PREVENTION OF INFECTION IN HOSPITALS

The first hospitals to care for the sick were recorded in Asia, Egypt, Palestine and Greece several thousand years before the birth of Christ. Although available treatments for disease were limited, these hospitals had high standards of hygiene and many of the principles of infection control were in place, such as the isolation of infected patients, avoiding touching wounds and the use of cleaning and hot ovens to sterilise instruments. Unfortunately, standards deteriorated after the fall of the Roman Empire and in the Western world hospitals become overcrowded and unhygienic. By the end of the 19th century, more than half of patients were dying of infection following surgery, and infection after surgery or childbirth was considered inevitable by many clinicians (Simpson 1869). Doctors were difficult to convince of the significance of cleanliness in the prevention of infection, preferring to blame 'intrinsic defects' in their patients or 'the atmosphere'. Although some doctors recognised the importance of cleanliness, their opinions were largely disregarded. An American, Oliver Wendell Holmes, wrote about the importance of washing thoroughly and changing clothes after contact with a case of puerperal fever in 1843 (Holmes 1843).

The role of hands in the transmission of infection was clearly demonstrated by the work of Ignaz Semmelweis, an Austrian obstetrician, in 1847. He suspected that 'cadaveric particles' were responsible for causing puerperal fever in women in labour, and that these were carried by doctors and students, who would conduct post-mortem examinations in the mortuary on women who had died, and then examine women in labour or following delivery. Once he had instituted a policy that all should wash their hands in chlorinated lime between contact with cadavers and visiting women in labour, the incidence of puerperal fever dropped dramatically (Newsom 1993). Unfortunately, this work was not published for many years and Semmelweis's abrasive personality meant that he was largely ignored by his colleagues.

In the latter part of the 19th century Florence Nightingale began to have a major influence on the provision of care for the sick. Her *Notes on Nursing: What It Is and What It Is Not*, published in 1859, emphasised the importance of cleanliness and ventilation and also promoted a healthy diet and safe storage of food. However, even in the 1960s, the significance of hands in the transmission of infection was not fully appreciated and airborne transmission was considered more important. Mortimer et al (1966), in a study on babies in a special care nursery, was able to demonstrate that staphylococci were transmitted between babies during the period when staff were instructed not to wash their hands between contacts, but were rarely transmitted when staff were instructed to wash their hands. It is perhaps a measure of the progress made in our understanding of the transmission of infection in hospital that such a study would now be considered too hazardous to repeat.

THE NEW SCIENCE OF MICROBIOLOGY

Most of the early progress in understanding the spread of disease was made in the absence of knowledge about bacteria as the cause of infection. Indeed, many of the pioneers such as Chadwick and Florence Nightingale firmly believed in the theory of miasmas. The suggestion that diseases could be caused by some agent that could then be transmitted to others was put forward as early as 1546, when an Italian clinician, Fracastoro, published a paper called *De contagione*. He proposed that each disease was caused by a particular 'seed' or germ, and that these could be transmitted by direct contact with sick people, by contact with their excreta, clothing or bedding, or through the air. However, these ideas were ignored for many years, even when the Dutchman Antonie van Leeuwenhoek observed bacteria under his primitive microscope 100 years later. Small creatures such as grubs and fleas were considered to arise through spontaneous generation and it was not until the mid-19th century, and the studies of Louis Pasteur in France and Robert Koch in Germany, that bacteria were clearly demonstrated as a cause of disease.

Prior to the work of Pasteur, it had been suggested that microbes might be involved in the process of fermentation. However, Pasteur clearly demonstrated that this was the case and that some microbes could cause fermentation in the absence of oxygen. He then went on to link specific microbes with particular forms of fermentation and found microbes responsible for the souring of milk. Another major discovery was that heating could be used to prevent harmful microbes from spoiling the fermentation process, and these principles of 'pasteurisation' are a key feature in the control of microbial contamination today. Pasteur then moved his attention to infectious disease, demonstrating that anthrax was caused by a microorganism and subsequently developing vaccines for anthrax, chicken cholera and rabies.

Joseph Lister, working in Scotland, was interested in whether Pasteur's discoveries could explain gangrene and the death of his patients following compound fracture or amputation. He applied carbolic acid to compound fractures and used phenolic dressings on wounds in an attempt to prevent the growth of bacteria. The resulting reductions in mortality were dramatic but, although they were published in 1867, it was many years before they were accepted.

Major progress in the science of microbiology was made possible by the work of Robert Koch, a doctor of medicine and a contemporary of Pasteur, who was responsible for developing the techniques that form the basis of modern diagnostic microbiology. He developed liquid and solid culture media and noted that the organisms grew in clusters called colonies, which eventually became visible to the naked eye. He saw that these colonies were characteristic and had defined requirements for growth. He was concerned about anthrax in sheep and cattle, and showed that the large, sporing bacillus always present in the blood of the animals who died could be cultured, used to re-infect other animals and then recovered again. These observations formed the basis of *Koch's postulates*, which can be used to establish the causative relationship between a microorganism and disease:

- the microbe must be regularly isolated from cases of the illness
- it must be grown in pure culture
- the typical illness must result when a pure culture is inoculated into a susceptible animal
- it must be possible to isolate the microbe from animals in which the illness has been induced.

These postulates could prove the causes of many bacterial and fungal infections but have to be modified for application to other infections, particularly those caused by viruses, which cannot be grown in culture. Koch identified and isolated many microbes using these methods, including tuberculosis. The same methods were also adopted by other workers and the causative microorganisms of many diseases began to be identified.

Towards the end of the 19th century, Roux and Yersin demonstrated that the effects of the diphtheria bacillus were caused by a toxin that it secreted, and this led to the development of the diphtheria antitoxin in 1896. A former colleague of Koch's, Paul Ehrlich, started work on standardising preparations of diphtheria toxin and then began a search for chemicals that could be used to treat infectious diseases. In 1910, he discovered Salvarsan 606, which was used successfully for many years as a treatment for syphilis. Following this lead, the search for chemotherapeutic agents intensified and in 1935 the dye Prontosil was found by Domagk to have antimicrobial activity. This dye was in fact broken down in the body to form the effective compound sulphonamide. Other sulphonamides were subsequently developed and widely used in the treatment of infection.

The treatment of infectious disease was transformed by the development of antimicrobial agents, in particular penicillin. This naturally occurring antimicrobial agent was discovered by Sir Alexander Fleming (Figure 1.3), who noticed that colonies of staphylococci were unable to grow next to a fungus, *Penicillium notatum*, which was inadvertently contaminating the culture plate. Considerable further work was required before the antibacterial substances were purified by Florey and Chain in the 1940s, but penicillin finally went into commercial production soon afterwards. The next few decades saw the discovery of many other naturally occurring antimicrobial agents and chemical modifications of their structure enabled a wide range of different drugs with activity against a variety of bacteria to be developed.

The study of viruses has developed more slowly because their small size meant they were not visible under conventional light microscopes and they could not be cultured in the absence of living cells. Tissue culture techniques were developed in the 1950s and from that time considerable advances in the development of viral vaccines were made. Unlike antibacterials, antiviral agents have been difficult to find, since a successful agent must be able to destroy the virus inside a host cell without damaging the tissues of the host.

CHALLENGES FOR THE FUTURE

In the developed countries of the world there has been a dramatic fall in the number of deaths caused by infectious disease since the beginning of the 20th century. These changes have been possible because of widespread immunisation programmes against a range

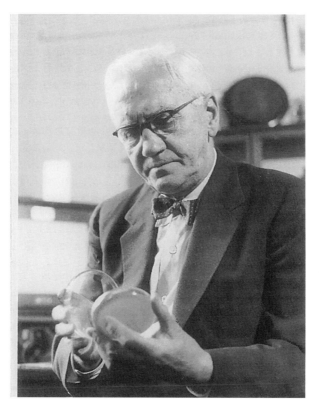

Figure 1.3 Sir Alexander Fleming (1881–1955).

of diseases and the availability of effective antimicrobial agents with which to treat infection. Some diseases have been completely eradicated as a result. The last outbreak of smallpox in the UK occurred in 1901 and the last naturally occurring case in the world occurred in Somalia in 1977; by 1980 the disease was considered to have been completely eradicated (Department of Health, 1996). Immunisation against other diseases, for example polio and diphtheria, has resulted in their virtual eradication from developed countries. Other infections, for example measles, at the peak of outbreaks in the 1950s and 1960s caused over 800 000 infections annually in England and Wales. Many of these patients would have developed complications related to the infection and some would have died. Since the introduction of the measles vaccine in

1968, and later the combined measles, mumps and rubella (MMR) vaccine in 1988, the incidence of measles infection has gradually reduced and now fewer than 1000 cases of the infection are reported annually (Department of Health 1996).

Improvements in living conditions and general health have also led to the decline of other infections, most notably tuberculosis, which previously thrived in debilitated people living in overcrowded conditions (Figure 1.4)

However, we should not be complacent about our ability to prevent and control infectious disease. In developing countries infectious disease still accounts for a high proportion of mortality, with infantile diarrhoea remaining the single most important cause of death. New infections such as the human immunodeficiency virus (HIV) are having particularly devastating effects in these countries, where access to education and healthcare is limited.

Even in developed countries new threats are emerging. The 1990s have seen the emergence of bovine spongiform encephalopathy and evidence that this prion, highly resistant to normal methods of eradication, can be transmitted to humans in food (Haywood, 1997). There is also increasing concern that many of the antimicrobial agents that have been available to us for less

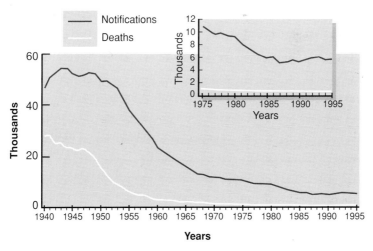

Figure 1.4   Notifications of tuberculosis and deaths in England and Wales (1940–1995). Reproduced from Department of Health (1996) *Immunisation against Infectious Disease*. HMSO, London.

than a century may lose their value because of the widespread emergence of resistant pathogens (Livermore 1998). Perhaps one of the greatest challenges for the future is controlling the use of the antimicrobial agents, which have become such a valuable tool in the fight against infection.

REFERENCES

Coleman, V. (1985) *The Story of Medicine*. Robert Hale, London.
Department of Health (1996) *Immunisation Against Infectious Disease*. HMSO, London.
Haywood, A.M. (1997) Transmissible spongiform encephalopathies. *N. Engl. J. Med.*, **337**(25), 1821–1828.
Holmes, O.W. (1843) The contagiousness of puerperal fever. *N. Engl. J. Med.*, **1**, 503–530.
Livermore, D. (1998) Multi-resistance and the 'superbugs'. *Comm. Dis. Public Health*, **1**(2), 74–76.
Mortimer, E.A., Wolinsky, E., Gonzaga, A.J. *et al.* (1966) Role of hands in the transmission of staphylococcal infections. *Br. Med. J.*, **1**, 319–322.
Newsom, S.W.B. (1993) Ignaz Philip Semmelweis. *J. Hosp. Infect.*, **23**, 175–188.
Simpson, J. (1869) Some propositions on hospitalism. *Lancet*, **16 Oct**, 535–538.

FURTHER READING

Calman, K. (1998) The 1848 Public Health Act and its relevance to improving public health in England now. *Br. Med. J.*, **317**, 596–598.
Kiple, K.F. (ed.) (1993) *The Cambridge World History of Human Disease*. Cambridge University Press, Cambridge.
Morgan, D. (ed.) (1989) Infection Control. *The British Medical Association Guide*. Edward Arnold, London.
Parker, L. (1990) From pestilence to asepsis. *Nurs. Times*, **86**(49), 63–67.
Selwyn, S. (1991) Hospital infection – the first 2500 years. *J. Hosp. Infect.*, **18**(Suppl. A), 5–65.

2

Microorganisms and their properties

INTRODUCTION

Microorganisms are living forms that are too small to be seen without the aid of a microscope, and include bacteria, fungi and protozoa. Two other organisms are also usually considered as microorganisms; viruses, which are not true living cells, and helminths, the parasitic flukes, round and flat worms, many of which have quite complex structures and are large enough to be seen by the naked eye. List 2.1 summarises the main types of microorganism.

All living material is made up of similar structures called cells. The most primitive forms of life consist of single cells, while higher plants and animals are made up of millions of cells, which form into groups to perform particular functions. All cells consist of a nucleus and cytoplasm enclosed in a semipermeable membrane, and in some cases a cell wall. There are two basic cell types: eukaryotic cells, found in higher forms of life such as animals and plants, and the more primitive prokaryotic cells, unique to bacteria.

THE STRUCTURE AND PROPERTIES OF EUKARYOTIC CELLS

Eukaryotic cells have a complex structure, with a range of distinct organelles in the cytoplasm (Figure 2.1), each of which carries out a particular function for the cell. Special transport proteins carry molecules from one organelle to another as required (Table 2.1). The nucleus contains the genome in the form of deoxyribonucleic acids (DNA) arranged into several chromosomes and surrounded

List 2.1 Microorganisms – a simple classification

Eukaryote
- Fungi, e.g. yeasts, moulds

Microscopic animals
- Protozoa (unicellular), e.g. amoebae, malarial parasites
- Helminths (multicellular), e.g. tapeworms, flukes, roundworms

Microscopic plants
- Algae (all non-pathogenic)

Prokaryotes
- Bacteria
- Actinomycetes (filamentous bacteria), e.g. *Streptomyces*
- Rickettsias (parasitic intracellular bacteria)
  - Rickettsias
  - Chlamydias
- Mycoplasmas (bacteria without cell walls)
- Phototrophic bacteria (produce oxygen in sunlight)
  - Cyanobacteria, e.g. blue-green algae
  - Photosynthetic, e.g. purple, purple sulphur bacteria

Viruses: non-cellular microorganisms

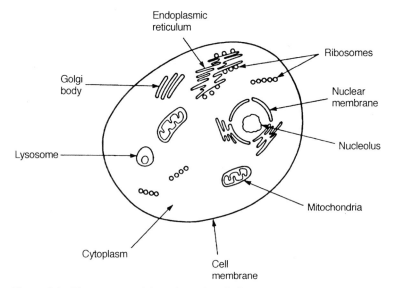

Figure 2.1 The structure of the eukaryotic cell. Source: Wilson, 1995.

Table 2.1   Eukaryotic cell organelles and their function

Organelle	Function
Nucleus	Contains genetic information. Site of DNA synthesis
Plasma membrane	Controls the movement of substances into and out of the cell and responds to external signals
Endoplasmic reticulum	Synthesises lipids, directs movement of lipids and proteins through the cell
Golgi apparatus	Modifies and sorts proteins and lipids
Cytoskeleton	Internal framework of the cell, provides transport structure
Ribosomes	Translate sequences of RNA into protein
Mitochondria	Oxidise glucose and fatty acids to make energy (ATP)
Lysosomes	Contain enzymes that break down unwanted molecules

by a nuclear membrane. The DNA determines what proteins can be made in the cell. It is composed of a series of nucleotides; sugar and phosphate molecules attached to a base molecule, and two strands of DNA are held together by weak bonds, which form between the bases (see Figure 2.2). The sequence of base molecules forms the genetic code, each set of three bases corresponding to a particular amino acid. An average protein contains 400 amino acids and each section of DNA that codes for a single protein is called a gene.

Eukaryotic cells are enclosed by a plasma membrane, which controls the entry of nutrients into, and the discharge of waste products out of, the cell and responds to signals in the environment, such as hormones. Usually there is no outer cell wall, although plant cells have a simple cell-wall structure composed of cellulose and some fungi have walls made of chitin or other carbohydrates.

THE STRUCTURE AND PROPERTIES OF PROKARYOTIC CELLS

Prokaryotic cells are much smaller and less complex than eukaryotic cells (Figure 2.3). They do not have internal organelles; instead the cytoplasmic membrane carries out most of the functions of the

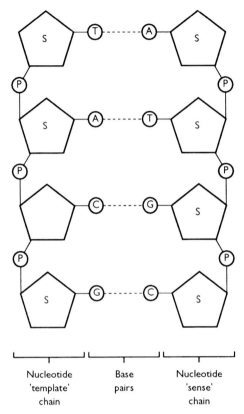

Nucleotide 'template' chain	Base pairs	Nucleotide 'sense' chain

Figure 2.2   The structure of deoxyribonucleic acid (DNA). S = sugar molecule; P = phosphate molecule; C = cytosine; G = guanine; A = adenine; T = thymine; dotted line = hydrogen bond. Source: Wilson, 1995.

cell. It transports required nutrients into the cell, synthesises cell components and generates energy. The surface area of the membrane can be increased by areas of folding called mesosomes. The cytoplasm contains inclusion bodies for the storage of lipids and ribosomes where proteins are synthesised. Unlike eukaryotic cells, bacteria have a single circular DNA chromosome, which is not surrounded by a nuclear membrane but lies in a nuclear region of the cytoplasm.

The size and shape of the cell is determined by a rigid cell wall, which includes a substance called peptidoglycan, unique to bacteria. The wall also helps the cell to withstand differences in osmotic pressure between the interior and exterior of the cell.

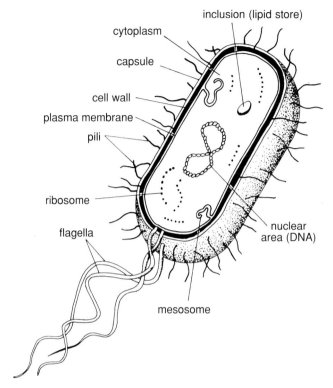

Figure 2.3 The structure of the prokaryotic cell. Source: Wilson, 1995.

Properties of bacteria

In the 300 years since the invention of the microscope a great deal has been learned about bacteria. They vary in shape and range in size from 0.3–14 μm (Figure 2.4). They can survive in almost every type of environment and can utilise almost any substance as a source of energy. Most bacteria are not harmful and many have a valuable role: some release nutrients by decomposing organic matter, others fix atmospheric nitrogen in soil making it available for use by plants. We have harnessed the activity of some microorganisms to produce foods such as cheese and yoghurt. Many bacteria live on and in our bodies without causing us any harm; indeed some are essential for health, protecting us against invasion by other harmful microorganisms and facilitating the degradation of food in the bowel. However, microorganisms can also be harmful; they can spoil foodstuffs and a few species are capable of causing disease. Fortunately, we have also learnt a great deal about preventing and treating infection, we have devised methods of preserving foods, appreciate the importance of sanitation and have a range of vaccines and antimicrobial agents to combat infectious disease.

Like other living things different types of bacteria are defined by two names, the generic name, e.g. *Staphylococcus*, and the specific or species name, e.g. *aureus*. Bacteria can be distinguished by differences in their shape and surface structure, response to stains and nutritional requirements.

The shape of bacterial cells is an important clue to their identity. There are three main shapes; round (cocci), rods (bacilli) and spirals (Figure 2.5). Cocci can occur in clumps, when they are called staphylococci, chains (streptococci) and pairs (diplococci). Bacilli can occur singly or in chains, some are curved (e.g. vibrios) and some are very short, called coccobacilli. Spiral-shaped bacteria are not very common but include the spirochaetes and Spirilla.

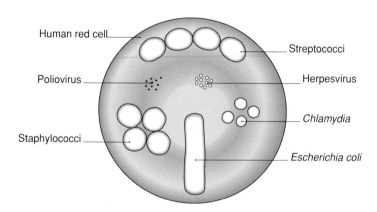

Figure 2.4 Relative sizes of microbes. The human red cell is 7–8 μm in diameter. Cocci are about 1 μm in diameter; *E. coli* is also about 1 μm in diameter and 3–5 μm long. Chlamydia cells are 0.2–0.5 μm in diameter and viruses are smaller again. It would take 700 red cells side by side to cover the width of the full stop at the end of this sentence. Source: Ackerman & Dunk-Richards, 1991.

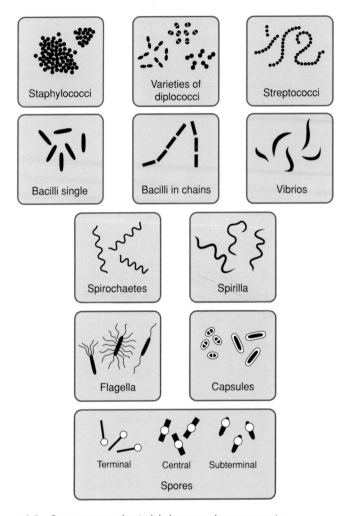

Figure 2.5   Some common bacterial shapes and arrangements.

Cell wall

The shape of the bacterial cell is determined by its cell wall which is made of a substance called peptidoglycan, a network of carbohydrates and amino acids. Although the basic structure of the cell wall is the same in all types of bacteria its thickness and complexity varies. A special method of staining cells, the Gram stain, is used to distinguish between Gram-positive and Gram-negative bacteria (Box 2.1).

Box 2.1 The Gram stain

The Gram stain was developed in 1884 by a physician, Christian Gram, and is an important technique used in diagnostic microbiology. The bacteria to be stained are spread on to a glass slide. Methyl violet, followed by iodine, is applied at this stage; the cells are stained blue; they are then treated briefly with acetone. Gram positive bacteria retain the methyl violet, but Gram-negative bacteria are decolorised by the acetone. Another dye, safranin, is applied and is taken up by the Gram-negative bacteria. When viewed under the microscope, Gram-positive cells appear blue and Gram-negative cells are stained red.

Gram-negative cells have a plasma membrane, a thin layer of peptidoglycan and an outer membrane made of proteins, phospholids and lipopolysaccharide (LPS). Transport proteins and special protein pores allow nutrients to be taken into the cell but other molecules cannot pass through the membrane. The LPS is toxic to mammals and, because it is integral to the cell, is called an *endotoxin* (page 39). It is responsible for many of the symptoms and signs associated with infection by Gram-negative bacteria: it stimulates the hypothalamus to cause a fever and can have a range of adverse effects on the vascular system, impairing the circulation of blood and inducing shock and damage to organs.

Gram-positive cells have a plasma membrane and a very thick layer of peptidoglycan but no outer membrane. Although large molecules are unable to penetrate the mesh of peptidoglycan, small molecules can pass through, so that substances that can harm the cell (e.g. dyes, antibiotics) are able to reach the cytoplasmic membrane relatively easily. The peptidoglycan is also vulnerable to attack by enzymes, such as lysozyme, but the thick layer does confer additional protection against attack by the immune system. Gram-positive cells secrete enzymes out of the cell; these *exotoxins* can damage the tissues of their host (page 39). Exotoxins cause important features of some infections, notably diphtheria and scarlet fever.

Capsules and slime

Many bacteria, including some of the most important pathogens, have a starchy or gelatinous structure around the cell called a capsule; these help to protect the cell from phagocytosis by white blood cells. Some bacteria produce a loose network of material, usually polysaccharides, outside the cell called extracellular slime or glycocalyx. This enables bacteria to adhere to hard surfaces such as teeth and intravascular devices.

Flagella

These are hollow hair-like structures that protrude from the surface of the cell and are often much longer than the cell itself. Flagella act like a propeller, enabling the cell to move towards nutrients or away from harmful substances. The number and arrangement of flagella varies according to the species, although not all bacteria have them and they rarely occur on cocci.

Fimbriae or pili

These are similar to flagella but thinner and shorter. They are present on many Gram-negative bacteria and enable the organism to adhere to specific host cells. For example, the pili of strains of *Escherichia coli* responsible for urinary tract infections assist adhesion to epithelial cells in the bladder. Special fimbriae called sex pili are used to join two cells together so that they can exchange genetic information.

Spores

Some species of bacteria, particularly those of the genera bacillus and clostridium, which are a significant cause of infection in humans, develop highly resistant structures called spores when they are exposed to adverse conditions, such as a lack of nutrients or water. The shape (ovoid or spherical) and position of the spore within the cell vary between species (Figure 2.5). Spores are resistant to disinfectants and to high or low temperatures. They may remain viable for many years but when the environmental conditions improve the spores germinate and the bacterial cell inside starts to multiply again.

Growth and multiplication

Just as all other living creatures, bacteria need food and water for growth and multiplication. Most will not survive for long on clean, dry surfaces but will readily multiply on poorly cleaned equipment, dirty water and even solutions of disinfectant. Many bacteria can synthesise a large proportion of the substances that are needed to build and operate the cell and can therefore grow in very simple media containing very few nutrients. Other bacteria have more complex requirements, needing specific minerals that they are unable to synthesise. All bacteria need water, a source of carbon to make the structure of the cell and for energy, nitrogen to make proteins and nucleic acids, and various inorganic ions including phosphate, sulphur, calcium and iron to make amino acids and to promote enzyme activity.

For each species of bacterium there is a definite temperature range within which growth takes place. The optimum temperature for human commensals and pathogens is about 37°C; most are only able to multiply very slowly below 10°C. Under moist conditions, most non-sporing bacteria are killed between 50°C and 65°C; spores are destroyed at temperatures between 100°C and 120°C.

Each species has an optimum pH for growth, but most prefer neutral or slightly alkaline pH. The body uses the mechanism of adverse pH to discourage potentially harmful bacteria. For example, the pH of the vagina, usually between 4 and 5 because of the lactic acid produced by the lactobacilli that normally live there, discourages the growth of other organisms.

Bacteria differ in their requirements for oxygen according to the mechanism they use to make energy. Some species can only grow in the presence of oxygen and are called *obligate aerobes*; others are *obligate anaerobes* and die rapidly if exposed to air. Anaerobes are present in large numbers in the human intestines, (e.g. *bacteroides, clostridium*) and can cause infection if the intestinal contents contaminate other organs, for example during surgery. They are infrequently associated with infection in contaminated, traumatic injuries where dead tissue is present, or when a large wound has a poor blood supply and therefore low levels of oxygen.

Many human pathogens and commensals can change the process they use to make energy according to the prevailing conditions and can therefore grow in either the presence or absence of oxygen. These are called *facultative anaerobes*.

Multiplication: the process of cell division

In prokaryotic cells, multiplication takes place by binary fission. The cell grows in size, elongating to about twice its original length, and then divides into two identical cells. In the right environmental conditions growth and division can occur very rapidly, with cells dividing every 20 minutes.

The chromosome contains all the information necessary for the activity of the cell and to enable it to replicate itself. When the cell divides, a second copy of the chromosome is made; the cell wall and cytoplasmic membrane grow inwards forming a new cell wall across the inside of the cell and separate the two copies of the chromosome (Figure 2.6).

Bacteria often carry extra genetic material in the form of small circular pieces of DNA called plasmids. These are replicated and transferred into each cell during binary fission, but they can also replicate independently.

In eukaryotic organisms, sexual reproduction is used to mix the genetic material from two individuals of the same species and involves the fusion of two cells, one from each individual. Bacteria do not use cell fusion, but have several methods of exchanging fragments of genetic material between cells of the same or different species (Figure 2.7):

Transformation. Fragments of DNA released from damaged bacterial cells can be absorbed into other cells and incorporated into their chromosome, although usually only those of closely related species.

Transduction. Viruses that infect bacteria (bacteriophages) sometimes copy part of the host-cell DNA by mistake, take it out of the cell with the newly constructed viruses and introduce it into the genome of other bacteria that the virus infects.

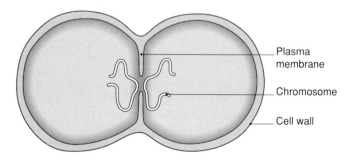

Plasma membrane

Chromosome

Cell wall

Figure 2.6 Binary fission in prokaryotic cells. The chromosome replicates and the daughter copy is separated into a new cell by the growth of a plasma membrane between them.

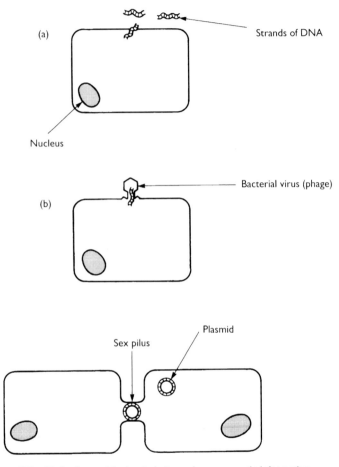

(a) Strands of DNA

Nucleus

(b) Bacterial virus (phage)

Sex pilus   Plasmid

Figure 2.7 Methods used by bacteria to exchange genetic information. A. Transformation. B. Transduction. C. Conjugation. Source: Wilson 1995.

Conjugation. The special fimbria called a sex pilus extends from one bacterial cell and adheres to another cell. A copy of plasmid DNA in one cell is transferred via the tube into the second cell. Sex pili can be formed between cells of the same species and of different species but, because the genetic information required to make the sex pili and DNA transfer proteins are carried on a plasmid, conjugation can only occur when the cell carries one of these plasmids. Bacteria can have between one and six plasmids, which often contain genetic information that enables the cell to adhere to tissue, to produce toxins or make enzymes which inactivate antimicrobial agents.

Genetic recombination techniques

Experimentation with the transfer of DNA between different bacteria has seen the development of a range of specialised techniques for gene manipulation. A range of enzymes which cut DNA strands at specific points have been identified. These restriction nucleases can be used to separate individual genes and incorporate them into a plasmid, which can then be transferred into another prokaryotic or eukaryotic cell. Viruses that infect bacteria (bacteriophages) have also been used extensively in recombinant DNA technology.

These recombinant techniques have been applied in a wide variety of plants and animals, including humans, to study genes and identify specific DNA sequences. They have been used to develop synthetic drugs and vaccines, such as insulin and hepatitis B vaccine, to modify plants and animals used in agriculture and may ultimately prove useful in the treatment of genetic disorders.

Atypical bacteria

There are a few species of bacteria that, although similar to typical bacteria in most respects, have a number of important differences and are therefore referred to as atypical bacteria.

Mycoplasmas and ureaplasmas

These are very small bacteria, smaller than a large virus. They vary in size and shape and because they do not have peptidoglycan cell walls they cannot be Gram-stained. They need special techniques to grow them in the laboratory: they only grow slowly and have exacting nutrient requirements. Many are parasites of animals, insects or plants. *Mycoplasma pneumoniae* causes atypical pneumonia in humans and *Ureaplasma urealyticum* is thought to be associated with some forms of sexually transmitted urethritis.

Chlamydias

These resemble very small Gram-negative bacteria: they contain DNA, RNA and a rigid cell wall but, as they do not have a full range of metabolic enzymes, they can only multiply inside other living cells. They cause infections in a variety of animals and birds and some also infect humans, e.g. *Chlamydia trachomatis*, which causes eye infections and sexually transmitted urethritis.

Rickettsias

These are small Gram-negative bacteria that multiply inside cells. They live in an animal host, such as rodents, cattle and sheep, and are transferred from animal to animal by biting insects such as fleas, lice and ticks. They cause a range of diseases in humans; for example, *Rickettsia typhi*, which causes murine typhus, is carried by rats and transferred to humans by fleas.

THE STRUCTURE AND PROPERTIES OF VIRUSES

Viruses are completely different from other organisms. They are simply a piece of genetic material inside a coat of protein (Figure 2.8). They have no structures for making their own constituents or for metabolism and are therefore entirely dependent

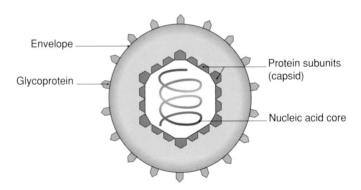

Figure 2.8 The structure of a virus.

on a host cell for their replication. The living host cell provides the energy, synthetic machinery and materials required for the synthesis of viral proteins and nucleic acids.

Viruses can infect plants, animals and even bacteria, and are responsible for a wide range of infections. Infection can occur at the site of entry to the body, e.g. gastroenteritis, or at a distant site, e.g. the polio virus, which enters via the gastrointestinal tract but infects motor neurones.

Viral structure

Viruses vary considerably in size and shape but all are too small to be visible under an ordinary light microscope; instead they are identified and studied under far more powerful microscopes, called electron microscopes.

The protein coat or *capsid* is made up of many identical polypeptides, which can be assembled into a variety of symmetrical shapes. Viruses can be grouped into three types, based on their shape: cubic with 20 faces (icosahedral); helical with the capsid wound round the nucleic acid; or complex (Figure 2.9). Some viruses also have an outer lipid membrane, which is acquired from the host cell as new viruses leave it by budding through the cell membrane. All viruses have a protein receptor binding site on their surface which reacts with corresponding receptors on the surface of a host cell. Viruses are able to invade only those cells that carry the appropriate receptors on their surface; this is the reason why many viruses affect a particular host and even target particular tissues. The human immunodeficiency virus, for example, binds to the CD4 receptor on T-helper lymphocytes. Other cells, including macrophages and brain cells, have some CD4 receptors and thus are also affected.

The genome of a virus is contained inside the capsid and is made of either DNA or RNA; viruses never contain both types of nucleic acid. This is a major difference from other living cells, which contain both DNA and RNA, the former for storing genetic information and the latter for translating the DNA code into protein. Most viruses have just one molecule of nucleic acid; it can be double- or single-stranded and linear or circular. In the smallest viruses the nucleic acid will code for fewer than 10 proteins, while in a large virus it may code for several hundred.

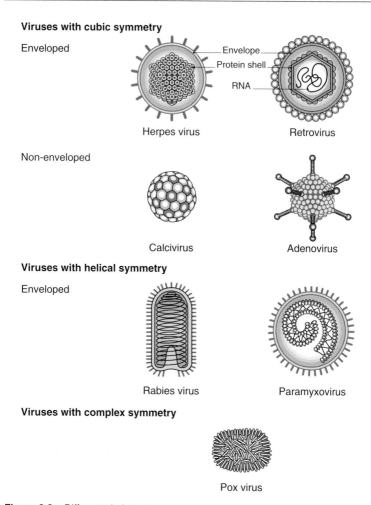

Viruses with cubic symmetry

Enveloped

Envelope
Protein shell
RNA

Herpes virus

Retrovirus

Non-enveloped

Calcivirus

Adenovirus

Viruses with helical symmetry

Enveloped

Rabies virus

Paramyxovirus

Viruses with complex symmetry

Pox virus

Figure 2.9   Different viral structures.

Viral replication

The virus attaches to a specific receptor on the host cell surface, then enters through the plasma membrane; the capsid is removed and the nucleic acid is released. The virus then takes control of the protein production structures in the cell, which start to make the proteins coded for on the viral nucleic acid. One of the first sections to be transcribed makes enzymes, which then direct the rest of the process. DNA viruses are transcribed into messenger RNA (mRNA) before translation into protein. In RNA viruses transcription of the nucleic acid occurs in one of three ways. In some viruses the RNA acts directly as mRNA. In others, the RNA is copied to make a mirror image, which then acts as mRNA. In the third group, the retroviruses, the RNA is first transcribed into double-stranded DNA by the enzyme reverse transcriptase. The DNA is then incorporated into the host genome as a proviral DNA before being transcribed into mRNA and protein.

Once all the viral proteins have been made, they are assembled into capsids and copies of the nucleic acid are inserted into each one (Figure 2.10). The new viruses are then released either by lysis of the host cell (e.g. poliovirus) or, in the case of enveloped viruses, by budding out of the cell membrane, acquiring their envelope in the process. Some viruses continue to be manufactured and bud out of the cell for prolonged periods.

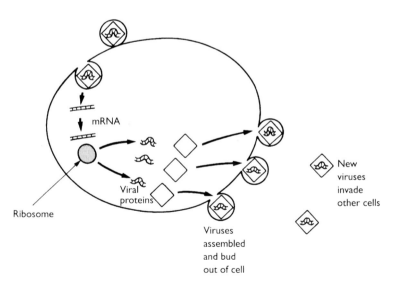

Figure 2.10 The replication of viruses within a host cell. The virus enters the host cell. Its genome moves to a ribosome, where it is transcribed to make many copies of viral proteins and genome. The protein coats and genomes are assembled and then bud out of the cell, collecting part of the cell membrane of the host cell on the way out. Source: Wilson 1995.

Effects of viral infection

The disease resulting from a viral infection depends on the type of cell infected and the number destroyed. Destruction of the cells may be brought about either by the virus itself or by the host immune system. Following an acute episode of infection, some viruses can remain dormant in the host cell. During this time the virus does not kill the cell, induce an immune response or replicate. Later, in response to some sort of stimulus, the virus is reactivated and starts to replicate once more. This type of latent infection is seen with herpesvirus infections, e.g. cold sores.

Sometimes, the viral nucleic acid is inserted into the DNA of the host cell and becomes latent; reactivation then causes the production of infective virus. DNA inserted into the genome can also interfere with the normal controls on cell division, causing the cell to be transformed into a malignant tumour cell and multiply rapidly. The best-known example of such transformation is Burkett's lymphoma, which is caused by the Epstein–Barr virus. There is also evidence of an association between hepatoma and the hepatitis B virus.

Since viruses use the metabolism of the host cell to replicate, finding drugs that will interfere with viral replication but not damage the host cell is difficult and only a limited range of antiviral therapies is currently available.

PRIONS

These are self-replicating pieces of protein and do not contain either DNA or RNA. Most affect the nervous system, causing chronic, degenerative disease, e.g. Creutzfeldt–Jakob disease (CJD) and (in cattle) bovine spongiform encephalopathy (BSE). The prions are highly resistant to normal methods of destroying microorganisms. They can withstand high temperatures and many of the conventional chemical disinfectants.

FUNGI AND YEASTS

These are eukaryotic organisms, formerly regarded as plants without the green pigment chlorophyll but now considered as a separate group. They range in size from the large, macroscopic forms such as mushrooms to microscopic moulds and yeasts.

Most are found in soil, where they decompose and recycle organic material. Only a few species cause disease in humans; some produce toxins that are occasionally associated with food poisoning.

Structure of fungi

Mycelial fungi grow as long filaments or hyphae, which branch and interlace to form a mycelium (Figure 2.11). They have rigid cell walls made of chitin and, although they cannot move, the cytoplasm can stream along the inside of the filaments. They reproduce asexually by forming spores at the end of tubes. These are released, germinate and grow into a new mycelium. The mycelium will continue to grow as long as a supply of nutrients is available and can often become large enough to be visible. Some, such as the mushroom, form a mycelium in the soil and specialised spore-bearing structures above ground. Most fungi can also reproduce sexually.

Yeasts are unicellular fungi which occur as single, spherical cells. They multiply by forming buds on the side of the cell which, when large enough, breaks away to form a new daughter cell. *Cryptococcus neoformans* is the only important pathogen. Yeast-like fungi, such as *Candida albicans*, grow partly as yeasts and partly as long, filamentous cells or pseudo-mycelium.

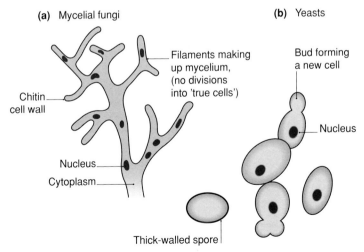

Figure 2.11 The structure of fungi. A. Mycelial fungus. B. Yeasts.

Dimorphic fungi grow in either a filamentous or yeast form, depending on the cultural conditions. For example, *histoplasma* grows in the filamentous form at room temperature but as a yeast form when growing in the body at a temperature of 37°C.

Fungal infections

Diseases caused by fungi and yeasts are called mycoses. They are usually not affected by antibacterial drugs, but a few therapeutic antifungal agents are available. There are three forms of fungal infection:

- **Superficial mycoses** occur in the surface layer of skin, nails or hair. They are caused by fungi called dermatophytes, which need keratin as a source of nutrients; e.g. ringworm.
- **Deep mycoses** are caused by fungi that normally live in soil or decomposing matter but which, if introduced into subcutaneous tissues, usually as a result of trauma, are able to spread through the tissue. Most infections are asymptomatic, but they can produce chronic skin ulcers or abscesses and may spread into the lymphatics to cause systemic infection; e.g. histoplasmosis.
- **Opportunistic mycoses**: some fungi are present in small numbers in the normal flora of mucous membranes in the respiratory, gastrointestinal and female genital tract. If they are able to multiply in an uncontrolled way local infection results and if the person has predisposing factors, e.g. reduced immunity, debility, diabetes mellitus, may invade the bloodstream and cause infection in other organs. Examples of opportunistic mycoses include candidosis, cryptococcosis and aspergillosis.

PROTOZOA

These are eukaryotic, single-celled, microscopic organisms, which occur in a variety of shapes and sizes. Most live in water and some are obligate parasites of animals (Figure 2.12).

Structure of protozoa

Although single cells, protozoa have all the structures associated with eukaryotic cells: they have a cytoplasmic membrane, one or more nuclei and mitochondria. Some groups are motile through

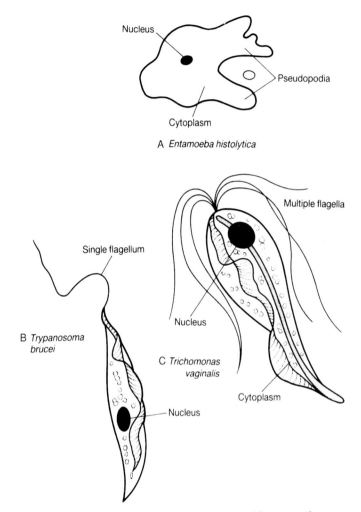

Figure 2.12 Examples of some pathogenic protozoa (diagrammatic representation). A. *Entamoeba histolytica*. B. *Trypanosoma brucei*. C. *Trichomonas vaginalis*.

possessing flagella, cilia or pseudopodia. They obtain nutrients by enclosing solid particles of food, pouring on digestive enzymes and then absorbing the soluble substances into the cytoplasm.

Protozoa reproduce asexually by dividing into two, but some also have sexual reproductive cycles involving different stages in more than one host. An important protozoal pathogen is plasmodium, the cause of malaria. It multiplies asexually in human red blood cells, producing male and female forms that are ingested by the mosquito when it bites and reproduce sexually in the mosquito before being inoculated into a new host.

Some protozoa can form cysts by secreting a protective coat around the cell. This enables them to survive outside the host until they can enter a new host.

FURTHER READING

Ackerman, V. and Dunk-Richards, G. (1991) *Microbiology – An Introduction for the Health Sciences*. W.B. Saunders/Baillière Tindall, London.

Duerden, B.I. Reid, T.M.S. and Jewsbury, J.M. (1993) *Microbial and Parasitic Infection*, 7th edn. Edward Arnold, London.

Wilson, J. (1995) *Infection Control in Clinical Practice*. Baillière Tindall, London.

3

The epidemiology of infection

INTRODUCTION

In its strictest sense, the term 'epidemiology' means the study of things that happen to people, but it is commonly applied to the study of the occurrence and distribution of disease. The analysis of which people acquire a particular infection and the factors associated with it, contributes to our knowledge of who is at risk of infection, how it spreads and how transmission may be prevented.

OUR RELATIONSHIP WITH MICROORGANISMS

There are thousands of different species of microorganisms, which inhabit almost every conceivable environment. Many species play an essential role in our survival. They form crucial links in the food chain by releasing nutrients through the breakdown of dead plants and animals and by converting atmospheric nitrogen into a form which can be used by plants.

Microorganisms that usually populate the human body are called the *normal flora*; they are commensals, do not harm their host and may even be beneficial. The species present in different parts of the body vary according to the local supply of nutrients, oxygen, pH and temperature. The normal flora of the warm, moist and oxygen-free environment of the gut will be quite different from that of the cool dry environment of the skin (Table 3.1).

Microbes that are normally resident at a particular site on the body can help to prevent invasion by harmful species. Lactobacilli

Table 3.1 The normal flora of the human body (from Wilson 1995)

Site	Common commensals
Skin	Staphylococci, streptococci, corynebacteria (diphtheroids), *Candida*
Throat	α-haemolytic streptococci, neisseria, corynebacteria (diphtheroids)
Mouth	α-haemolytic streptococci, moraxella, actinomyces, spirochaetes
Respiratory tract	α-haemolytic streptococci, moraxella, corynebacteria (diphtheroids), micrococci
Vagina	Lactobacilli, corynebacteria (diphtheroids), streptococci, yeasts
Intestines	Bacteroides, anaerobic streptococci, enterococci, clostridrium, E. coli, klebsiella, proteus

in the vagina produce acid from glycogen, making the environment inhospitable for other microorganisms. Some commensals
play a more active role; for example, bacteria in the gut are involved
in the degradation of food material passing through.

Pathogenicity

The few microbial species that are able to invade and then damage
tissue to cause disease are called *pathogens*. The capacity of a
microorganism to cause disease is referred to as *pathogenicity*.
Some microorganisms cause a single characteristic disease, e.g.
Clostridium tetani, which causes tetanus. Other microorganisms
can cause a wide range of different diseases. For example, *Staphylococcus aureus* can cause skin infections such as abscesses and
wound infection, pneumonia and osteomyelitis.

Some pathogens invariably cause infection if they gain access
to a host, although the severity of the disease may depend on host
susceptibility. For example, *shigella* causes dysentery, an acute
diarrhoeal illness, which tends to be most serious in debilitated
people. Other microorganisms are able to cause disease only in
individuals with impaired defences and are called *opportunistic
pathogens*. For example, the protozoon *Pneumocystis carinii* lives in
the respiratory tract of healthy people without causing adverse
effects, but can cause a very serious form of pneumonia in individuals who have an impaired immune system.

Susceptibility to infection

The body has a range of defences designed to protect it against invasion by pathogens (p. 52). Susceptibility to infection depends on the effectiveness of these defences. For example, bacteria cannot penetrate intact skin but will enter via damaged skin. Likewise, in a healthy person the respiratory tract is protected by cilia and the cough reflex; if these responses are damaged or breached by drugs or intubation, microorganisms may gain access more easily.

Microorganisms that are present normally as commensals at a particular site of the body can cause infection if they are introduced elsewhere. For example, *Escherichia coli*, found normally in the large bowel, causes urinary tract infection if it enters the bladder. Infections caused by the transfer of microorganisms from one site on the body to another are called *endogenous*. They are commonly associated with the use of invasive devices, which provide microorganisms with an opportunity to enter the body, especially at sites that do not normally have a commensal population, e.g. the pleural cavity, the bladder.

Pathogens can be present on the body without invading the tissues or infection. This is described as *colonisation*. While colonisation has no adverse effects on the individual concerned, it provides a source from which the pathogen can be readily transferred to another person and subsequently cause infection. Infection acquired through the transfer of microorganisms from one person to another is called *exogenous infection* or *cross-infection*.

STAGES IN THE DEVELOPMENT OF INFECTION

There are a series of stages in the process of infection, beginning with penetration of the tissues at a particular site (List 3.1).

List 3.1 Stages in the development of infection

- Acquisition
- Adhesion to host cells
- Penetration of cells
- Multiplication in tissues
- Damage to tissues
- Spread to other tissue
- Resolution or death

Penetration of tissue

This is dependent on the microorganism being able to resist the host defences, such as gastric acid in the stomach or secretions from sebaceous glands on the skin. In addition, to invade the tissue the microorganism must first be able to adhere to the cells. Bacteria use a variety of methods to facilitate adherence. Some have special hairs on their surface called fimbriae or pili, some secrete sticky substances such as dextran (e.g. α-haemolytic streptococci in the mouth) and others produce slime (e.g. *Staphylococcus epidermidis*). Viruses recognise specific molecules on the surface of their target host cell and by binding to these receptors are able to gain entry to the cell.

Multiplication in the host

To establish infection the microorganism must be able to multiply. This is determined by the availability of nutrients and oxygen, a temperature appropriate to the needs of the particular microorganism, and, in the case of viruses, the ability to switch the metabolism of the cell to the production of viral components.

The number of microorganisms introduced can have a crucial effect on whether or not infection develops. A few microorganisms introduced on to the surface of a wound may be unable to compete with the normal commensal population and be easily overpowered by the host's defences, preventing infection from becoming established. In outbreaks of food poisoning, a range of symptoms, from very mild to extremely severe, can occur following consumption of the same contaminated food, the severity of symptoms largely reflecting the quantity of microorganisms consumed.

Spread to other tissues

Some infections remain at the site of invasion, causing symptoms related to invasion of the epithelial tissue at that particular site. For example, *shigella* invades the epithelial tissue of the gut, causing diarrhoea. Once infection has been established at a particular site, microorganisms may spread to adjacent tissues or may be carried in the bloodstream to other parts of the body. For example, in typhoid the causative bacterium, *Salmonella typhi*, initially infects the intestine but causes generalised symptoms of fever by invading the bloodstream.

Tissue damage

Pathogenic microorganisms cause disease by damaging the host. Damage may result from the release of enzymes that destroy cells or tissue in the local area (e.g. proteases, colleganases) and toxins that have specific local or systemic effects (Box 3.1). Sometimes damage to tissues is caused by the host's immune system: the permeability of blood vessels is increased in response to the microorganisms, allowing plasma proteins and white blood cells to flood into the area but resulting in inflamed, swollen tissue. In chronic infections e.g. *Mycobacterium tuberculosis*, the prolonged immune response can cause permanent changes in the surrounding tissue.

Box 3.1   Bacterial toxins

Toxins are substances released by microbial cells, which, by damaging or destroying specific tissues, are responsible for some or all of the disease processes. There are two types of toxin.

Exotoxins are usually protein enzymes secreted by bacteria into their local environment. They may be transported in the bloodstream and cause damage in parts of the body remote from the site of infection. Even minute amounts can cause serious damage to specific tissues. Botulinum toxin, released by *Clostridium botulinum*, is a powerful neurotoxin: ingestion of a tiny amount starts to cause paralysis 12–36 hours later. Other exotoxins include *enterotoxins*, released by some intestinal pathogens such as *Vibrio cholerae* and *Escherichia coli*, stimulate mucosal cells in the gut causing profuse diarrhoea.

Endotoxins are lipopolysaccharides contained in the outer cell membrane of Gram-negative bacteria. They are not actively secreted by the cell but are released when it is destroyed and is broken open. They do not have enzymatic activity but have profound systemic effects on the host, including induction of high fever, reduction in blood pressure and disruption in coagulation causing bleeding into the tissues. These effects, termed *septic* or *endotoxic shock*, are associated with septicaemia caused by Gram-negative bacteria and are frequently fatal.

In viral infections, the function of the cell may be disrupted or the cell may be destroyed when new viruses are released. The effects depend on the particular virus and the location of the infected cells. For example, the polio virus infects motor neurone cells and shuts down protein synthesis, causing the death of neurones and paralysis of the muscles that they innervate. Some viruses affect only cells at the site of invasion, while others migrate to other tissues. For example, herpes simplex travels from the skin along sensory nerves to the ganglia.

Virulence

The term *virulence* is used to describe the ability of a microorganism to cause disease. Virulence depends on the microorganism's ability to invade, multiply in and damage the host and is mediated by factors in both the host and the microorganism. The ability of a microbe to cause disease depends on factors that: assist adhesion (e.g. fimbriae, slime); enable invasion of tissues (e.g. extracellular enzymes); protect against the immune system (e.g. capsules); and determine toxin production. These virulence factors may not be carried by all the microorganisms of a particular species; thus some strains may be virulent while others are not. For example, some strains of *Streptococcus pyogenes* can produce an erythrotoxin, and throat infections caused by these strains result in scarlet fever. *Corynebacterium diphtheriae* can cause infection of the upper respiratory tract, but only those strains with DNA coding for the diphtheria toxin are associated with neurological and cardiac effects of the disease.

A particular microorganism may be able to live in more than one animal host, but only able to cause disease in one. An example of this is *Mycobacterium tuberculosis*, which can infect cattle as well as humans but only causes serious disease in humans.

SOURCES AND RESERVOIRS OF MICROORGANISMS

The site where a microorganism usually lives is called a *reservoir* and is where it finds nutrients, moisture and the environmental conditions necessary for its growth. A reservoir may be in the environment, humans or other animals (Table 3.2). To cause infection, microorganisms need a means of transferring to a susceptible host. When this occurs, the reservoir becomes a source of infection. For example, the reservoir of *Legionella pneumophila* is water. In an air-conditioning system it becomes a source of infection if droplets of water are inhaled by people in the building. Identifying the source of an infection is important when an outbreak of infection occurs, but it is important to recognise that not all reservoirs of microorganisms are sources of infection. In clinical settings moist environments such as the waste pipes of sinks and washbasins support the growth of a wide range of bacteria, in particular Gram-negative species, which flourish in a moist envi-

Table 3.2   Examples of microbial reservoirs

Reservoir	Microorganism	Disease
Environment		
Soil	*Clostridium tetani*	Tetanus
Water	*Legionella pneumophila*	Legionnaires' disease
Animals		
Cattle	*Escherichia coli* (toxogenic strains)	Gastroenteritis
Poultry	*Salmonella spp.*	Gastroenteritis
Humans		
Respiratory tract	Rhinovirus	Common cold
Gut	Rotavirus	Gastroenteritis

ronment. These sites are an unlikely source of infection since the organisms are not readily transferred to susceptible sites such as wounds and invasive devices in the patients, and the strains found are rarely the same as those found in patients (Levin et al 1984, Orsi et al 1994). Invasive equipment such as surgical instruments, endoscopes, urine and intravenous catheters present a much greater risk, if inadequate decontamination enables them to become a source of infection (National Nosocomial Infection Surveillance system 1991, Das et al 1997).

More commonly, the sources of microorganisms are patients themselves, their body fluids or skin lesions. Infection may be readily transmitted from individuals who are suffering from or recovering from infection. During the incubation period between acquisition of the microorganism and the development of overt symptoms, such as a rash or increase in respiratory secretions, the microorganism will be released in excreta or secretions and may subsequently infect another person. Likewise, even after the symptoms of infection have resolved, the causative microorganisms may still be present, in reduced numbers, in secretions and excretions for a few days or weeks and be unwittingly transferred to other people. Some affected individuals may completely recover from the illness but retain the pathogen, becoming carriers of the disease for prolonged periods. *Salmonella typhi*, for example, causes a systemic intestinal illness but sometimes, following recovery, the bacteria remain in the gall bladder or kidneys from where they are intermittently released into the faeces or urine for many months or years. Outbreaks of infection can result from such carriers, the most well-known example, Typhoid Mary, was a cook who became a carrier of *S. typhi* and over a period of 10 years infected over 50 people. Similarly, a small proportion of individuals infected by hepatitis B do not completely clear the virus from their bloodstream and, although they recover from the acute infection, become carriers of the virus.

Sometimes, microorganisms are carried by one person who does not develop the infection but who acts as a source of infection for others who are susceptible to the organism. A good example of this is the meningococcus. Many people carry this organism asymptomatically in their upper respiratory tract; occasionally it is transferred to a susceptible person, who subsequently develops meningococcal meningitis. Such asymptomatic carriage is a common feature in outbreaks of infection caused by antibiotic-resistant strains of bacteria, such as methicillin-resistant *Staphylococcus aureus* (MRSA).

ROUTES OF MICROBIAL TRANSMISSION

To cause disease microorganisms must have a means of gaining access to the tissues of the host. Common points of access are the respiratory tract, by inhalation, or gastrointestinal tract, by ingestion. Some microorganisms use several different routes of transmission; for example, varicella zoster virus, which causes chicken-pox, can be acquired by inhalation of respiratory droplets as well as through contact with fluid seeping from skin lesions. Other infections rely on a single route of transmission; for example, *Treponema pallidum*, the cause of syphilis, is only transmitted by sexual intercourse.

Once the microorganisms have entered the body they may spread to other sites (Figure 3.1). To transmit to another host the pathogen must also have a means of leaving the body, a portal of exit. Usually, microorganisms leave in excreta or secretions, which are therefore an important source of pathogens.

Transmission by direct contact

Microorganisms can be physically transferred from one person to another by direct contact between body surfaces. Infection spread by sexual intercourse and transplacentally from mother to fetus transmit by this type of route. Many other infections are

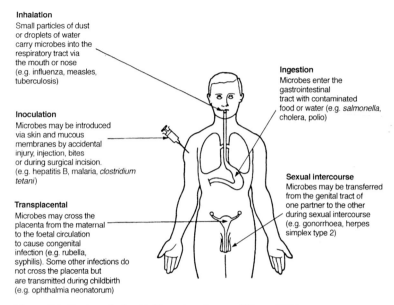

Inhalation
Small particles of dust or droplets of water carry microbes into the respiratory tract via the mouth or nose (e.g. influenza, measles, tuberculosis)

Inoculation
Microbes may be introduced via skin and mucous membranes by accidental injury, injection, bites or during surgical incision. (e.g. hepatitis B, malaria, *clostridium tetani*)

Transplacental
Microbes may cross the placenta from the maternal to the foetal circulation to cause congenital infection (e.g. rubella, syphilis). Some other infections do not cross the placenta but are transmitted during childbirth (e.g. ophthalmia neonatorum)

Ingestion
Microbes enter the gastrointestinal tract with contaminated food or water (e.g. *salmonella*, cholera, polio)

Sexual intercourse
Microbes may be transferred from the genital tract of one partner to the other during sexual intercourse (e.g. gonorrhoea, herpes simplex type 2)

Figure 3.1 Routes of microbial invasion. Source: Wilson 1995.

spread by direct contact with respiratory secretions, (e.g. colds, which are caused by rhinoviruses; Epstein–Barr virus, which causes glandular fever).

Transmission by indirect contact

Many infections are transferred from one host to another on animate or inanimate objects. Common vehicles are:

- airborne particles
- hands
- equipment and other inanimate objects (fomites)
- food and water
- insects.

Airborne particles

Although microorganisms cannot travel through the air on their own, they can be carried on airborne particles such as dust, water and respiratory droplets.

Dust is largely composed of skin squames, 10–20 µm in diameter, which are constantly shed from the surfaces of the skin. In addition, droplets of moisture are expelled from the respiratory tract during talking, sneezing or coughing. Most of these are fairly large and drop rapidly to the floor. Others evaporate into minute particles called droplet nuclei, which are less than 10 µm in diameter and can remain airborne for several hours (Sandford 1986). Many of these dust particles or droplet nuclei carry microorganisms, which could establish infection if they are inhaled or settle in open wounds, e.g. during surgery (Whyte et al 1982).

Most particles fall harmlessly to the floor or other surfaces and are then unlikely to be disturbed sufficiently to become airborne again. In most circumstances the risk of inhaling particles carrying pathogenic microorganisms is low and this route of infection is uncommon. Many respiratory infections are more likely to be transmitted directly by contact with respiratory secretions transferred on to hands or tissues during sneezing or coughing (Ansari 1991).

Hands

Pathogenic microorganisms are readily acquired on hands though contact with contaminated surfaces, secretions, excreta or open skin lesions. Most are not able to survive for long on the skin but in the meantime can be transferred on to the next object or person that is touched (Mackintosh & Hoffman 1984). Transmission on hands is probably responsible for a considerable amount of cross-infection in health care settings, since staff have regular contact with both patients and their body fluids (Reybrouck 1983, Sanderson & Weissler 1992, Larson 1988).

Equipment and inanimate objects (fomites)

Inanimate objects can act as a vehicle for the transmission of pathogens, but the risk of infection depends on the extent to which they become contaminated during use, how well they support their growth and the type of contact with the potential host. Equipment that is clean and dry does not usually support the growth of microorganisms. However, body fluids are an important source of microorganisms and equipment in contact with them can readily transmit infection if not decontaminated between each use. The risk of transmission depends on how the equipment is used. A few microorganisms introduced into a sterile body cavity on surgical instruments may be able to establish infection easily, while many introduced on to intact skin are unlikely to. Many bacteria survive and multiply more easily in moist environments, and equipment such as humidifiers, baths and washbowls, which contain fluids, are particularly susceptible to contamination (Cefai et al 1990, Greaves 1985). In assessing the potential of such equipment to cause infection it is important to distinguish between reservoirs and sources of microorganisms. A washbasin may be an important reservoir for microorganisms but is an unlikely source of infection, while a contaminated respiratory humidifier provides an ideal means of transmitting microorganisms directly into the respiratory tract.

Food and water

Gastrointestinal pathogens use food and water as a means of transmission from one host to another. Some foods are contaminated with pathogenic microorganisms in their raw state and if they are not cooked properly the organisms are not destroyed and can cause infection when eaten. For example, raw chicken is frequently contaminated with *Salmonella* or *Campylobacter*, which are readily destroyed during the cooking process but can cause infection if not thoroughly cooked or transferred to other food in the kitchen. Food may also be contaminated after it is cooked by contact with microorganisms on equipment, hands or other uncooked, contaminated food. Food handlers with a gastrointestinal infection can transmit infection via their hands if these are not properly washed after defaecation.

Water may also act as a source of infection if it is contaminated by pathogens and not treated to remove them before drinking. *Vibrio cholerae*, the bacterium that causes cholera, and the protozoa *giardia* and *cryptosporidium* are common causes of water-borne infection.

Insect and animal vectors

Insects can be involved in the transmission of infection both passively, (e.g. the transfer of pathogens from faeces to food on the feet of flies) and actively, by supporting part of the life cycle of the parasite. In active transmission, the parasite is transferred from the human host into the insect when it bites and sucks blood. Protozoan parasites often undergo stages in their development while in the insect before being injected, in a mature form, into the next human host when the insect bites – e.g. malaria, trypanosomiasis (sleeping sickness). As well as protozoa, species of bacteria, rickettsiae, viruses and worms can all be transmitted by insects (Tables 3.3, 3.4). Other parasites, particularly worms, use animals as part of their life cycle. Eggs or cysts

Table 3.3 Examples of insect-borne infections

Microorganism	Species	Disease	Insect involved in transmission
Protozoa	*Plasmodium malariae, P. ovale, P. falciparum, P. vivax*	Malaria	Mosquito
	Leishmania donovani	Leishmaniasis	
	Trypanosoma gambiense,	Sleeping sickness	Sandfly
	T. rhodesiense		Tsetse fly
Bacteria	*Yersinia pestis*	Bubonic plague	Rat flea
Rickettsiae	*Rickettsia prowazekii,*	Epidemic typhus	Human louse
	R. typhi	Murine typhus	Rodent flea
Viruses	Flaviviruses	Dengue, yellow fever	Mosquito
Helminths (worms)	*Wuchereria bancrofti*	Bancroftian filariasis	Mosquito
	Onchocerca	'River blindness'	Black fly

Table 3.4 Examples of animal vectors of helminths

Helminth	Species	Disease	Vector
Trematodes (flukes)	*Schistosoma mansoni, S. japonicum, S. haematobium*	Schistosomiasis	Water snail
Cestodes (tapeworms)	*Taenia solium*	Tapeworm – cysticercosis	Pig
	T. saginata		Cattle
	Echinococcus granulosus	Tapeworm – hydatid cyst	Sheep (also goats, cattle, horses)

are passed out of the human host in faeces and are then swallowed by animals such as cows and pigs. New human hosts are then infected by ingesting meat that has not been properly cooked and contains viable cysts.

Animals can also be involved in the transmission of infection. Some microorganisms that normally live in animals can be accidentally transferred to humans, for example *brucella* from cows. Infections caused by these pathogens are called zoonoses and people who have considerable direct contact with animals,

Table 3.5 Examples of zoonoses

Disease	Causative microorganism	Animal host	Mode of transmission
Anthrax	*Bacillus anthracis*	Cattle	Contact with infected hides/tissue, inhalation of spores
Brucellosis (undulant fever)	*Brucella abortus* B. melitensis B. suis	Cattle Sheep, goats Pigs	Contact with infected tissues, ingestion of infected milk
Contagious pustular dermatitis	Orf virus	Sheep, goats	Contact with infected animals
Lassa fever (West Africa)	Arenavirus	Rats	Direct contact with infected urine
Leptospirosis Weil's disease canicola fever	*Leptospira icterohaemorrhagiae* *Leptospira canicola* *Leptospira hardjo*	Rats Dogs Cattle	Contact with water, soil or vegetation contaminated with infected urine
Lyme disease	*Borrelia burgdorferi*	Deer	Tick bite from infected animal host
Psittacosis	*Chlamydia psittaci*	Parrots	Contact with infected birds, inhalation
Q fever	*Coxiella burneti*	Cattle, sheep, other animals	Contact with infected tissues, inhalation
Rabies	Rhabdovirus	Foxes, dogs	Bite of infected animal
Toxoplasmosis	*Toxoplasma gondii*	Cats (ingested by sheep, pigs, goats, cattle)	Ingestion of faecally contaminated soil or infected meat
Tuberculosis	*Mycobacterium bovis*	Cattle	Ingestion of unpasteurised milk

such as agricultural or abattoir workers and veterinary surgeons, are at greatest risk of acquiring them. Examples are given in Table 3.5.

EPIDEMICS OF INFECTION

The prevalence of a disease within a community can vary at different times. Some diseases are always present and are described as *endemic*; a marked, but temporary, increase in the occurrence of a disease is called an *epidemic* and where this affects communities throughout the world, a *pandemic*.

Some epidemics are seasonal, with the number of cases increasing in the winter months, e.g. influenza and chickenpox. Others are associated with susceptibility within the community. For example, epidemics of rotavirus tend to occur among the very young, who have not been previously exposed and who are therefore not immune, and the elderly, who have diminished immunity. Epidemics of whooping cough have been associated with decreased level of immunisation against the disease.

Single-point epidemics, such as those caused by food poisoning, occur when many people are exposed to the infection at the same time, causing a sudden increase in the disease followed by a rapid fall. Later cases may then occur as a result of cross-infection from infected individuals (Figure 3.2). The measures used to describe the occurrence of disease in a population are shown in Box 3.2.

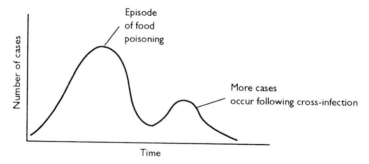

Figure 3.2 A single-point epidemic with secondary spread by cross-infection. Source: Wilson 1995.

Box 3.2   Measuring the occurrence of disease

Prevalence: a measure of the number of infections present in a particular population at a particular time, e.g. the proportion of patients in a hospital with infection on a particular day.

Incidence: the number of new infections that occur in a defined population during a specified period of time. It is commonly expressed as a ratio, e.g. the number of urinary tract infections per 100 catheterised patients, or a rate, e.g. the number of bloodstream infections per 100 patient days in hospital.

REFERENCES

Ansari, S.A. Springthorpe, S., Sattar, S.A. *et al.* (1991) Potential role of hands in the spread of respiratory infections: studies with human parainfluenza virus 3 and rhinovirus 14. *J. Clin. Microbiol.* **29**, 2115–2119.

Cefai, C., Richards, J., Gould, F.K. *et al.* (1990) An outbreak of *Acinetobacter* respiratory tract infection resulting from incomplete disinfection of ventilatory equipment. *J. Hosp. Infect.*, **15**, 177–182.

Das, I., Philpott, C., George, R.H. *et al.* (1997) Central vascular catheter-related septicaemia in paediatric cancer patients. *J. Hosp. Infect.*, **36**(1), 67–76.

Greaves, A. (1985) We'll just freshen you up, dear. *Nurs. Times*, 6 March (Suppl.), 3–8.

Larson, E. (1988) A causal link between handwashing and risk of infection? Examination of the evidence. *Infect. Control Hosp. Epidemiol.*, **9**(1), 28–36.

Levin, M.H., Olsen, B., Nathan, C. *et al.* (1984) *Pseudomonas* in the sinks of an intensive care unit: relation to patients. *J. Clin. Pathol.*, **37**, 424–427.

Mackintosh, C.A. and Hoffman, P.N. (1984) An extended model for the transfer of micro-organisms via the hands: differences between organisms and the effect of alcohol disinfection. *J. Hyg.*, **92**, 345–355.

National Nosocomial Infection Surveillance system (1991) Nosocomial infection rates for interhospital comparison: limitations and possible solutions. *Infect Control Hosp. Epidemiol.*, **12**, 609–621.

Orsi, G.B., Mansi, A., Tomao, P. *et al.* (1994) Lack of association between clinical and environmental isolates of *Pseudomonas aeruginosa* in hospital wards. *J. Hosp. Infect.*, **27**(1), 49–60.

Reybrouck, G. (1983) Role of hands in the spread of nosocomial infections. *J. Hosp. Infect.*, **4**, 103–110.

Sanderson, P.J. and Weissler, S. (1992) Recovery of coliforms from the hands of nurses and patients: activities leading to contamination. *J. Hosp. Infect.*, **21**, 85–93.

Sandford, J.P. (1986) Lower respiratory tract infections. In: *Hospital Infections* (eds Bennett, J.V. and Brachman, P.S.). Little, Brown, Boston, MA.

Whyte, W., Hodgson, R. and Tinkler, J. (1982) The importance of airborne bacterial contamination of wounds. *J. Hosp. Infect.*, **3**, 123–135.

Wilson, J. (1995) *Infection Control in Clinical Practice*. Baillière Tindall, London.

FURTHER READING

Garner, J.S. (1996) Hospital Infection Control Practices Committee. Guideline for isolation precautions in hospital. *Infect. Control Hosp. Epidemiol.*, **17**, 53–80.

Rhame, F.S. (1998) The inanimate environment. In: *Hospital Infections*, 4th edn. (eds Bennett, J.V. and Brachman, P.S.). Little, Brown, Boston, MA.

4

The immune response

INTRODUCTION

This chapter is concerned with the mechanisms that protect the body from foreign substances and microorganisms. Some of these defences are non-specific: they do not recognise and act against particular microorganisms but affect any foreign substance. They include physical barriers that protect points of entry into the body, such as the cilia lining the mucosal surfaces of the respiratory tract and circulating phagocytic cells which remove foreign substances from the blood and tissues. Other defences are triggered when they recognise specific foreign molecules (antigens). Any foreign material, including bacteria, viruses or toxins, that induces an immune response is termed an *antigen.*

These specific immune defences are formed by the B and T lymphocytes that circulate in the bloodstream and lymphatic system. The B lymphocytes produce antibodies, proteins that bind to specific antigens and promote their ingestion by phagocytic cells. The T lymphocytes deal with host cells that have been invaded by microorganisms or have become malignant, and coordinate the activity of all the different components of the immune system's response to invasion. If the B and T lymphocytes have encountered a particular antigen before, they can mount a very rapid response to it and prevent infection from becoming established. Thus, once exposed to a particular infection, an individual can develop immunity against subsequent infection by the same microorganism.

NON-SPECIFIC DEFENCES AGAINST INFECTION

These can be separated into external defences, which protect points at which microorganisms or foreign substances enter the body, and internal defences, which confine and destroy any invaders that do manage to penetrate the external defences.

External defences

The body is surrounded by microorganisms and foreign substances and therefore needs a number of physical barriers to protect it against invasion (Figure 4.1).

Skin

Intact skin presents a hostile environment for many microorganisms and cannot be penetrated by them, except by trauma, needle or

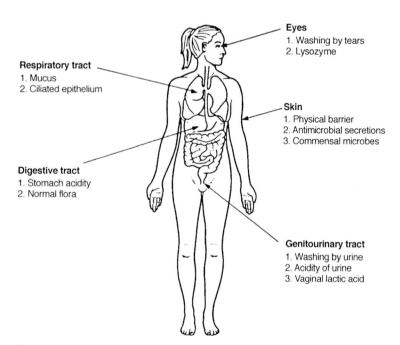

Eyes
1. Washing by tears
2. Lysozyme

Respiratory tract
1. Mucus
2. Ciliated epithelium

Skin
1. Physical barrier
2. Antimicrobial secretions
3. Commensal microbes

Digestive tract
1. Stomach acidity
2. Normal flora

Genitourinary tract
1. Washing by urine
2. Acidity of urine
3. Vaginal lactic acid

Figure 4.1 External defences that protect against invasion by microorganisms. Source: Wilson 1995.

insect bite. Lactic and fatty acids secreted by sebaceous glands can result in a low pH on the surface of the skin, facilitating the growth of harmless bacteria such as diphtheroids and discouraging the growth of other pathogens. However, hair follicles, sweat and sebaceous glands in skin harbour microorganisms and enable invasion from these sites, e.g. abscesses. Cuts, abrasions or areas of epithelium destroyed by burns are vulnerable to invasion by microorganisms, which may also be inoculated through the skin by a traumatic injury or insect bite.

Respiratory tract

The membranes lining the surfaces of the respiratory tract secrete mucus, which traps microorganisms and prevents them from adhering to and invading the tissues. The bones of the nose are arranged so that inhaled air is directed against them and bacteria stick to the mucus. Large particles are filtered out by hairs in the nose or expelled by the cough reflex. In the wider bronchial passages the speed of air flow is considerably reduced. The few remaining microorganisms are trapped in the mucus, which is gradually moved upwards, out of the respiratory tract, by fine hairs (cilia) that line the mucous membranes. When the mucus reaches the pharynx it is swallowed.

Gastrointestinal tract

The surface of the gastrointestinal tract is also protected from adherence and invasion of microorganisms by mucous membranes. In addition, the normal flora of the bowel discourages invasion by pathogens though the production of inhibitory substances and effective competition for nutrients. Acid secreted in the stomach produces a pH of between 2 and 3, in which most bacteria are unable to survive, and the alkaline bile secreted into the duodenum is also antibacterial.

Vagina

The lactobacilli that normally inhabit the vagina produce lactic acid as a by-product of their metabolism and create a local pH of between 4 and 5. This is low enough to inhibit other bacteria.

Other mucosal surfaces

Tears, nasal secretions and saliva contain an enzyme called lysozyme, which destroys bacterial cells; these fluids also protect the mucosal surfaces by washing them.

Internal defences

Microorganisms that manage to penetrate the external defences trigger a number of responses intended to destroy as many invaders as possible and confine them to the point of entry. Although these defences have a general effect against any foreign material or microorganisms, they also interact with the specific immune responses (Figure 4.2).

Phagocytic cells

These are white blood cells which ingest antigens and then digest them with enzymes (Figure 4.3). They are attracted to the site of an infection by damaged tissue cells, products from bacterial cells, antibodies and complement proteins. There are two main types of phagocytic cell: polymorphonuclear neutrophils and macrophages, both derived from stem cells in the bone marrow; eosinophils play a role in some infections (Figure 4.4).

Polymorphonuclear neutrophils are the main white cells in the blood. They have a short life span, only circulating for 6–8 hours, and a high affinity for antibodies and complement proteins, attaching to and digesting microorganisms that have been coated by them.

Macrophages, unlike neutrophils, are long-lived, and are mainly present in the lung, spleen, connective tissues and lymph nodes. They are scavenger cells, which engulf microorganisms and degrade infected or diseased cells. They play a key role in attacking organisms causing chronic infection and microorganisms that invade host cells, and are attracted to the site of an infection by damaged tissue cells, products from bacterial cells, antibodies and complement proteins. Some microorganisms, e.g. *Mycobacterium tuberculosis*, are ingested by macrophages but can prevent the release of enzymes, and are therefore able to survive and multiply within the cell.

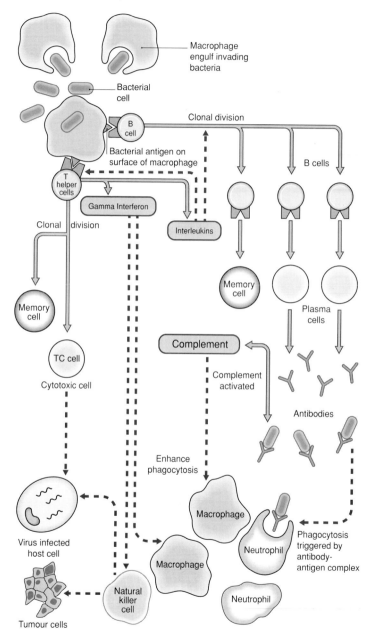

Figure 4.2   The relationship between different components of the immune system. Source: adapted from Wilson 1995.

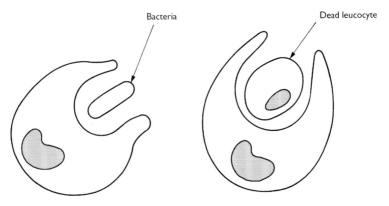

Bacteria   Dead leucocyte

Figure 4.3   Phagocytosis. Source: Wilson 1995.

After a macrophage has engulfed a microorganism, antigens from the microorganism are transported to and displayed on the surface of the macrophage. Helper-T lymphocytes, which recognise these surface antigens, are triggered to proliferate and initiate the cell-mediated immune response to the invaders.

Eosinophils are similar to neutrophils, but their role is to attack large microorganisms such as parasitic protozoa and helminths. They are triggered to release their enzymes by complement proteins that bind to the surface of the parasites.

Complement

This is a complex set of around 20 proteins, which plays an important role in enabling microorganisms or other antigens to be ingested by phagocytic cells. The complement proteins circulate in the blood in an inactive form, but when the first protein in the series encounters an antigen–antibody complex, or microorganism, a series of reactions are triggered, with the product of one reaction catalysing the next (Figure 4.5). The product of these reactions, a protein called C3b, coats the surface of the microorganism and is recognised by receptors on phagocytic cells, which can then bind to and ingest the microorganisms. Other complement proteins are involved in lysing the cell and triggering the release of histamine from mast cells (p. 62).

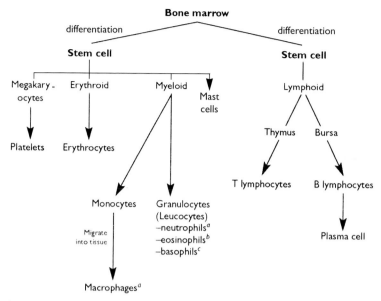

a Phagocytic cells
b Active against parasites, important in allergic reactions
c Unknown activity

Figure 4.4 Differentiation of blood cells. Source: Wilson 1995.

Natural killer (NK) cells

These lymphocytes monitor the body for parasites and malignant cells, binding to them and then releasing enzymes that make holes in the membrane of the cell, destroying it.

Interferon

These are a group of proteins that prevent viral replication and belong to a family of molecules called cytokinins, which carry signals locally between cells. All cells can produce type I interferons (alpha- or beta-interferon) when they are invaded by a virus. These interferons interfere with viral replication by binding on to specific receptors on neighbouring cells, trigger-ing them to produce enzymes that degrade viral mRNA and reduce the rate at which it is translated into protein. T lymphocytes and NK cells

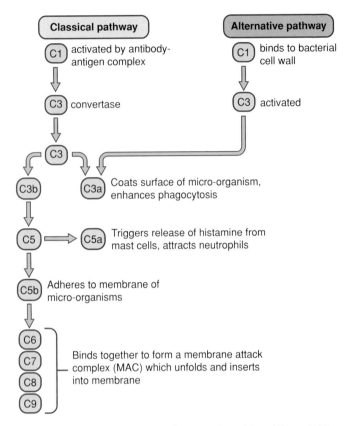

Figure 4.5 The complement system. Source: adapted from Wilson 1995.

produce type II interferon (gamma-interferon) in response to the presence of microorganisms inside other cells, or to malignant cells. Gamma-interferon then coordinates the activity of other parts of the immune system, facilitating macrophage to engulf more pathogens and display their antigens for recognition by other T lymphocytes, and controlling the production of antibodies by B lymphocytes.

The ability of interferon to enhance the destruction of tumour cells by NK cells has led to its use in the treatment of certain types of cancer (e.g. hairy-cell leukaemia, Kaposi's sarcoma) and many clinical trials are under way to test other potential uses. Beta-interferon is now used to treat multiple sclerosis, an autoimmune disease, and alpha-interferon to treat chronic Hepatitis B and C infection. Unfortunately, interferons are associated with severe side-effects, including bone marrow depression, and can only be used in low doses (Johnson et al 1994).

SPECIFIC IMMUNE RESPONSE

The non-specific defences provided by complement, interferon and phagocytic cells cannot destroy all invaders, but are assisted by that part of the immune response that recognises and targets its activity against specific antigens. Two types of cell make up the specific immune response. B lymphocytes produce antibodies, proteins that bind to specific antigens, and provide the humoral immune response. T lymphocytes recognise specific antigens from malignant cells or cells invaded by pathogens. They coordinate other cells involved in the immune response through the production of messenger proteins and destroy infected or malignant cells. They form the cell-mediated immune response.

Humoral immune response

Antibodies are Y-shaped proteins called *immunoglobulins*, which have three important regions as part of their structure (Figure 4.6).

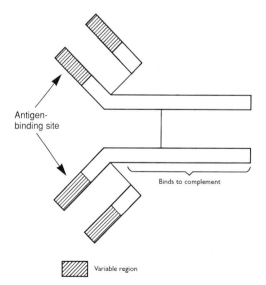

Figure 4.6   The structure of immunoglobulin. Source: Wilson 1995.

The two regions in the stem of the Y are the same in all antibodies; one attaches to complement, the other to phagocytes. The third region is on the two arms of the Y and attaches to an antigen with a complementary shape, rather like a lock and key. The structure of this region varies between antibodies and enables each to recognise and attach to a different antigen.

Antibodies are made by B lymphocytes. B lymphocytes are formed in the bone marrow and each is programmed to make a unique antibody, which is displayed on the outer surface of

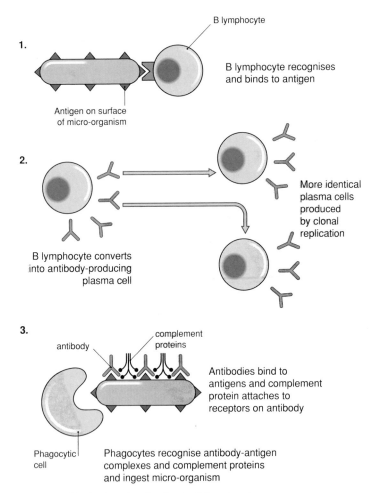

Figure 4.7 Production of antibodies by B lymphocytes.

the cell, acting as a receptor for passing antigens. When an antigen with a complementary shape binds to the receptor, it triggers the lymphocyte to convert into a plasma cell. This secretes large quantities of antibody identical to the one on the surface of the lymphocyte. The plasma cell divides rapidly to create a pool of identical plasma cells, called clones, all producing the same antibody. This mechanism enables the body to produce large quantities of antibody in response to a specific antigen (Figure 4.7).

When an antibody binds to an antigen, it activates the first protein in the complement series and triggers phagocytic cells to ingest the antigen. B lymphocytes also have surface receptors for the messenger proteins produced by T lymphocytes, which influence their activity.

Classes of immunoglobulin

There are five classes of immunoglobulin produced by B lymphocytes; each has a slightly different structure and a different role in the immune response (List 4.1). The first immunoglobulin to be produced by the plasma cell is IgM; after a few days T lymphocytes mediate a switch in production to IgG. Newborn infants only have maternal IgG, since this is the only class that can cross

---

List 4.1: Classes of immunoglobulin

- **IgG**, the most abundant type of immunoglobulin, is able to diffuse from blood vessels into tissue fluids and cross the placenta in the last 3 months of pregnancy. It coats bacteria, facilitating phagocytosis and neutralising toxins.
- **IgM**: this large immunoglobulin molecule is the first to appear in the immune response but is confined to the blood. It assists phagocytosis by coating the antigen and binds with complement very efficiently.
- **IgA** is found in the secretions of the respiratory, gastrointestinal and reproductive tracts, where it coats microorganisms and prevents them from adhering to the epithelial cells.
- **IgE** is mainly found attached to mast cells. If it encounters an antigen it triggers the release of histamine from the mast cell. It is associated with allergic response, e.g. hay fever, but is also thought to be involved in the destruction of parasites.
- **IgD**: maximum levels of this immunoglobulin are detected during childhood, but its exact function is unknown.

the placenta, but it disappears from the baby's blood within about 6 months. Soon after birth they begin to synthesise their own IgM, but adult levels of IgG will not be achieved until 5–7 years of age and IgA not until 10–12 years.

Mediator cells

These cells influence the response of the immune system by releasing vasoactive chemicals such as histamine. Vasoactive chemicals increase the permeability and dilation of local arterioles, causing an increase in flow of blood to the area and enabling lymphocytes from the bloodstream to reach the site of invasion. Mediator cells include basophils and platelets, which circulate in the blood, and mast cells, which are found in the tissues of the skin, lungs and gastrointestinal tract. The histamine is contained in specialised granules in their cytoplasm and is released when IgE bound to their surface is activated by binding to an antigen.

Cell-mediated immune response

T lymphocytes are formed in the bone marrow but develop in the thymus, a gland situated behind the sternum, which is large in children but gradually shrinks with age. There are two types of T lymphocyte; T-helper (CD4) cells, which regulate the activity of both B lymphocytes and phagocytic cells, and cytotoxic T cells, which destroy cells invaded by intracellular pathogens and malignant cells. Each T lymphocyte carries a different surface receptor, which recognises a specific antigen on the surface of an infected cell, or a phagocytic cell that has engulfed a pathogen. All cells constantly degrade proteins into small fragments, which are then carried to the surface of the cell. This process also applies to foreign proteins from invading microorganisms, which are then available for recognition by a passing T lymphocyte with an appropriate receptor. When cytotoxic T cells bind to an antigen on the surface of a cell they are triggered to release lysosomal enzymes and destroy the cell. When a T-helper cell binds to one of these surface antigens it secretes messenger proteins, *interleukins*, which activate and promote the proliferation of B lymphocytes and other T lymphocytes, and gamma-interferon, which activates macrophage and NK cells to engulf and destroy pathogens. Gamma-interferon can also switch off antibody production by activating T-suppressor cells. This may be necessary where the presence of an intracellular pathogen requires activity to be concentrated on the cell-mediated immune response rather than antibody production (Figure 4.8).

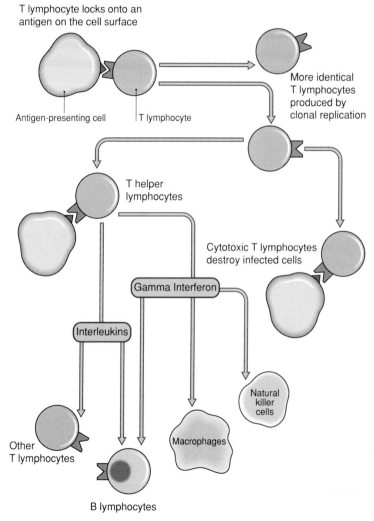

Figure 4.8   Activity of T lymphocytes.

Memory lymphocytes

Following exposure to a particular antigen, some of the B and T lymphocytes produced in response become memory cells. These are ready to respond rapidly should the same antigen be encountered again, and can protect against subsequent infection by the same pathogen. This mechanism explains the protective effect of immunisation.

The effect is illustrated by the levels of immunoglobulin that are detectable in the blood. On the first exposure to a particular antigen, specific antibodies against it can be measured in the blood after about 5 days: initially IgM, which is then replaced by IgG. A second exposure to the same antigen results in specific antibodies produced by memory cells, with both IgM and IgG appearing within 3 days and IgG in concentrations 10–15 times higher than in the initial response (Figure 4.9).

ORGANS OF THE IMMUNE SYSTEM

The immune response originates from lymphoid tissue located at points susceptible to invasion by microorganisms – the liver, gut (Peyer's patches and appendix), spleen, tonsils and adenoids –

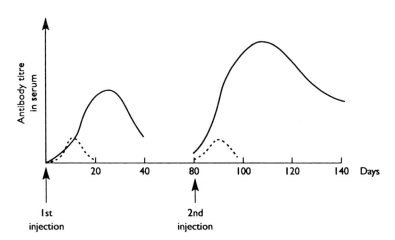

Figure 4.9 Immunisation – the primary and secondary response. After the first injection a small amount of IgG (solid line) and IgM (dotted line) are produced, but rapidly disappear. After the second injection the levels of IgG are much higher and persist for longer. Source: Wilson 1995.

and are connected by the small vessels that comprise the lymphatic system (Figure 4.10). Lymphoid tissue is also present in the lymph nodes, small glands located at the junctions between lymph and blood vessels, which filter out circulating antigens.

The cells of the immune system are made in the bone marrow and, following differentiation, migrate to the lymphoid tissue. There the macrophages trap microorganisms, ingest them and display their antigens on the surface of the cell for recognition by T lymphocytes. Once the invading pathogens have been destroyed, memory B and T lymphocytes circulate round the body in blood and lymph vessels, ready to mount a rapid response should the same pathogen invade again.

Recognition of 'self'

For the body to effectively defend itself against invaders, it must be able to distinguish between its own cells, 'self-cells', and those of the invader. During their development in the thymus, any T lymphocytes that recognise 'self' molecules are eliminated.

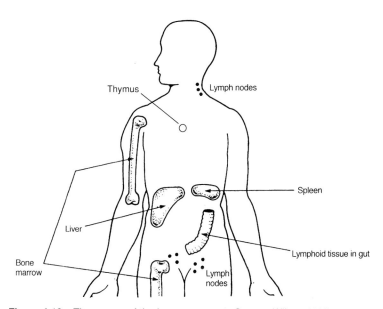

Figure 4.10   The organs of the immune system. Source: Wilson 1995.

Cells are marked as 'self' by the presence of a group of molecules on their surface called the major histocompatibility (MHC) marker. These molecules vary between individuals so that tissue transplanted from another individual will have different MHC markers and will be recognised and destroyed by the immune system as 'non-self'. Tissue-typing is used to identify potential donors whose MHC markers are similar to those of the recipient. Since the MHC marker is determined by specific genes, similarity is more likely among close family members.

INFLAMMATORY RESPONSE

Cells damaged by injury or infection release prostaglandins. These proteins increase the permeability of local blood vessels, enabling lymphocytes and plasma proteins to pass into the tissues. Prostaglandins also induce fever by stimulating the temperature control centre in the hypothalamus of the brain (Watson 1998). The exact purpose of an increase in body temperature is unknown, but it may potentiate the immune response and disadvantage the pathogens, which grow best at 37°C (Mackowiak 1994). Children have immature temperature control mechanisms and if pyrexia develops rapidly may experience febrile convulsions. Aspirin inhibits prostaglandins and can be used to reduce fever in adults. Cooling the skin by sponging with water may reduce the body temperature but can increase the discomfort of the patient (Kinmouth et al 1992).

The inflammatory response is also mediated by IgE, bound to mast cells and basophils. This recognises and attaches to specific antigens, triggering the release of granules from the cell. These contain vasoactive amines (e.g. histamine), which cause dilation of local arterioles, increasing the flow of blood to the area. These vascular changes enable lymphocytes, phagocytic cells, coagulase and complement proteins to be concentrated in the affected area and to repel invading microorganisms. The visible signs of this response on the skin include redness and heat caused by vasodilation, swelling from the increased influx of plasma and pain induced by the swollen tissue affecting local nerve endings.

A dense mesh of fibrin is formed around the site of injury or invasion and helps to confine the infection. An abscess forms if pus, which comprises dead bacterial cells, lymphocytes and dead tissue, becomes trapped inside this mesh.

IMMUNISATION

Immunity, conferred by memory lymphocytes, is acquired naturally following an infection or artificially through inoculation. The principle of immunisation is to administer sufficient antigen to induce a specific immune response without causing the actual disease. Whole communities can be protected from infectious disease, provided that sufficient numbers of the population are inoculated to prevent a pool of susceptible hosts remaining. A variety of methods are used to make vaccines.

Killed organisms

These are made from whole cells, which are killed before being incorporated into the vaccine. This method is used to make vaccines against typhoid and whooping cough (pertussis). Generally, three doses are required to achieve an adequate immune response.

Live attenuated organisms

These are microorganisms that have been altered so that they infect and multiply in the host in the same way as the original organisms but are unable to cause disease. They induce a greater immune response than killed organisms because the dose of antigen is much greater if the microorganism continues to multiply after inoculation. Another advantage is that live attenuated organisms multiply at the normal sites of infection and therefore mimic the local immune response induced by the real pathogen. Polio, measles, mumps, rubella and BCG are all live attenuated vaccines. Strains are attenuated by changing growth conditions, e.g. increasing or decreasing growth temperature, removing part of the genome or using strains that can infect humans but are virulent only in animals. In many people these vaccines produce a long-lasting antibody response after one dose. Live poliomyelitis vaccine requires three doses to confer sequential immunity to all three polio virus types present in the vaccine.

There is a small risk of an attenuated strain reverting to the virulent form of the microorganism, although when this does occur, symptoms are usually mild. Some of these vaccines are contra-indicated for people with impaired immune systems (Department of Health 1996).

Purified components

This method is used to make vaccines based on toxins. The toxin is treated with formaldehyde so that it will induce an immune response without causing symptoms. Absorption of the toxin on to an adjuvant such as aluminium hydroxide stimulates macrophage activity and prevents dispersal of the vaccine from the site of inoculation. Diphtheria and tetanus vaccines are prepared using this method.

Genetic recombination

The specific antigens involved in inducing an immune response can be identified and incorporated into an artificial vaccine. Hepatitis B vaccine is made by inserting an antigenic part of the viral genome into a yeast, this synthesises large amounts of the antigen, which is then purified and recovered.

Specific immunoglobulins

Specific antibodies against a particular infection can be collected from the blood of people who have recently become infected or who have high levels of antibody after vaccination. These can be used to provide immediate protection to a susceptible person who is at risk of acquiring a particular infection. For example, hepatitis B immunoglobulin can be administered to a non-immune member of staff following a needle-stick injury. This type of immunity is described as passive and confers protection only during the lifespan of the immunoglobulin. Infants have passive immunity for the first few months of their life through the maternal IgG that crosses the placenta. IgA is secreted in breast milk and will continue to provide passive immunity while the infant's immune system is maturing.

Vaccination programmes

In developed countries, widespread immunisation programmes have had a dramatic impact on infant mortality and are recognised as a key part of disease prevention. Many vaccines require several doses to induce effective immunity (Figure 4.9) but after a full course the level of antibody will remain high for many years.

The Department of Health recommends a programme of immunisation for all children in the UK (Table 4.1). This programme is aimed at protecting children from the most serious infectious diseases to which they are vulnerable, which may carry a significant risk of severe illness or mortality. For an immunisation programme to be effective, it is important that at least 60% of the population are protected, thus preventing the pathogen from spreading to susceptible hosts. This is called *herd immunity* and high rates of immunisation must be maintained to achieve this effect. This was clearly demonstrated in the 1970s, when the uptake of pertussis vaccine fell from 80% to 30% amid concerns about its safety. As a result notification of whooping cough increased from around 2400 cases in 1973 to over 100 000 between 1977 and 1979 (see Figure 8.8).

Manufacturers must extensively test the quality and safety of vaccines before they can be licensed, and samples of each batch must undergo independent potency, safety and purity tests. Adverse reactions to vaccines are reported by doctors to the Medicines Control Agency. The risks of serious complications following immunisation need to be balanced against the risks associated with acquiring the infection (Department of Health 1996). In addition, with increasing worldwide travel both adults and children may require protection against infections that, while rare in the UK, are endemic in other countries. Although it is rare for an infection to be eradicated completely, worldwide immunisation programmes have effectively eradicated smallpox and have eliminated polio from many countries throughout the world.

Table 4.1   Schedule for routine immunisation (UK) (Source: Department of Health 1996)

Vaccine	Age	Dose
Diphtheria, tetanus, pertussis (DTP)	2 months	
Polio, *Haemophilus influenzae* (Hib)	3 months	Primary course
	4 months	
Measles, mumps, rubella (MMR)	12–15 months	1st dose
Diphtheria, tetanus and polio	3–5 years	Booster
MMR		2nd dose
Tuberculosis (BCG)	10–14 years or infancy	1st dose
Diphtheria, tetanus and polio	13–18 years	Booster

DISEASES OF THE IMMUNE SYSTEM

The ability of the immune system to respond to infection may be affected by a variety of disease processes, including genetic abnormalities, autoimmune disease, drugs or infection.

Congenital disorders

Abnormal development of stem cells in the bone marrow can affect the production of B lymphocytes, T lymphocytes or both. The latter results in a disease called severe combined immunodeficiency syndrome (SCIDS), in which the child is susceptible to overwhelming infection caused by bacteria, fungi or viruses. In the past most children died while very young, but SCIDS can now be treated by bone-marrow transplant.

Hypersensitivity reactions

These sometimes occur when the immune system, primed by an initial exposure to an antigen, produces an excessive reaction, often within minutes, when exposed for a second time. The effects can range from relatively mild (e.g. hay fever caused by pollen allergy), to a severe, frequently fatal, systemic anaphylactic reaction. A common cause is insect stings (e.g. those of bees and wasps), in people who are highly sensitive. Hypersensitivity reactions are mediated by rapid releases of vasoactive amines from basophils and mast cells, which increase local vascular permeability and cause oedema. If released into the bloodstream in excessive amounts they can cause hypotensive shock, cardiac and respiratory failure. Other hypersensitivities are associated with antibody– antigen complexes – for instance, haemolytic anaemia, which occurs when a drug binds to red blood cells, antibodies are formed against them and the cells are destroyed by the activity of complement.

Hypersensitivity reactions often only affect the point of entry of the allergen; for instance, inhalation of animal fur or pollen causes asthma or hay fever, allergenic foods cause gastrointestinal disturbances. Delayed hypersensitivity reactions occur 24–48 hours after exposure to an intracellular microorganism and are mediated by T-helper cells and macrophages. The delayed hypersensitivity reaction to the tuberculin antigen is used to establish whether an individual is immune to *Mycobacterium tuberculosis*, by inoculation of the antigen into the skin (Heaf or Mantoux test).

Autoimmune diseases

These occur when the mechanism for recognising 'self cells' is defective, and appears to be of genetic origin. They result in antibodies being formed to tissues, which are subsequently destroyed. A variety of tissues can be affected. In juvenile onset diabetes mellitus the pancreatic islet cells, which produce insulin, are gradually destroyed and eventually this results in diabetes. Other common autoimmune diseases are listed in Table 4.2.

Acquired immune deficiency syndrome

Immune deficiencies can be caused by a variety of viruses. The human immunodeficiency virus (HIV), which causes AIDS, is now recognised as a major human pathogen. The virus is able to invade cells in the body that have a particular receptor, called CD4; these include the T-helper lymphocytes and macrophages. Although the immune system may be able to control virus replication for many years, T lymphocytes in the lymph nodes are gradually destroyed until they are so depleted that the immune system can no longer mount a response to intracellular pathogens such as mycobacteria, cryptosporidia, toxoplasmas and viruses. The virus is able to evade the immune system because its enzyme, reverse transcriptase, which converts the viral RNA genome into DNA, tends to copy inaccurately and the viral progeny may vary sufficiently to evade memory cells produced previously.

Table 4.2 Examples of autoimmune diseases

Autoimmune disease	Self-antigen recognised by T cells
Pernicious anaemia	Gastric parietal cells
Juvenile insulin-dependent diabetes	Pancreatic islet cells
Multiple sclerosis	Central nervous system myelin
Lupus erythematosus	DNA, red blood cells, lymphocytes, platelets
Rheumatoid arthritis	IgG

REFERENCES

Department of Health (1996) *Immunisation Against Infectious Disease*. HMSO, London.

Johnson, H.M., Bazer, F.W. Szente, B.E. *et al.* (1994) How interferons fight disease. *Sci. Am*, **270**, 40–47.

Kinmouth, A.L. Fulton, Y. and Campbell, M.J. (1992) Management of feverish children at home. *Br. Med. J.*, **305**, 1134–1136.

Mackowiak, P.A. (1994) Fever: blessing or curse? A unifying hypothesis. *Ann. Intern. Med.*, **120**, 1037–1040.

Watson, R. (1998) Controlling body temperature in adults. *Nurs. Stand*, **12**(20), 49–53.

Wilson, J. (1995) *Infection Control in Clinical Practice*. Baillière Tindall, London.

FURTHER READING

Nowak, M.A. and McMichael, A.J. (1995) How HIV defeats the immune system. *Sci. Am.*, **273**, 42–57.

Roitt, I. (1991) *Essential Immunology*, 7th edn. Blackwell Scientific, Oxford.

Roitt, I., Broscoff, J. and Male, D. (1996) *Immunology*, 4th edn. Times Mirror, International Publishing Ltd, London.

Von Boehmer, H. and Kisielow, P. (1991) How the immune system learns about self. *Sci. Am.*, **265**, 50–59.

5

Antimicrobial chemotherapy

HISTORICAL CONTEXT

Although the concept of infectious or transmissible diseases has been accepted for at least 2000 years, their treatment by destroying invading microorganisms within the body was virtually unknown before the pioneering work of Ehrlich in the early 20 century. In 1904, Ehrlich succeeded in curing trypanosomiasis (sleeping sickness) by using a dye (trypan red), and then introduced organic antimicrobial agents based on arsenic compounds, which he used to treat trypanosomiasis and syphilis. After these early developments, specific drug therapy remained unchanged for the next 25 years. Then in 1935, Domagk reported some success with the dye Prontosil, which he used to treat infections caused by β-haemolytic streptococci. The success of this agent was that it was able to prevent the growth of bacteria without harming the patient. The active compound, sulphonilamide, was formed in the body when Prontosil was broken down. Its antimicrobial effect was due to its resemblance to a substance called p-aminobenzoic acid (PABA), which many bacteria require to synthesise folic acid, an essential co-enzyme in the production of DNA. Mammals obtain their DNA from their diet and therefore do not use PABA. A range of related drugs called sulphonamides were subsequently developed to provide a wider range of activity, greater potency, less toxicity and different absorption and excretion characteristics. Some of these early antimicrobials are still in limited use today.

The efficacy of the sulphonamides prompted others to search for similar antimicrobial agents. The next major development came with the discovery of penicillin. This began in 1928, when Alexander Fleming noticed that colonies of staphylococci were 'dissolved' around a mould of *Penicillium notatum* that was growing by accident on a culture plate. He published his findings in 1929, showing that substances produced by the mould destroyed several kinds of bacteria without being toxic to animals. However, the substance was difficult to extract and purify and it was not until 1940 that Florey and Chain managed to produce sufficient penicillin for the treatment of infection. By the end of the Second World War, penicillin was being produced commercially and was in widespread use, particularly for the treatment of Gram-positive infections caused by staphylococci and streptococci.

The search for antimicrobial substances continued throughout the 1940s. Many were isolated from microorganisms present in soil, notably from the genus streptomyces, of which streptomycin was the first. Then followed chloramphenicol, which was derived from a species found in mulch in a Venezuelan stubble field, and tetracycline, both broad-spectrum antibiotics able to kill a wide range of both Gram-positive and Gram-negative microorganisms. In the 1950s erythromycin, gentamicin and rifampicin were discovered and in the 1960s fucidic acid, all from soil microorganisms.

Soon after penicillin came into commercial production, strains of staphylococcus resistant to it were noticed. The emergence of resistance drove forward the development of existing antimicrobial agents and the search for new ones. Experimentation in the laboratory established that small alterations to the chemical structure of naturally occurring antibiotics could change the range of microorganisms against which they were active, their duration of effect, and characteristics of absorption and excretion from the body. A new type of penicillin called methicillin, effective against resistant strains of staphylococci, was developed in this way and introduced in 1960. Unfortunately, with the increasing exposure of bacteria to a wide range of antimicrobial agents, the emergence of resistance remains a continuing problem, especially in hospitals, where serious, life-threatening infections may become difficult to treat. Resistance to antimicrobial agents is discussed in more detail later in this chapter.

In the early years of antimicrobial development, chemical agents with the ability to destroy microorganisms without being toxic were called *chemotherapeutic agents*. These include the sulphonamides, trimethoprim, metronidazole, nalidixic acid and the fluoroquinolones. The agents derived from naturally occurring substances produced by one microbial species to inhibit the growth of another were called *antibiotics*. However, the distinction between the two has been blurred by the development of many agents derived from the original antibiotic but synthesised in the laboratory. The term 'antibiotic' is now widely applied to all drugs capable of destroying bacteria.

A few drugs are available that will treat fungal infections, but antibiotics cannot be used to treat viral infections, since viruses do not have the structures against which antibiotics exert their effect.

MECHANISMS OF ACTION

Antibiotics are either *bactericidal*, i.e. they kill the bacteria, or are *bacteriostatic*, preventing their growth and replication, allowing the immune system time to destroy them.

There are four main mechanisms involved in the action of antimicrobial drugs against microorganisms (Figure 5.1).

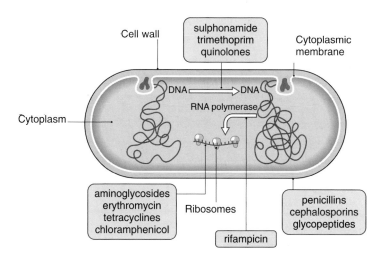

Figure 5.1   Sites of action of antibiotics on the bacterial cell.

Interference with cell wall synthesis

Bacterial cells differ from mammalian cells in that most have a cell wall made of peptidoglycan (p. 19). Some antibiotics affect the synthesis of peptidoglycan, either by preventing the cell wall from forming or by making a faulty wall. The contents of the cell cannot be protected from osmotic pressures outside with a defective cell wall, causing the cell to swell and break open. The groups of antibiotics which act in this way are:

- penicillins
- cephalosporins
- glycopeptides, e.g. vancomycin.

Disruption of cell membrane

The cell membrane in bacterial cells has an important role in maintaining the correct solute concentration in the cytoplasm. Some antibiotics, such as the polymixins, selectively damage bacterial cell membranes, causing the cells to break open. Amphotericin B and nystatin disrupt cell membranes which have a high cholesterol content, and therefore act selectively against fungal eukaryotic cells. The groups of antibiotics that act in this way are:

- polymixins, e.g. colistin
- polyenes, e.g. amphotericin B, nystatin.

Inhibition of nucleic acid synthesis

A number of antibiotics affect different stages in the synthesis of nucleic acids. The sulphonamides and trimethoprim interfere with the synthesis of folic acid, and essential co-enzyme in the synthesis of nucleic acids for DNA production. Mammalian cells, and some bacterial cells, do not synthesise folic acid, relying on dietary sources instead, and are therefore not affected by these antibiotics. The quinolones, such as ciprofloxacin, disrupt the gyrase enzyme, which controls coiling and uncoiling of DNA strands during synthesis. Rifampicin prevents DNA being transcribed into RNA. The groups of antibiotics that act in this way are:

- sulphonamides
- trimethoprim
- quinolones

- rifamycins, e.g. rifampicin
- metronidazole.

Inhibition of protein synthesis

The ribosomes of bacterial cells are smaller than, and structurally different from, ribosomes in eukaryotic cells. Antibiotics that recognise and bind to bacterial ribosomes can therefore inhibit bacterial protein synthesis while not affecting the ribosomes of the host cells. Some, such as tetracycline and chloramphenicol, bind reversibly to the ribosome and therefore have a bacteriostatic action. Fusidic acid also interferes with protein synthesis and is bacteriostatic or bactericidal depending on the type and number of bacteria and concentration of the drug. Erythromycin affects the early stage of protein synthesis and the aminoglycosides affect both protein synthesis and membrane permeability and are bacteriostatic. The groups of antibiotics that inhibit protein synthesis in this way are:

- aminoglycosides, e.g. gentamicin
- macrolides, e.g. erythromycin
- tetracyclines
- chloramphenicol
- fusidic acid.

THE PRINCIPLES OF ANTIMICROBIAL THERAPY

The review of antimicrobial agents provided in the latter part of this chapter illustrates the vast numbers of drugs available and the subtle variations between drugs in their activity within the body and range of microorganisms affected. In the UK, specialist advice on the treatment of infection and the most appropriate antimicrobial agent to use is provided by medical microbiologists. These are doctors who are based in the microbiology laboratory and who have undergone training in microbiology and the principles of antimicrobial therapy.

There are a number of factors that need to be taken into account when selecting an appropriate treatment for a particular infection.

Reason for treatment

An assessment of the signs and symptoms in the patient to ensure that they are consistent with the presence of infection and cannot be explained by another disease process is the first step in establishing whether antibiotic treatment is required. Many sites on the body are colonised by a variety of bacteria, in particular the skin, gastrointestinal and respiratory tracts, and the isolation of microorganisms from these sites in the absence of any overt signs of infection does not warrant the use of antimicrobial therapy. In some circumstances, although an infection may be present, antibiotic therapy is inappropriate, since the causative organism is unlikely to respond; such infections include upper respiratory tract infections, which are usually viral in origin, and most cases of gastroenteritis.

Causative microorganism

Sometimes the signs and symptoms of infection give sufficient clues about the causative microorganism to enable appropriate treatment to be commenced immediately. This is the case where the symptoms are characteristic of a particular infection and the causative organism is susceptible to a specific antibiotic. An example is a rapidly spreading, painful red erythema of the skin caused by a haemolytic streptococcus, for which treatment with penicillin is indicated. The characteristic rash of meningococcal meningitis similarly indicates the need for high doses of systemic penicillin.

Meningitis, urinary tract and wound infections are likely to be caused by one of a small number of bacteria, enabling the clinician to choose one, or sometimes more than one, appropriate antibiotic. Microbiological specimens should be taken when signs of infection first become apparent and before any treatment is commenced, which may make the causative organism more difficult to detect. In other situations the help of the microbiology laboratory in establishing the causative organism and antibiotics to which it is sensitive are essential.

Susceptibility to antimicrobial agents

Once the causative microorganism has been identified, an antibiotic that will treat the infection can be selected. Each type of antibiotic has a slightly different range of microorganisms against which it is effective; this is referred to as its *spectrum of activity*. Some, such as the cephalosporins, quinolones, tetracyclines and aminoglycosides, can be used to treat a wide range of both Gram-positive and Gram-negative infections and are therefore described as *broad-spectrum antibiotics*. Others, such as benzyl penicillin, cloxacillins and macrolides, are active against only a few types of bacteria and are considered to be *narrow-spectrum antibiotics*. Broad-spectrum drugs have advantages for treating infection where the causative organism is unknown, since they will work against many of the likely culprits. They can also be useful for the treatment of infections in which more than one pathogen is involved. Their disadvantage is that they will kill not only the pathogen in question, but also the body's normal flora, which has an important role in protecting against invasion by more harmful species (p. 35) and the elimination of which may encourage resistant microorganisms to take over the site.

Combination of antibiotics

Occasionally, a combination of more than one antibiotic is required to treat an infection. This may be because resistance to one drug is likely to develop during treatment. In the case of tuberculosis, treatment continues for weeks and if the organism becomes resistant, the patient is effectively not being treated. If two drugs are given some of the organisms may become resistant to one or other drug but it is unlikely that they would become resistant to both at the same time. To minimise the risk of resistance three drugs are prescribed for the treatment of tuberculosis. Combinations are also indicated where more than one pathogen is causing the infection (e.g. peritonitis), or when a complete bactericidal effect is required and two antibiotics given together will enhance each other's activity (e.g. the treatment of endocarditis caused by *Enterococcus faecalis*).

Pharmacodynamics

Different drugs are absorbed to a greater or lesser extent and excreted from the body by different routes; these factors can be very important in determining their efficacy as a form of treatment. Not all drugs are able to pass unaltered through the acidic environment of the stomach. Some can be protected by capsules that dissolve only in the small intestine; others are not absorbed well from the gut and are given parenterally. Once in the blood, the antibiotic must be able to reach the infected tissues; lipophilic drugs, such as ciprofloxacin, can pass particularly well into the bronchial mucosa, hence their suitability as a form of treatment for pseudomonal infections in the lungs of people with cystic fibrosis; clindamycin and fucidin penetrate bone well and are therefore an effective treatment for osteomyelitis. In some cases, antibiotics can only pass across membranes (or tissues) during an infection; for example, penicillin can only penetrate the meninges when they are inflamed.

The route of excretion can also influence the efficacy of a drug. Some are excreted mostly by the kidneys (e.g. sulphonamide) and are therefore useful for treating infections of the urinary tract.

The dose prescribed and route of administration chosen may depend on the severity of the infection, the age of the patient and any underlying conditions that may alter its efficacy or toxicity.

Prophylactic treatment

Antimicrobial therapy may be indicated to prevent a patient acquiring an infection in situations that markedly increase their vulnerability. This type of treatment is called *prophylaxis*. Prophylactic antibiotic treatments include:

- operations involving the intestine, where normal flora may contaminate the operative site
- extensive burns
- dental treatment in people with abnormal heart valves, who are at risk of developing endocarditis
- travel to countries where malaria is endemic.

To minimise the risk of resistant microorganisms emerging, prophylactic antibiotics should be given only at the time the patient is exposed to the risk of infection. In the case of surgical prophylaxis, they should be started at the time surgery commences and stopped after a maximum of 12 hours.

ANTIMICROBIAL RESISTANCE

The terms *sensitive* and *resistant* are used to distinguish when a microorganism is susceptible to or unaffected by a particular antibiotic. A sensitive microorganism is killed or its growth inhibited by the drug, while a resistant one survives in its presence. Resistance may be the result of intrinsic factors that prevent the antibiotic attacking the species or genus, such as a cell wall or membrane impermeable to the drug, absence of specific surface proteins that the drug needs to attach to, or lack of a specific intracellular target such as a ribosomal protein. These factors influence the range of microorganisms susceptible to a particular drug.

Acquired resistance

This type of resistance is of particular concern because it reduces the range of antibiotics available to treat specific infections. The mechanisms involved include:

Enzymes that inactivate the antibiotic

This is one of the most common mechanisms of acquired resistance. The most prevalent enzymes are the beta-lactamases, which inactivate drugs in the penicillin and cephalosporin groups. Some microorganisms produce them continuously but in others their production can be switched on when exposed to an antibiotic. Other drugs inactivated by enzymes include aminoglycosides and chloramphenicol.

Alteration to the target site of the antibiotic

This involves structural changes at the point where the antibiotic attaches to the bacterium or where it exerts its effect. In the case of *Staphylococcus aureus*, penicillin binds to a particular protein on the surface of the bacterial cell. Methicillin-resistant strains of this organism (MRSA) are resistant to a range of beta-lactam antibiotics because they have altered penicillin-binding proteins that prevent the drugs attaching to the cells.

Alteration to transport systems

Some antibiotics use the active transport system of the bacteria to enter the cell. Alterations that decrease the entry of the drug enable the bacteria to develop resistance. This mechanism contributes to resistance in aminoglycosides and tetracycline.

Alteration to metabolic pathways

Where a drug acts on a particular metabolic pathway the bacteria may be able to avoid harmful effects by switching to a different pathway. This occurs in resistance to trimethoprim.

Using these mechanisms, previously susceptible microorganisms can develop resistance to one or several antibiotics. The resistance is secured either through mutation of genes or by acquisition of resistance genes.

Mutation and selection of resistance

In a population of microorganisms exposed to a particular antibiotic, a few mutate, rendering them resistant to the drug. Although the sensitive bacteria will be prevented from growing, the mutants that are resistant will continue to multiply and build up a population of bacteria not affected by the drug.

Transfer of resistance genes

The capacity of bacteria to exchange genetic information has led to the widespread transfer of genes determining resistance between different strains of the same species and even between different species of bacteria. Genes can be transferred by bacterial viruses – bacteriophages – but by far the most common route of transfer is by a process called *conjugation* (p. 24), where small circular pieces of DNA called *plasmids* are transferred along special tubes that form between two cells. Plasmids can carry genetic information determining resistance to several different types of antibiotic so that, when exposed to one of them, microorganisms resistant to the other drugs to which the patient has not been exposed will emerge. Plasmid transfer of resistance factors is particularly prevalent among Gram-negative bacteria and the enterobacteria that harmlessly colonise the gut to provide an important source for the transfer of genetic material to other pathogenic strains or species. This problem is exacerbated when antibiotics are used as growth promoters in animal feeds, causing antibiotic-resistant intestinal flora to emerge in animals and be disseminated to humans.

Clinical problems associated with antibiotic resistance

Resistance to antibiotics is increasing in many pathogens as a result of both selection through antimicrobial usage and spread of resistant microorganisms between patients (Livermore 1998,

Pillay 1998). The unnecessary or inappropriate use of antimicrobial agents has been recognised as a widespread and international problem for many years (World Health Organization 1983, 1995). Exposure to antibiotics exerts a selective pressure on microbial populations, encouraging the emergence of microorganisms resistant to the most commonly used drugs. This is a particular problem in hospitals, where a high proportion of patients receive antibiotics, frequently without evidence of infection (Greenwood 1995a). Patients in high-dependency or intensive-care units are especially vulnerable to colonisation and infection as a result of impaired immune defences and exposure to various invasive devices (McGowan, 1994). In addition, more than 60% of patients in these units are likely to receive antibiotics and organisms resistant to a broad range of antibiotics can readily become endemic (Chadwick et al 1996, Sanyal et al 1993). There is also increasing concern about the potential of resistant strains to emerge in the community through the excessive prescription of antibiotics in general practice or community healthcare facilities. Avason et al (1996) showed a strong association between the total consumption of antibiotics in a community and the carriage of penicillin-resistant *Streptococcus pneumoniae* in children. The use of antibiotics as growth promoters in animal feeds is also thought to contribute to the problem (Greenwood 1995b). Resistant microorganisms of particular concern in hospitals in the UK are methicillin-resistant *Staphylococcus aureus* and vancomycin-resistant enterococcus. Multi-drug-resistant tuberculosis is causing significant problems in some countries, although so far the prevalence in the UK is low.

Antibiotic policies

In the past we have depended on the introduction of new antibiotics to deal with resistance problems but, with the current costs of drug development, new products are being introduced at a much slower rate. In addition to measures designed to control the spread of resistant microorganisms, a key factor in controlling the problem is improving the way in which antimicrobial agents are used (McGowan, 1994). A number of strategies to control the indiscriminate use of antibiotics have been suggested, including written policies defining recommended treatments and prophylactic regimens, restricting access to certain drugs and education campaigns to encourage more discriminating use of drugs. The medical microbiologist and pharmacy department may undertake audit to establish the effectiveness of antibiotic policies and the incidence of antibiotic-resistant strains. In addition, microbiology laboratories frequently report only a limited number of antibiotic sensitivities to encourage doctors to select the most effective and narrow-spectrum drug (BSAC Working Party 1994).

Nursing staff have an important role to play by carefully observing and recording signs and symptoms of infection and alerting medical staff to patients who may be receiving inappropriate or prolonged treatment.

METHICILLIN-RESISTANT *STAPHYLOCOCCUS AUREUS* (MRSA)

Staphylococci have been particularly successful in developing resistance to anti-microbial agents designed to defeat them (Table 5.1). Beta-lactamase producing strains of *S. aureus* appeared very soon after penicillin was introduced and now nearly all isolates of *S. aureus* in hospitals are resistant to penicillin. A modified penicillin resistant to the action of beta-lactamases, called methicillin, was introduced in 1960 and a related drug, flucloxacillin, became the drug of choice for the treatment of staphylococcal infection. However, strains of *S. aureus* to which flucloxacillin cannot bind and which are also resistant to a number of other antibiotics emerged, causing major outbreaks of infection in hospitals through-

Table 5.1 The emergence of antibiotic-resistance in *Staphylococcus aureus* (Source: Wilson, 1995)

Date	Event
1960	Methicillin introduced
1961	Methicillin-resistant *S. aureus* (MRSA) reported
1970	5% of *S. aureus* isolates methicillin-resistant
1976	*S. aureus* resistant to gentamicin and methicillin reported
1980	New penicillins and cephalosporins introduced
	Epidemic strains of MRSA reported in London
	Incidence of MRSA increases
1990	MRSA affecting most parts of the UK; many different strains responsible

out the world. Now, several distinct strains of MRSA are recognised, many of which also have the capacity to spread readily from person to person and cause serious infection, particularly among hospital patients (Communicable Disease Report 1997). Vancomycin is usually used to treat serious infections caused by MRSA. The recent report of a vancomycin-resistant strain of MRSA raises concerns about future treatment strategies (Hiramatsu et al 1997).

S. aureus is a common cause of pyogenic infection of the skin, taking advantage of wounds or hair follicles to form boils, carbuncles and abscesses, but can also cause osteomyelitis, bronchopneumonia and endocarditis. Between 20% and 30% of people carry S. aureus in their noses and may also carry the organism on their skin (Boyce 1996). Methicillin-resistant strains cause the same infections as sensitive strains but are particularly associated with hospitalisation, exposure to invasive procedures and treatment in intensive care (Humphries & Duckworth 1997). Resistant microorganisms are more likely to emerge in patients who have previously received antibiotics and the use and abuse of antimicrobials is also recognised as an important contributory factor in the emergence of MRSA (Péchere, 1994). Where outbreaks of MRSA occur, colonised or infected patients act as the major reservoir, with transmission from patient to patient via the hands of healthcare staff. Although healthcare workers sometimes acquire infection caused by MRSA, carriage of the organism is usually transient (Cookson et al 1989). The environment and airborne particles are rarely involved in the transmission of MRSA, except in special circumstances such as exist in burns units (Mylotte 1994, Barrett et al 1993). The risk of both transmission and serious infection caused by MRSA is greatest amongst hospital patients and the control measures required will be different from those recommended for the management of patients infected or colonised with MRSA in community settings. (Working Party Report 1995, 1998). The approach to controlling MRSA in hospitals may also vary according to its prevalence and the particular clinical areas affected. More extensive control measures are likely to be implemented in some surgical areas, e.g. orthopaedic, vascular and cardiothoracic, and specialist units such as intensive care units, special care baby unit and burns units, where the risk of invasive infection is high (Working Party Report, 1998). The key components of MRSA control are summarised in List 5.1.

List 5.1 Control measures for hospital patients colonised or infected by methicillin-resistant *Staphylococcus aureus*

Isolation
- Affected patients should be nursed in a single room, where available
- Gloves and aprons should be used for contact with the patient and discarded after use. They should also be changed between procedures
- Hands should be washed after contact with the patient or his/her environment

Cohorting
- A group of several affected patients can be isolated together in a designated part of the ward. This can help to reduce workload for staff and improve adherence to the control measures

Cleaning
- Isolation rooms should be kept clean during use, especially the horizontal surfaces, where dust may settle
- Rooms can be cleaned with detergent and water after isolation has been discontinued

Treatment of affected patients
- Apply antistaphylococcal cream to open skin and intranasally (Mupirocin three times per day for 5 days, naseptin four times a day for 7 days). To prevent resistance to mupirocin emerging, a maximum of two courses of treatment only should be given in any one admission
- Bathe daily for 5 days using antiseptic detergents (e.g. chlorhexidine) to eliminate skin colonisation
- Wash hair with antiseptic detergent
- Isolation can be discontinued when three sets of negative swabs from all previously positive sites have been obtained
- Clinical infections will require treatment with antibiotics, usually vancomycin or teicoplanin

Re-admission
- Previously colonised/infected patients should be re-screened on re-admission to hospital as the resistant strain may persist in small numbers
- Notes can be labelled and records flagged in computer-held records to indicate patients who have had MRSA

Screening of other patients
- Other patients can be sampled for MRSA carriage by taking swabs from the nose, perineum or groin, skin lesions and invasive device insertion sites. This can enable early identification, isolation and treatment of MRSA carriers and help to limit spread
- The extent of screening will depend on the type of clinical area and the number of patients affected

Screening of staff contacts
- This is usually only necessary in high-risk areas (e.g. ICU) or where the organism continues to spread despite the control measures and a staff carrier may be contributing to transmission
- Swab nose and skin lesions of staff in contact with affected patients
- Staff who are colonised with MRSA should be treated with mupirocin. In high-risk wards exclusion from work for 48 hours may be necessary

VANCOMYCIN-RESISTANT *ENTEROCOCCUS* (VRE)

Enterococci are normal commensals of the gut but in recent years have become an increasingly common cause of infection in hospital, particularly in specialist units. They can cause a range of serious infections including septicaemia, abdominal abscesses, urinary tract infection, meningitis and endocarditis. The increase in prevalence of enterococci has been associated with the use of invasive devices and the increase in the number of seriously ill and immunocompromised patients, although person-to-person spread and ability to survive in the environment are also important factors (Bonilla et al 1996).

While enterococci have some intrinsic resistance to a number of antibiotics, including some beta-lactams and the aminoglycosides, strains that not only have increased resistance to these drugs but have also acquired resistance to new drugs are becoming more common and are seriously reducing the options for treatment of infection (Murray 1990).

The emergence of these resistant strains of enterococci has been associated with the use of antibiotics, such as cephalosporins, that have no activity against enterococci, but which eliminate other bacteria, leaving the enterococci to multiply. These resistant strains colonise the gut from where they can cause infection in the same patient or be transferred to another patient. Of particular concern are strains resistant to vancomycin, which is a valuable form of therapy for enterococcal infection. The incidence of vancomycin-resistant enterococci (VRE) has increased markedly in the last few years and infections are associated with a high mortality (Weber & Rutala, 1997). VRE was detected in the UK in 1987 and, although the incidence is still low, outbreaks of infection have occurred in a number of liver, renal and intensive care units and there is evidence of spread between hospitals (Morrison et al 1996).

MULTI-DRUG-RESISTANT TUBERCULOSIS (MDRTB)

The incidence of tuberculosis infection and the mortality associated with it has been gradually declining in developed countries during this century with the improvements in living conditions and introduction of immunisation and antituberculous therapy.

However, many developed countries have seen a significant rise in notifications of the disease during the last decade, related to migration, overcrowding and, in some part, to the AIDS epidemic (Communicable Disease Report, 1997). The ability of *Mycobacterium tuberculosis* to develop resistance to treatment was recognised very soon after the first antituberculosis drugs were introduced. To combat this problem treatment regimes using combinations of drugs over a prolonged period were established. Unfortunately, in recent years strains of *M. tuberculosis* resistant to the two most effective antituberculosis drugs, rifampicin and isoniazid, have emerged. Infections caused by these multi-drug-resistant strains (MDRTB) can be very difficult to treat and prolonged infectiousness of the patient increases the risk of spread to others. While the incidence of MDRTB in the UK is still low, accounting for less than 2% of isolates, outbreaks of MDRTB infection have occurred among HIV patients. Breathnach et al (1998) reported an outbreak in an HIV unit where a multi-drug-resistant strain was transmitted from an index case to seven other HIV-positive patients, two of whom, together with the index case, died.

Resistant strains of tuberculosis emerge where patients default on therapy. Close monitoring of treatment, including directly observed therapy (DOT) have been used to ensure compliance with treatment (Morse 1996). Health visitors and specially trained respiratory nurses play a key role in tracing contacts of infected patients and monitoring the treatment programme (Cowle 1995).

In the UK, MDRTB is more likely to be found among some immigrant groups exposed to *M. tuberculosis* in their country of origin, where the incidence of resistance may be very high as a result of poor access to proper treatment and, in some countries, the practice of adding low levels of isoniazid to cough medicines (Department of Health 1997). Where MDRTB is suspected the patients should be nursed in an isolation room with negative pressure ventilation, and the use of filter masks by staff caring for the patient has also been recommended (McGowan 1995, Interdepartmental Working Group on Tuberculosis 1998).

MAIN GROUPS OF ANTIMICROBIAL AGENTS

The clinical applicability of the main groups of antibiotics is described below and summarised in the appropriate tables.

Penicillins

These antibiotics are based on a structure called the beta-lactam ring (Figure 5.2), which prevents cell-wall synthesis by binding to an enzyme that makes peptidoglycan. Penicillin is an extremely effective bactericidal drug. The naturally occurring penicillins, benzyl penicillin and penicillin V, are mainly active against Gram-positive bacteria, in particular streptococci, and some Gram-negative bacilli, such as the neisserias. Benzyl penicillin is destroyed by acid in the stomach and must therefore be given parenterally. The range of species against which penicillin is effective, and its pharmacology, have been extensively modified by changing the side-chain of the beta-lactam ring. A whole range of semi-synthetic penicillins are now available with different spectrums of activity, absorption and bacterial penetration characteristics (Table 5.2).

Resistance to penicillin was recognised very soon after commercial production of the drug began and is due to a beta-lactamase enzyme (penicillinase), which is able to break open the beta-lactam ring and destroy the antibiotic. Resistance to penicillin is widespread in some species, notably in staphylococci and increasingly in others, e.g. *Streptococcus pneumoniae, Neisseria gonorrhoeae*. Penicillinase-resistant penicillins (methicillin and flucloxacillin) were introduced in the 1960s. Treatment with methicillin was discontinued because of its toxicity but it is used in antibiotic sensitivity testing as a marker of flucloxacillin resistance. Flucloxacillin, which can be taken orally and is well absorbed, is of considerable value in the treatment of staphylococcal infection. However, outbreaks of staphylococcal infection resistant to flucloxacillin have been reported since the 1970s and are becoming an increasing problem in hospitals (Table 5.1). Other penicillinase-resistant drugs have been developed using combinations of clavulanic acid, a beta-lactam that inactivates beta-lactamases,

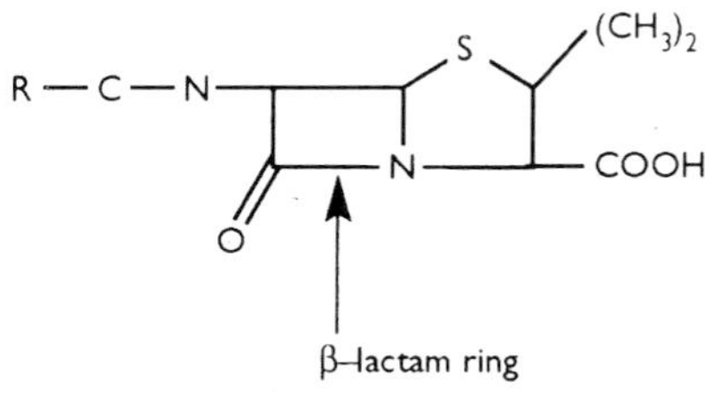

Figure 5.2   The beta-lactam ring. Source: Wilson, 1995.

Table 5.2 Penicillins (P = parenteral administration; O = oral administration)

Antibiotic	Route	Indications
Natural penicillins		
Benzyl penicillin (penicillin G)	P	Gram-positive infections including streptococcal, pneumococcal, meningococcal meningitis, clostridia, diphtheria, tetanus, gonorrhoea, syphilis
Penicillin V	O	Same spectrum as penicillin G but used for mild infections, e.g. tonsillitis, otitis media
Penicillinase-resistant penicillins		
Flucloxacillin	P	Same spectrum of activity as penicillin G but mainly used to treat staphylococcal infections because of widespread resistance to penicillin. Flucloxacillin preferred as better absorbed in the gut.
Oxacillin	O	
Broad-spectrum penicillins		
Ampicillin	O or P	Gram-positives, enterococci, *H. influenzae* and some enterobacteria. Middle ear infections and UTI. Amoxycillin penetrates sputum well and therefore particularly useful for respiratory infections.
Amoxycillin	O or P	
Co-amoxiclav (augmentin)		Combination of clavulanic acid and amoxycillin, for penicillinase producers
Anti-pseudomonal penicillins		
Piperacillin	P	Used to treat serious Gram-negative infections, especially in immunocompromised. Usually in combination with an aminoglycoside. Azlocillin particularly effective against pseudomonas.
Azlocillin	P	
Mezlocillin	P	

with other penicillins. The most commonly used is co-amoxiclav (Augmentin), a combination of clavulanic acid and amoxycillin.

Adverse reactions to the penicillins are rare and are related to hypersensitivity rather than toxicity. However, a patient who is sensitive to one type of penicillin is likely to be sensitive to other drugs in the group.

Cephalosporins

Like penicillin, cephalosporins have a beta-lactam ring with side-chain molecules that can be altered to produce drugs with differing biological and biochemical activities (Table 5.3). The first cephalosporin, cephalothin, was derived from a mould, *Cephalosporium acremonium*, in the mid-1960s. The early, or first-generation, cephalosporins have a similar spectrum of activity to ampicillin and the oral preparations, such as cephradine, are still widely used. In the years after the introduction of cephalosporins resistance became increasingly common, particularly amongst the enterobacteria. Resistance was due to a range of beta-lactamase enzymes, some with activity against penicillin alone, others that act against both penicillins and cephalosporins. The second-generation cephalosporins, which came into use after 1975, are not affected by most beta-lactamases and are active against various Gram-negative bacteria and staphylococci. The third-generation cephalosporins were developed in the 1980s; they have enhanced activity against Gram-negative bacteria but are less active against some Gram-positive species, such as *S. aureus* and pneumococci. They penetrate cerebrospinal fluid well and are therefore useful in the treatment of meningitis. However, their use has been linked to increased resistance, especially in pseudomonas, enterobacteria and serratia. They are frequently misused when a cheaper, less broad-spectrum antibiotic would be more suitable and have been implicated in pseudomembranous colitis, a diarrhoeal illness

Table 5.3 Cephalosporins (P = parenteral administration; O = oral administration)

Antibiotic	Route	Indications
First-generation		
Cephradine	O or P	Active against a broad range of Gram-negative and Gram-positive bacteria but not pneumococci, streptococci or pseudomonas. Similar spectrum to ampicillin but better resistance to some beta-lactamases
Ceflacor	O	
Cephalexin	O	
Cefadroxil	O	
Second-generation		
Cefuroxime	O or P	Active against a wide range of Gram-negative bacteria and staphylococci; less susceptible to inactivation by beta-lactamases than first-generation cephalosporins
Cefamandole	P	
Cefoxitin	P	
Third-generation		
Cefotaxime	P	Considerably better activity against Gram-negative bacteria, including acinetobacter and pseudomonas (ceftazidime). Not so effective against Gram-positives. Tend to encourage Gram-negative bacteria to develop resistance to beta-lactams
Ceftazidime	P	
Ceftizoxime	P	
Fourth-generation		
Cefepime	P	Broad spectrum of activity, less susceptible to beta-lactamases than previous generations
Cefpirome	P	

caused by the overgrowth of toxogenic strains of *Clostridium difficile* in the gut (p. 16). The latest, fourth-generation, cephalo-sporins, such as cefepime, which have a broad spectrum of activity and are stable against beta-lactamases, are now available but are not yet in widespread use.

About 10% of people who are hypersensitive to the penicillins are also hypersensitive to cephalosporins.

Other beta-lactam antibiotics

Carbapenems are very broad-spectrum beta-lactams, active against most Gram-negative and Gram-positive bacteria, including anaer-obes. They are sometimes used to treat serious infection in hospi-talised patients if the causative organism is resistant to the more commonly used antibiotics. The *monobactams* are highly effective against aerobic bacteria, including *Pseudomonas*, and do not cause hypersensitivity reactions in patients who are sensitive to peni-cillin or cephalosporin.

Aminoglycosides

These antibiotics were originally derived from *streptomyces*, a bacterium found in soil. Their bactericidal effect is caused by binding to bacterial ribosomes, preventing messenger RNA from being accurately transcribed into protein. The first to be produced in 1944, streptomycin, was the earliest form of treatment against tuberculosis. Gentamicin and tobramycin are effective against a broad range of organisms, including enterobacteria, but not anaer-obes. Resistance through the production of enzymes that can degrade the drug is becoming increasingly common. Aminogly-cosides cannot be mixed in solution with other drugs and all are associated with oto- and nephrotoxicity, so that renal function and serum levels must be closely monitored (Table 5.4).

Quinolones

These drugs are synthesised from nalidixic acid. They act by inhibiting DNA gyrase, the enzyme responsible for supercoil-ing of DNA, and have no effect on the corresponding mam-malian enzyme. They are rapidly bactericidal, with activity against a wide range of microorganisms, including enterobacteria,

Table 5.4 Aminoglycosides (P = parenteral administration; O = oral administration)

Antibiotic	Route	Indications
Gentamicin	P	Broad spectrum of activity against Gram-negative and Gram-positive bacteria. Used to treat serious Gram-negative infections and, in conjunction with penicillin and metronidazole, infections suspected to originate from the gut or urinary tract. Amikacin useful for gentamicin-resistant organisms. Blood levels must be checked regularly to avoid oto- and nephrotoxicity
Amikacin	P	
Tobramycin	P	

Haemophilus influenzae, neisseria and Gram-positive organisms, but little activity against anaerobes. They are well absorbed orally and resistance is uncommon. The original quinolones had little activity against pseudomonas, but the addition of a fluorine into the molecule has produced a new range of drugs, the fluoroquinolones (e.g. ciprofloxacin), which are active against pseudomonas. They are particularly useful for the treatment of bacteria resistant to unrelated antibiotics and are used to treat acute gastrointestinal infections such as *shigella.* Their activity against *pseudomonas* means they have become a useful form of treatment of lung infections in people with cystic fibrosis. They are not recommended in children, or in pregnant or lactating women, because of potential effects on the cartilage of weight-bearing joints of infants.

Nalidixic acid has no activity against Gram-positive bacteria or pseudomonas. It concentrates in urine and, although it is used for the treatment of urinary tract infection, resistance amongst urinary pathogens is common.

Tetracycline

Chlortetracycline was introduced in 1948 from a species of *streptomyces.* Tetracyclines exert a bacteriostatic effect by reversibly binding to ribosomes, preventing transfer RNA from attaching to messenger RNA. They have activity against a broad range of Gram-negative and Gram-positive bacteria, mycoplasmas, ureaplasmas, rickettsiae and chlamydiae. They can be given orally but tend to irritate the gut and are erratically absorbed. Resistance is common, especially among streptococci. The newer tetracyclines, e.g. demeclocycline, are better absorbed and more slowly excreted.

Tetracycline should not be given to children of under 12 years as it causes permanent yellow staining of teeth (Table 5.5). The fetus may also be affected and therefore tetracycline should not be given during the late stages of pregnancy.

Metronidazole

This was once regarded solely as an antiparasitic agent used for the treatment of trichomonas infection, giardiasis and amoebiasis. It was then discovered that it was effective against anaerobic bacteria and it is now widely used as an effective form of treatment for infections caused by anaerobes, especially *Bacteroides fragilis*; it is also used prophylactically prior to bowel and gynaecological surgery to minimise the risk of postoperative infection. It is used in combination with other drugs to treat *Helicobacter pylori* infection of the stomach. It is rarely associated with resistance or adverse reactions, although it should not be taken with alcohol.

Sulphonamides

These drugs are synthetic chemicals that resemble para-aminobenzoic acid, a co-enzyme in the production of folic acid, and have a bacteriostatic effect by interrupting the synthesis of folic acid. They were the first group of antimicrobials found to be effective against many different pathogens but, while inexpensive and of low toxicity, they are not in common use now because of widespread resistance and the availability of newer, more effective drugs. They are concentrated in the urine and, in combination with trimethoprim, are a useful treatment for urinary tract infection.

Table 5.5   Tetracyclines (P = parenteral administration; O = oral administration)

Antibiotic	Route	Indication
Tetracycline	O (usually)	Broad spectrum, but poor absorption and increased resistance has reduced use.
Oxytetracycline	O	Useful for treatment of non-specific urethritis, exacerbations of chronic bronchitis, mycoplasmal and chlamydial infections. Can cause nausea and diarrhoea; stains teeth in young children. Contraindicated in pregnancy
Doxycycline	O	Better absorbed and can be used where renal function impaired

Trimethoprim and co-trimoxazole

Trimethoprim, like the sulphonamides, disrupts folic acid production, but at a different point in its synthesis. It has a broader spectrum of activity than the sulphonamides and, since it penetrates sputum well, can be used to treat respiratory as well as urinary tract infection. Concerns about the potential of bacteria developing resistance to trimethoprim led to the introduction of a combination of trimethoprim and sulphamethoxazole called co-trimoxazole. This combination is used to treat urinary tract infection, chronic bronchitis, pneumocystis, toxoplasmosis and, because it can penetrate host cells, infections caused by intracellular pathogens, such as typhoid and brucellosis.

Macrolides

The first macrolide, erythromycin, was isolated from a species of *Streptomyces*, and is active against the same range of organisms as benzyl penicillin. It is only bactericidal at high concentrations. Its main disadvantages are irregular absorption from the gut and gastrointestinal disturbance. However, because it is non-toxic and can be made into an oral suspension, it is widely used for the treatment of infection in children and as an alternative to penicillin in people who are hypersensitive. It is also the main drug used in the treatment of campylobacter and legionella, and as an alternative in the treatment of mycoplasmas, ureaplasma, rickettsias and chlamydias. Newer macrolides are now available, such as azithromycin and clarithromycin, which are better absorbed and are active against a wider range of organisms.

Other antimicrobial agents

Other, smaller groups of antimicrobial drugs include:

• **Clindamycin**, derived from lincomycin, a drug isolated from a streptomyces and similar in activity to the macrolides but well absorbed orally and particularly useful for the treatment of osteomyelitis since it penetrates bone well.
• **Vancomycin**, a glycopeptide, isolated from a streptomyces and with a high level of activity against staphylococci. It is used intravenously to treat staphylococcal infections associated with implants (e.g. hip prostheses) and serious infections caused by

strains of staphylococcus resistant to other antibiotics. Serum levels need to be monitored to prevent side-effects, which include renal damage and deafness. Taken orally, it is the main treatment for pseudomembranous colitis and staphylococcal enteritis.

• **Rifampicin** is a synthetic derivative of a streptomyces antibiotic. It is useful for the treatment of tuberculosis but, although it is effective against staphylococci and streptococci, resistance develops rapidly. At high doses it is excreted in the urine and tears, which it colours red.

• **Fucidin** is a steroid derived from a fungus. It is particularly effective against *S. aureus* and, since it penetrates bone well, is used to treat osteomyelitis. However, resistance can develop rapidly during the course of treatment and it must therefore always be used in combination with another antistaphylococcal antibiotic.

• **Chloramphenicol** was originally derived from *streptomyces venezuelae* but is now produced synthetically. It exerts a bacteriostatic effect by binding reversibly to the ribosomes, preventing protein synthesis. It has a dose-related, reversible depressant effect on the bone marrow and even at low doses can cause a fatal aplastic anaemia. Consequently, it should never be prescribed for minor infections and its main use is in the treatment of typhoid fever.

Antituberculosis therapy

Mycobacterium tuberculosis grows extremely slowly and a long period of antimicrobial therapy is therefore required to treat the infection. In addition, the mycobacterium may be protected by closed cavities in the lung or macrophages. Treatment with a combination of drugs is therefore used to prevent resistant organisms emerging and to kill intracellular bacteria (Table 5.6). Three drugs, rifampicin isoniazid and pyrazinamide, are usually given for 2–3 months, followed by several months of rifampicin and isoniazid. Second line antituberculosis drugs are used when the organism is resistant to one or more of the first-line drugs (p. 88).

Antifungal agents

Antibiotics used to treat bacterial infections are not effective against fungi, which have a more complex, eukaryotic cell structure. There are, however, a few antifungal agents available. Griseofulvin is derived from a penicillium fungus and disrupts cell formation in

Table 5.6 Antituberculosis agents (P = parenteral administration;
O = oral administration)

Agent	Route	Indication
First-line drugs		
Isoniazid	O or P	Only used for the treatment of tuberculosis; highly effective, although resistant strains common. Peripheral neuritis and hepatitis may occur at high doses
Rifampicin	O or P	Most potent of the antituberculosis drugs; causes failure of low-dose oestrogen contraceptive pill, colours urine and tears red, may cause liver damage
Pyrazinamide	O	Good penetration of tissues and meninges; useful for treatment of tuberculosis meningitis. Hepatotoxic
Second-line drugs		
Ethambutol	O	Reserved for treatment of resistant strains and atypical mycobacteria; can cause visual impairment
Streptomycin	P	Effective, but has to be used parenterally
Cycloserine	O	Used only when bacteria resistant to several first-line drugs
Thiacetazone	O	Rarely used in developed countries

some fungi; the polyene antifungals (e.g. nystatin, amphotericin B), disrupt the cell membrane of fungi by interfering with its sterol content; flucytosine is an analogue of a nucleic acid, which is incorporated into RNA and disrupts protein synthesis; and the imidazoles (e.g. clotrimazole, miconazole), selectively inhibit fungal cell-wall synthesis by interfering with ergosterol production. The characteristics of the main antifungal drugs are summarised in Table 5.7.

Antiviral agents

Viruses are obligate intracellular parasites and use the metabolic processes of their host cell to replicate. An antiviral agent must therefore be able to target viral replication without damaging the host cell. Most of the agents currently available interfere with the synthesis of viral nucleic acids.

Table 5.7   Anti fungal agents (P = parenteral administration;
O = oral administration; T = topical administration)

Anti fungal	Route	Indications
Polyenes		
Nystatin	T	Superficial candidiasis, too toxic for parenteral use
Amphotericin B	P	Broad antifungal spectrum, main form of treatment for deep mycoses. Nephrotoxic
Flucytosine	O or P	Active against yeasts (eg. candida, cryptococci); can be used to treat systemic infections. Blood levels need to be monitored to avoid neutropenia and thrombocytopenia
Imidazoles		
Clotrimazole	T	Superficial candidiasis (e.g. vaginal thrush)
Miconazole	T or P	Second-line treatment for systemic candidiasis. Adverse reactions common
Fluconazole	O or P	Treatment of and prophylaxis against systemic candidiasis and cryptococcus. Minimal toxicity
Itraconazole	O	Treatment of systemic infections, including aspergillus
Griseofulvin	O	Concentrates in the skin and therefore used for treatment of ringworm
Allylamine		
Terbinafine	O or T	New antifungals active against candida and aspergillus

The first agent found to have an antiviral effect was interferon, which was discovered by the British virologist Alick Isaacs in 1956. The interferons are proteins, produced by cells infected by a virus and by lymphocytes in response to viral infection. They appear to protect susceptible surrounding cells from infection by blocking viral replication and help to switch on the cell-mediated immune response. Unfortunately, interferon therapy was found to be associated with severe flu-like side-effects and bone-marrow suppression and this has limited its use. However, it has been used to treat some chronic infections, such as hepatitis B and C.

The first specific antiviral drug to be developed was idoxuridine, a thymidine analogue, which was introduced in 1962 for the topical treatment of herpesviruses. In the 1970s, research concentrated on drugs for the treatment of infections caused by herpesviruses, resulting in the introduction of acyclovir and vidarabine. Since the emergence of AIDS in the 1980s, the research effort has been directed towards developing anti-HIV agents. The most successful drug developed so far is zidovudine (azidothymidine, AZT). Originally devised as a treatment for cancer, it has been found to inhibit viral DNA polymerases and to slow the progression of the disease. Unfortunately, side-effects of nausea and vomiting and bone-marrow depression, which results in neutropenia, limits the size of the dose. Other drugs that have less bone marrow toxicity, e.g. 2′,3′-dideoxycytidine (ddT), are also being developed. The most commonly encountered antiviral drugs are summarised in Table 5.8.

Table 5.8 Antiviral agents (P = parenteral administration; O = oral administration; T = topical administration)

Anti-viral agent	Route	Indication
Idoxuridione (IDU)	T	Herpes skin or corneal infection; too toxic to use systemically
Amantadine	O	Can be used prophylactically to prevent infection with influenza A virus.
Acyclovir	T, O or P	Herpes simplex, including ocular, skin, mucous membrane, genital infections and encephalitis. Also effective against varicella-zoster virus. Requires prompt administration to be effective and does not destroy latent virus
Gancyclovir	P	Similar to acyclovir but more effective against Cytomegalovirus, especially in immunosuppressed patients. May induce neutropenia
Vidarabine		Has been used i.v. for varicella-zoster in the immunosuppressed, herpes simplex (e.g. corneal lesions). Low toxicity
Ribovirin	P Aerosol	Blocks viral RNA production. Used to treat Lassa fever and, as an aerosol, severe RSV in children
Foscarnet		Inhibits DNA polymerases in herpesviruses and reverse transcriptase in retroviruses. Used to treat severe CMV infection
Zidovudine	O	Inhibits DNA polymerases, slows down viral replication and progression of disease in people infected with HIV. Nausea and vomiting common and also toxic to bone marrow, causing anaemia and neutropenia
2′3′-dideoxycytidine		Inhibits DNA polymerases in a similar way to zidovudine. Less bone marrow toxicity but can cause peripheral neuropathy.

REFERENCES

Avason, V.A. Kristinsson, K.G., Sigurdson, J.A. *et al.* (1996) Do antimicrobials increase the carriage rate of penicillin resistant pneumococci in children? Cross sectional prevalence study. *Br. Med. J.*, **313**, 387–391.

Barrett, S.P., Teare, E.L. and Sage, R. (1993) Methicillin-resistant *Staphylococcus aureus* in three adjacent health Districts of South-East England 1986–91. *J. Hosp. Infect.*, **24**, 313–325.

Bonilla, H.F., Zervos, M.J. and Kauffman, C.A. (1996) Long-term survival of vancomycin-resistant *Enterococcus faecium* on a contaminated surface. *Infect. Control Hosp. Epidemiol.*, **17**(12), 770–771.

Boyce, J.M. (1996) Preventing staphylococcal infections by eradicating nasal carriage of *Staphylococcus aureus*: proceeding with caution. *Infect. Control Hosp. Epidemiol.*, **17**, 775–779.

Breathnach, A.S., de Ruiter, A., Holdsworth, G.M.C. *et al.* (1998) An outbreak of multidrug resistant tuberculosis in a London teaching hospital. *J. Hosp. Infect.*, **39**(2), 111–118.

BSAC Working Party (1994) British Society for Antimicrobial Chemotherapy (BSAC) Hospital antibiotic control measures. Working party report. *J. Antimicrob. Chemother*, **34**, 21–42.

Chadwick, P.R., Chadwick, C.D. and Oppenheim, B.A. (1996) Report of a meeting on the epidemiology and control of glycopeptide-resistant enterococci. *J. Hosp. Infect.*, **33**(2), 83–92.

Communicable Disease Report (1997) Epidemic methicillin resistant *Staphylococcus aureus*. *Commun. Dis. Rep.*, **7**(22), 191.

Cookson, B.D., Peters, B., Webster, M. *et al.* (1989) Staff carriage of epidemic methicillin resistant *Staphylococcus aureus*. *J. Clin. Microbiol.*, **27**(7), 1471–1476.

Cowle, R. (1995) TB: cure, care and control. *Nurs. Times*, **91**(38), 29–30.

Department of Health (1997) *Resistance to Antimicrobial Agents*. House of Lords Select Committee on Science and Technology. HMSO, London.

Greenwood, D. (1995a) Sixty years on: antimicrobial drug resistance comes of age. *Lancet*, **346**(suppl), 1.

Greenwood, D. (ed.) (1995b) *Antimicrobial Chemotherapy*, 3rd edn. Oxford University Press, Oxford.

Hiramatsu, K., Hanaki, H. and Ino, T. (1997) Methicillin-resistant *Staphylococcus aureus* clinical strain with reduced vancomycin susceptibility. *J. Antimicrob. Chemother.*, **40**, 135–136.

Humphries, H. and Duckworth, G. (1997) Methicillin-resistant *Staphylococcus aureus* (MRSA) – a re-appraisal of control measures in the light of changing circumstances. *J. Hosp. Infect.*, **36**(3), 167–170.

Interdepartmental Working Group on Tuberculosis (1998) The prevention and control of tuberculosis in the United Kingdom. Department of Health, Stoves, Wetherby.

Livermore, D. (1998) Multiresistance and 'superbugs'. *Commun. Dis. Pub. Health*, **1**(2), 74–76.

McGowan, J.E. (1994) Do intensive hospital antibiotic control programs prevent the spread of antibiotic resistance? *Infect. Control Hosp. Epidemiol.*, **15**(7), 478–483.

McGowan, J.E. (1995) Editorial: preventing nosocomial tuberculosis – progress at last. *Infect. Control Hosp. Epidemiol.*, **23**, 141–145

Morrison, D., Woodford, N. and Cookson, B. (1996) Epidemic vancomycin-resistant *Enterococcus faecium* in the UK. *CMI*, **1**(2), 146.

Morse, D.I. (1996) Directly observed therapy for tuberculosis. *Br. Med. J.*, **312**, 719–720.

Murray, B.A. (1990) The life and times of the enterococcus. *Microbiol. Rev.*, **3**(1), 46–65.

Mylotte, J.M. (1994) Control of methicillin-resistant *Staphylococcus aureus*: the ambivalence persists. *Infect. Control Hosp. Epidemiol.*, **15**, 73–77.

Péchere, J.C. (1994) Antibiotic resistance is selected primarily in our patients. *Infect. Control Hosp. Epidemiol.*, **15**, 472–477.

Pillay, D. (1998) Emergence and control of resistance to antiviral drugs in herpes viruses, hepatitis B virus and HIV. *Commun. Dis. Publ. Health*, **1**(1), 5–13.

Sanyal, D., Williams, A.J., Johnson, A.P. *et al.* (1993) The emergence of vancomycin resistance in renal dialysis. *J. Hosp. Infect.*, **24**(3), 167–174.

Weber, D.J. and Rutala, W.A. (1997) Role of environmental contamination in the transmission of vancomycin-resistant enterococci. *Infect. Control Hosp. Epidemiol.*, 18: 306–9

Wilson, J. (1995) *Infection Control in Clinical Practice*. Baillière Tindall, London.

World Health Organization (1983) Control of antibiotic resistant bacteria. *Bull. WHO*, **61**, 423–433.

World Health Organization (1995) Scientific working group on monitoring and management of bacterial resistance to antimicrobial agents. *WHO/CDS/BVI/95.7*. WHO, Geneva.

Working Party Report (1995) Guidelines on the control of methicillin-resistant *Staphylococcus aureus* in the community. Report of a combined working party of the British Society for Antimicrobial Chemotherapy and the Hospital Infection Society *J. Hosp. Infect.*, **31**, 1–12.

Working Party Report (1998) Revised guidelines for the control of methicillin-resistant *Staphylococcus aureus* infection in hospitals. *J. Hosp. Infect.*, **39**(4), 253–290.

FURTHER READING

Cooksey, S. (1995) Managing chemotherapy for tuberculosis. *Nurs. Times*, **91**(35), 32–33.

Department of Health (1996) Methicillin-resistant *Staphylococcus aureus* in community settings. *PL(CMO)96*. HMSO, London.

Handysides S (1997) Editorial: Tuberculosis remains 'the captain of all these men of death' *CDR Rev.*, **7**(8), R105–106.

Hospital Infection Control Practices Advisory Committee (1995) Recommendations for preventing the spread of vancomycin resistance. *Am. J. Infect. Control*, **23**, 87–94.

Joint Tuberculosis Committee of the British Thoracic Society (1994) Control and prevention of tuberculosis in the United Kingdom: Code of Practice 1994. *Thorax*, **49**, 1193–1200.

Shaw, T. (1995) The resurgence of tuberculosis; current issues for nursing. *Nurs. Times*, **91**(40), 35–37.

Walters, J. (1988) How antibiotics work. *Prof. Nurse*, **3**(7), 251–254.

Walters, J. (1990) How antibiotics work: nucleic acid synthesis. *Prof. Nurse*, **5**(12), 641–643.

Wilson, J. and Richardson, J. (1996) Keeping MRSA in perspective. *Nurs. Times*, **92**(19), 58–60.

Wood, M.J. and Geddes, A.M. (1987) Antiviral therapy. *Lancet*, **ii**, 1189–1193.

6

Cleaning, disinfection and sterilisation

INTRODUCTION

Equipment used in healthcare can transmit infection from one person to another. Therefore, the physical and chemical processes required to remove microorganisms form an important part of infection prevention and control in the healthcare environment.

Selecting an appropriate method of decontamination for a particular piece of equipment should be based on an assessment of the risk of the particular item acting as a source or vehicle of infection, and take into account the processes that the item will withstand.

LEVELS OF DECONTAMINATION

The destruction of microorganisms on equipment is achieved by using a variety of physical or chemical processes to disrupt, destroy or remove the microbial cells. Physical processes, such as heat, tend to be more reliable than chemicals, since the latter have a variable effect on different microorganisms, may be unstable and are susceptible to inactivation.

Three different levels of decontamination are recognised and are described in Table 6.1. The highest level, sterilisation, aims to remove or kill all microorganisms, and to do this the process must be able to eliminate highly resistant bacterial spores (p. 21). The second level of decontamination, disinfection, removes most microorganisms but is not sufficient to destroy bacterial spores. Disinfected items cannot be described as 'sterile'. The third level of decontamination is cleaning, which relies on the use of deter-

Table 6.1 Levels of decontamination

Term	Definition
Sterilisation	The removal or destruction of all microorganisms, including bacterial spores
Disinfection	The reduction in number of microorganisms to a level at which they are not harmful. Spores are not usually destroyed
Cleaning	The use of detergent to remove contamination physically (blood, faeces, etc.) and with it many microorganisms

gent to physically remove microorganisms. Cleaning alone is a sufficient form of decontamination for many items of equipment; it is also an essential preparation for equipment prior to disinfection or sterilisation. These processes are more effective if organic material, together with many microorganisms, is first removed from the surfaces by cleaning with detergent.

On exposure to a decontamination process, the destruction of microorganisms does not occur immediately. The heat or chemical must first penetrate the cells, and in the case of spores this can take a considerable time. The longer the period of exposure the more cells will be destroyed, until the maximum number have been destroyed. The duration of the process is therefore an important determinant of the level of decontamination and varies according to the method employed.

SELECTING THE LEVEL OF DECONTAMINATION

The risk of equipment transmitting microorganisms depends on how it is used. Items, such as surgical instruments, that are used to penetrate the skin or mucous membranes or enter normally sterile body areas can introduce infection to these susceptible sites. Such high-risk equipment should be used sterile. Equipment in contact with less susceptible sites such as mucous membranes, but which may become contaminated by microorganisms that are easily transmitted to others, is considered to be medium-risk. This type of equipment should be disinfected as a minimum but sterilised where possible after each use (e.g. endoscopes, vaginal specula). Equipment that comes into contact with intact skin is unlikely to transmit infection and decontamination by cleaning is therefore sufficient. These categories of decontamination are summarised in Table 6.2.

Table 6.2 Categorisation of equipment by risk of transmitting infection

Category of risk	Indication	Level of decontamination	Method of decontamination
High	Items that penetrate skin/mucous membranes or enter sterile body areas	Sterilise	Autoclave and use sterile or sterile single-use disposable – e.g. surgical instruments, needles
Medium	Items that have contact with mucous membranes or are contaminated by readily transmissible microorganisms	Disinfect or sterilise	Autoclave, if possible – e.g. vaginal specula Chemically disinfect (thermolabile items) – e.g. endoscopes
Low	Items used on intact skin	Clean	Wash with detergent and hot water – e.g. washbowls, mattresses

It is important to ensure that the level of decontamination used routinely is sufficient to prevent cross-infection. In most situations it should not be necessary to use a higher level of decontamination if a patient is known to be infected with a particular pathogen. The main exception to this is where infection with *Mycobacterium tuberculosis* is suspected in a patient undergoing endoscopy, as prolonged immersion in disinfectant is required to destroy this organism.

METHODS OF DECONTAMINATION

CLEANING OF EQUIPMENT

In this process, detergent and water are used to remove organic material from a piece of equipment. It is important as a method of decontamination for a variety of low-risk equipment and prior to disinfection or sterilisation, to improve the efficacy of these processes. It is also required to remove protein in organic material such as blood, which is coagulated by heat and can be very difficult to remove from instruments after disinfection or sterilisation.

Detergent is necessary to loosen grease and dirt, enabling water to remove them more easily. At least 80% of microorganisms can be removed by simple cleaning with detergent and hot water (Ayliffe et al 1967), and probably more where automatic washing machines are used. These machines are useful for washing large amounts of equipment, e.g. surgical instruments in Central Sterile Supply departments (CSSD) or crockery and cutlery in catering departments. They also remove blood and body fluids from sharp items that may cause injury, enabling them to be decontaminated prior to handling.

Ultrasonic cleaning machines generate high-frequency sound waves in a tank containing water and detergent. The waves dislodge blood and dirt on instruments submerged in the water and are especially useful for cleaning delicate instruments with awkward crevices. Hollow tubing is particularly difficult to clean and is best achieved by using special brushes or high-powered water jets. This type of cleaning should not be attempted on single-use items such as nasogastric tubes, because of the risk of cross-infection (Anderton & Nwoguh 1991).

Low-risk items which have been decontaminated by cleaning should be dried, with disposable towels or by airing in a warm place, before storage. Damp equipment allows those bacteria remaining after cleaning to multiply: washing bowls left damp after use are more likely to be contaminated with Gram-negative bacteria than bowls thoroughly dried after use (Greaves 1985). Similarly, items should not be left immersed in a container of detergent as some bacteria are able to grow in these solutions.

DISINFECTION

Disinfection aims to remove most microorganisms, including all pathogens, although it cannot be relied upon to destroy bacterial spores. It should be used to minimise the risk of cross-infection from a range of non-surgical equipment, especially those instruments used in contact with mucous membranes, which are likely to have become contaminated with pathogens.

Disinfection can be achieved by physical methods involving heat, or by chemicals, although the former is the more reliable and preferable method. Whichever process is used, it should always be preceded by thorough cleaning.

Disinfection by heat

Heat is an excellent method of disinfection, being reliable, inexpensive, readily available and broad-spectrum. Disinfection by heat occurs most efficiently in water, because the moisture conducts the heat evenly to all parts of the object. The effectiveness of the process is dependent on the temperature and the duration of exposure. The time required to kill microorganisms decreases as the temperature is raised.

Heat is widely used as a method of disinfection in clinical settings. Bedpan washers disinfect by washing and then exposing the bedpan to a temperature of 80°C for at least 1 minute. Similarly, linen is disinfected during the wash cycle, by holding it at a temperature of 71°C for not less than 3 minutes (NHS Executive 1995). Other examples of decontamination by hot water include dishwashers and instrument or anaesthetic equipment washers.

Water boiler/disinfectors

A higher level of disinfection can be achieved by total immersion in boiling water. This method is used in water boilers and can be used to kill all microbes except bacterial spores. Instruments should be completely immersed and, once the water is seen to be boiling, timed for a period of 5 minutes before removal. Ideally, machines should have a device to prevent opening during this time to remove or add instruments. Forceps used to remove objects from the machine should not be stored in containers of disinfectant as they may become heavily contaminated. Instead they should be either kept in sterile packs or disinfected in the boiler and stored in a dry, covered container. The boiler must cleaned and descaled regularly. Sterilisation is therefore a preferable method and should be used instead of hot-water-boiler disinfection wherever possible. The availability of inexpensive, small autoclaves makes sterilisation a feasible option in most situations (Medical Devices Agency 1996).

Disinfection using chemical agents

A variety of chemicals are capable of killing microorganisms; most are not active against all microorganisms, particularly tubercle bacilli and bacterial spores, and some do not affect viruses. Also, the selection of an appropriate agent for a specific task is made more difficult because individual chemicals have different properties and are only effective at particular concentrations. They are frequently used when disinfection is not indicated and are prone to inaccurate dilution.

Other disadvantages as decontamination agents include:

- **corrosion** of metal components or equipment
- **damage** to plastics, rubber or lens cement
- **toxicity** to the skin and mucous membranes of staff and, if absorbed into plastic or rubber parts, they can leach out and affect the patient
- **instability**: dilute solutions decay and lose efficacy, particularly if stored in warm conditions
- **contamination**: solutions can become contaminated by microorganisms, especially Gram-negative bacteria
- **inactivation** by various substances, including body fluids, detergents and plastics, which then interfere with their antimicrobial activity
- **penetration**: the inability of some agents to penetrate blood or other body fluids on surfaces will affect the reliability of decontamination
- **exposure time**: the required period of exposure to the disinfectant varies according to the type of chemical and the target microorganism.

Choice of disinfectant

A simple approach to deciding whether chemical disinfection is appropriate has been proposed by Kelsey & Maurer (1967), who recommend that chemicals should not be used when:

- sterilisation is required
- disinfection by hot water or steam is possible
- cleaning alone is adequate.

Many pieces of equipment can be decontaminated more appropriately either by cleaning with detergent and water or by sterilisation in an autoclave. One exception to this formula is fibreoptic endoscopes. Many, particularly those used in the respiratory and gastrointestinal tract, are readily contaminated with microorganisms and when inadequately decontaminated have been implicated in the transmission of infection (Langenberg et al 1990, Akamatsu et al 1996). Their narrow channels and valves are difficult to clean prior to disinfection and they are usually damaged by heat, thus requiring chemical disinfection. The reliability of the process can be improved by using automated washer–disinfecter machines, which clean and then disinfect more thoroughly than manual methods (Ayliffe et al 1993).

If a chemical disinfectant is required for decontamination there are a number of factors that should be taken into account to ensure the efficacy and safety of the process. The Control of Substances Hazardous to Health Regulations (Health and Safety Executive 1988) require that the risk presented by hazardous substances such as chemicals should be assessed and prevented by defined measures such as use of ventilation or protective clothing (Box 6.1). After disinfection, equipment usually needs to be thoroughly rinsed with water to ensure that residual chemical does not cause subsequent corrosion or irritation. The principles of safe and effective use of chemical disinfectants are described in List 6.1.

List 6.1   Principles for the use of chemical disinfectants

- Check the Policy to ensure disinfection is necessary and the correct agent to use
- Check the appropriate COSHH assessment
- Clean equipment thoroughly with detergent first
- Make up the chemical in the correct dilution; do not guess
- Completely immerse the equipment for the correct time
- Discard disinfectant after use; clean and dry the container

---

Properties of common disinfectants

This section outlines the important properties of the disinfectants most commonly used in clinical areas. Their recommended uses are summarised in Table 6.3. More detailed information can be found in Ayliffe et al 1993.

Alcohol. Concentrations of 70% or more can destroy a wide range of bacteria and fungi, but not bacterial spores. They are effective against viruses, although not those without lipid envelopes. Since it does not penetrate organic matter well and is inflammable, alcohol is not generally useful for the disinfection of soiled equipment. The use of alcohol-impregnated wipes to disinfect a variety of surfaces is probably both ineffective and unnecessary (Thompson & Bullock, 1992). Alcohol is useful for skin disinfection where an agent that acts rapidly and dries quickly is required. When used as a surgical scrub, alcohol both markedly reduces resident skin flora and has a persistent effect over several hours (Rotter et al 1980).

Chlorhexidine has a greater effect against Gram-positive than against Gram-negative bacteria and no effect on tubercle bacilli, spores or some viruses. This limited spectrum of activity makes it

---

Box 6.1   Control of Substances Hazardous to Health (COSHH) Regulations

The COSHH regulations are aimed at ensuring that hazardous substances are handled safely in the workplace and that employers are protected from chemical, carcinogenic and microbiological hazards. The regulations require employers to systematically assess the risks presented by any hazardous substances in use and determine the control measures necessary to ensure that they are handled safely. The risk assessment should review the following:
- how the chemical is used and whether it is necessary
- potential harmful effects
- how exposure can be prevented and controlled, e.g. restricted use, ventilation, containers, protective clothing, management of spillages
- informing and training users
- health surveillance, if appropriate.

There is a hierarchy of methods, in order of preference and effectiveness, that should be used to reduce risk:
- elimination
- substitution
- enclosure (segregation of people)
- safe system of work that reduces risk to an acceptable level
- written procedures that are known and understood by all those affected
- adequate supervision
- identification of training needs
- information and instruction
- personal protective equipment

This hierarchy emphasises the importance of first assessing the need for the chemical and the importance of systems of work and training, rather than simply relying on protective clothing, which, if used alone, is the least effective method of risk reduction.

In the healthcare setting, many chemicals and treatments are covered by COSHH regulations, (e.g. disinfectants, detergents, radioactive material, chemotherapy agents). A careful risk assessment for each must be made, documented and made available to all staff who use or handle the substance. Blood and body fluids can be a microbiological hazard and a risk assessment of procedures that involve contact with these substances should also be made (Health and Safety Executive 1994, East 1992). The pharmacy and supplies departments and the infection control team can provide information and support in the development of risk assessment for clinical areas.

---

unsuitable for the decontamination of equipment. Aqueous solutions must be discarded immediately after use as they can become contaminated with micro-organisms and act as a source of infection (McAllister et al 1989, Oie & Kamiya 1996). Chlorhexidine is useful as a skin disinfectant in handwash solutions or preoperative skin preparations, either as an aqueous solution or with alcohol. It has a persistent effect, progressively killing resident skin flora over time and with subsequent applications (Lilly et al 1979). It is

Table 6.3 Properties of chemical disinfectants

Chemical	Recommended usage	Comment

Alcohol
  Ethanol
  Isopropyl
  IMS (industrial
   methylated spirit)
	Rapid disinfection of
	skin and clean surfaces.
	Handrubs, alcohol-
	impregnated wipes
		Usual concentration of 70%
		effective against bacteria/
		fungi; ethanol and IMS
		effective against viruses
		at 90%

Chlorhexidine
  Hibiscub/Hibisol
  Hibitane (with
   alcohol
  Savlon (with
   cetrimide)
  Savlodil
	Decontamination of intact
	skin as preoperative
	preparation or handwash
	solution. Wound
	cleansing
		Active against bacteria and
		fungi, but not tubercle bacilli,
		spores or viruses

Glutaraldehyde
  Cidex
  Asep
  Totocide
	Decontamination of
	fibreoptic endoscopes,
	which cannot be
	autoclaved
		Used in a 2% alkaline
		solution, activated before
		use. Prolonged exposure
		will destroy spores. Non-
		corrosive, but highly irritant

Hydrogen peroxide	Useful for some specialised equipment	Highly irritant and can be corrosive

Hypochlorites (chlorine
based compounds)
  Milton
  – 125 ppm av. Cl
  – 1000 ppm av. Cl
  – 10 000 ppm av. Cl
   (undiluted)
	
	Infant feeding bottles
	Contaminated surfaces
	Treatment of body fluid
	spills
		Active against a wide range
		of microorganisms, including
		tubercle bacilli and spores.
		Non-irritant but may be
		corrosive at high
		concentration

Domestos (50 000 ppm av. Cl)	Dilute before use	Good general purpose disinfectant for the environment (when diluted)

NaDCC
  (e.g. Presept,
   Haz-Tabs)
  – tablets
  – powder
	As Milton
	
	Absorbing spills of body
	fluid	

Iodine
  Aqueous iodine
  Povodone iodine*
   e.g. Betadine
	
	Skin preparation and
	handwash solutions
		Poor activity against viruses.
		Iodophors do not stain skin
		or cause allergic reactions

Peracetic acid	High level decontamination of complex medical equipment, e.g. endoscopes. Probably non-irritant and mostly non-corrosive	Rapidly bactericidal, virucidal, fungicidal and sporicidal

Table 6.3   Properties of chemical disinfectants (contd)

Chemical	Recommended usage	Comment
Peroxide compounds Virkon Hydrogen peroxide	Used for some specialised equipment, but may be irritant and corrosive (check with manufacturer)	Active against a wide range of microorganisms
Phenolics Hycolin Stericol Clearsol	Disinfection of contaminated environment. Agent of choice for tubercle bacilli	Poor activity against viruses. has caused then to be largely replaced by hypochlorites

also used for wound cleansing, although there is some evidence to suggest it is toxic to fibroblasts and may interfere with wound healing (Neider & Schöpf 1986).

Glutaraldehyde destroys bacteria, fungi and viruses within minutes, tubercle bacilli within 60 minutes and bacterial spores after 10 hours. Activated solutions have a shelf-life of between 14 and 28 days, depending on the brand. Glutaraldehyde is non-corrosive and not significantly inactivated by organic material. Unfortunately these advantages are counteracted by its toxicity. Repeated exposure has been associated with sensitisation, resulting in dermatitis, rhinitis and asthma (Russell 1994). Glutaraldehyde vapour is released from the solution, and it should be stored in a covered container in a room with exhaust ventilation; nitrile gloves and eye protection must be used to handle the chemical.

The use of glutaraldehyde should be restricted to high-level disinfection of equipment that presents a risk of cross-infection and cannot be decontaminated by heat, in particular fibre-optic endoscopes. These should be processed in automated washer–disinfecters to minimise contact with the chemical and its vapour. Equipment must be thoroughly rinsed after immersion in glutaraldehyde as chemical remaining in the channels may damage the intestinal epithelium and cause colitis (Ryan & Potter 1995). The rinse water in automatic washing machines must be changed regularly to prevent build-up of the chemical.

Peraceric acid has a wide range of activity against bacteria, fungi and viruses, which it kills rapidly. It is also highly sporicidal, killing spores within 10 minutes. It is supplied in a stabilised, buffered preparation (e.g. Nu-cidex) and appears to have minimal corrosion effects for decontamination of complex medical instruments such as flexible fibreoptic endoscopes, although damage to rubber and brass components may occur if immersion is prolonged. It decomposes into harmless products (carbon dioxide, water and oxygen) and there is currently no evidence of toxicity, although it has not been in widespread use for long enough to establish any adverse effects. It has a strong odour, which, although less noxious than glutaraldehyde, should be contained by using exhaust ventilation systems (Haythorne 1998).

Peroxygen compounds (e.g. hydrogen peroxide, Virkon) have activity against a wide range of bacteria, viruses and fungi, although their activity is greatly reduced by organic matter. Concentrated solutions are irritant to the skin and mucous membranes and vapours may affect the respiratory tract (Block 1991). They can be corrosive to some metals and manufacturers' approval should be sought before using them on equipment.

Hypochlorites and other chlorine-based compounds are probably the best general-purpose disinfectants, with activity against a wide range of bacteria, fungi and viruses, tubercle bacilli and bacterial spores. They work rapidly; dilute solutions are non-toxic and not corrosive but lose their activity rapidly and should be discarded daily. They do have a number of disadvantages: they corrode some metals and damage fabrics and furnishings if used in high concentration. The concentration of chlorine-based solutions is described in parts per million of available chlorine (ppm av. Cl). The recommended concentrations are shown in Table 6.3. Sodium dichlorisocyanurate is a chlorine-releasing agent, which can be supplied in a tablet or powder form and is useful for absorbing spills of blood or other body fluids (Coates & Wilson 1989, Bloomfield et al 1990) It should not be used on urine spills as chlorine gas is released if the urine is acidic (Department of Health 1990).

Iodine and iodophors are active against a wide range of bacteria, fungi and viruses and have some activity against spores. They are inactivated by organic material and can corrode metal. Their most common use is as a skin disinfectant. Iodophors are complexes of iodine and a carrier molecule and, unlike iodine alone, do not stain skin or induce allergic reactions.

Phenols are active against most bacteria, including tubercle bacilli, but have poor activity against non-enveloped viruses and bacterial spores. Concentrated solutions are stable but toxic. They have largely been replaced by hypochlorites which have greater activity against viruses, but are still widely used in laboratories where their anti-mycobacterial activity is an advantage. Hexachlorophane is a chlorinated phenolic compound which is used on intact skin as a pre-operative skin preparation, or as Ster-zac powder, in umbilical care of the newborn.

STERILISATION

Sterilisation destroys all microorganisms, including bacterial spores. This level of decontamination is required for equipment used in sterile body areas. 'The only method of sterilisation that is both reliable and widely applicable is by heating under controlled conditions sufficiently higher than 100°C to ensure killing even the most resistant micro-organisms and spores' (Kelsey 1967). Other methods are used to sterilise drugs or devices which would be damaged by heat (Table 6.4).

Sterilisation using heat

Either moist or dry heat can be used: dry heat in hot air ovens or incinerators and moist heat in autoclaves and pressure cookers. Moist heat is more effective than dry heat, requiring lower temperatures and shorter times.

Table 6.4 Methods of sterilisation

Method	Procedure	Common uses
Heat		
Moist	Steam under pressure (autoclave)	Surgical instruments
Dry	Hot air oven	Powdered drugs, glassware
	Incinerator	Disposal of infected waste
Gas	Ethylene oxide	Heat sensitive medical equipment/devices, drugs
Radiation	Gamma ions	Single-use plastics (large scale manufacturing), some foods
Filtration	Membrane filter	Heat-sensitive infusion fluids, drugs, laboratory media
	High-efficiency particulate air (HEPA) filters	Air, e.g. in preparation of pharmaceuticals

Sterilisation by moist heat – autoclaves

Vegetative bacteria are destroyed by moist heat below 100°C; however the destruction of spores requires much higher temperatures. At atmospheric pressure water boils at 100°C to produce water vapour or steam. When water is boiled in a closed vessel at increased pressure, the temperature at which it boils, and that of the steam it forms, will rise above 100°C. For example, at 1.03 bar (15 psi) water boils at 121°C and at 2.2 bar (32 psi) it boils at 134°C. When steam comes into contact with an article it condenses on the surface, releasing energy in the form of heat, which destroys any microorganisms present. The time taken to kill spores depends on the temperature so that at 121°C it takes 15 minutes and at 134°C, 3 minutes.

Autoclaves range from the simplest form, the pressure cooker, to complex, fully automatic machines. The basic structure is a chamber with an airtight door, constructed to withstand high internal pressures, a controlled steam inlet and outlet and a safety valve. The efficiency of sterilisation is improved by removing the air. A mixture of air and steam results in a lower temperature at the chosen temperature than steam alone; pockets of air prevent steam penetrating into all parts of the items in the chamber. There are two main types of autoclave.

Porous load autoclaves are large machines used in Central Sterilising Supply departments for sterilisation of prepacked instruments and equipment. They have electrically driven pumps that remove 98% of the air from the chamber prior to the introduction of steam. This removes air from the load, enabling steam to penetrate all parts of the load, including porous material such as paper or linen, rather than condensing on the surface of the pack. Sterilisation is followed by a drying cycle to ensure that packs do not leave the autoclave with wet wrappings that could allow microorganisms to pass through. Provided the autoclaved paper wrappings remain intact and do not become wet they will protect equipment from contamination indefinitely.

Bench-top sterilisers are much smaller and simpler autoclaves, which do not usually include a pre-vacuum stage in the cycle and cannot therefore be used to sterilise wrapped instruments, porous loads such as dressings or equipment with lumens (Figure 6.1). Instruments are sterilised as the steam condenses on their surface. They should be used immediately after sterilisation or protected

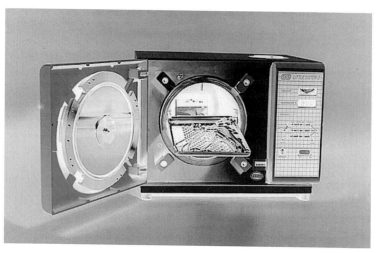

Figure 6.1   A bench-top autoclave. Source: Wilson 1995.

from re-contamination by placing in a sterile container or covering with sterile paper and using within 3 hours. A range of relatively inexpensive autoclaves suitable for processing unwrapped instruments in clinics and surgeries is available (Medical Devices Agency 1996) and the British Standard 3970 can be used to provide a guide to their suitability.

All autoclaves require proper maintenance to ensure that they sterilise equipment reliably and safely. Quarterly and annual tests should be carried out by specialist technicians and there should also be a planned and documented programme of maintenance (BS EN554:1994). The performance of new autoclaves must be validated by an authorised test person before they can be used (Health Technical Memorandum 2010, part 4). Advice on installation, testing and maintenance of autoclaves can be obtained from qualified authorised persons, who are registered with the Institute of Healthcare Engineering and Estate Management.

Sterilisation by dry heat

Hot air ovens

This is less efficient than moist heat as it relies on conduction of heat rather than the transfer of heat through condensation. It therefore requires higher temperatures and longer exposure times than an autoclave and is not suitable for fabrics or other materials that are damaged by high temperature, although it can be used to sterilise some oily or powdered pharmaceutical preparations. The recommended temperature for sterilisation is 170°C for 1 hour; however additional time is required for instruments to reach this temperature before commencing timing and to cool before removal. These prolonged times limit the use of hot air ovens to items that do not require a rapid turnround time. Instruments must be thoroughly cleaned with detergent prior to sterilisation since the high temperature will bake organic material on to the surface.

Ensuring effective heat sterilisation

The following principles should be adhered to when sterilising equipment in autoclaves or hot air ovens:

- Clean instruments thoroughly with detergent and water prior to sterilisation
- Wash cleaning brushes after use and store dry
- Do not exceed load specifications
- Use an autoclave or oven with automatic cycles
- Check the temperature and pressure gauges regularly
- Ensure regular servicing according to the manufacturer's recommendations and guidance in HTM2010 and BS EN554:1994.

Sterilisation without heat

Ethylene oxide

This gas sterilises at 55°C and is suitable for equipment that would be damaged by heat or other sterilisation processes. It is toxic by contact and inhalation to staff, and explosive. To achieve sterilisation the gas concentration, temperature, humidity and duration of exposure must be carefully controlled. Its use is therefore confined to industry, where it is an important process for the sterilisation of a range of medical devices, equipment and drugs.

Irradiation

This method of sterilisation uses machines to accelerate electrons to high energy levels. These penetrate microorganisms, releasing energy and disrupting the cells. They do not heat or wet materials significantly and are used for heat-sensitive equipment, but can affect some materials, so the process is not suitable for all items. The complexity and expense of irradiation means that it is only appropriate for commercial use. Many single-use disposable products such as needles, syringes and suture material are sterilised by this method.

Ultraviolet light radiation can also be used to kill microorganisms but it will only destroy spores at levels that cannot be practically achieved in clinical settings and is therefore not a useful sterilising agent.

Filtration

This method is used to sterilise pharmaceutical fluids and laboratory media that would be damaged by other methods. Membrane filters with very fine pores allow only very small particles to pass through but not bacteria. Filtration is also used to remove microorganisms from air. Cellulose or fibre filters can remove particles as small as 0.3 μm and are used to decontaminate air in cabinets used, for example, to prepare certain pharmaceutical products.

DECONTAMINATION POLICIES

All hospitals should have a policy to guide staff on the appropriate level of decontamination and on the choice of physical or chemical agent for instruments, equipment, skin, mucous membranes and the environment. These policies will be developed by a group of people with expertise in various aspects of decontamination, including the infection control nurse, infection control doctor, pharmacist and manager of the Central Sterile Supplies department. Wherever possible, physical methods of decontamination will be recommended and the range of chemicals may be restricted to minimise confusion, avoid misuse and to encourage compliance with the Control of Substances Hazardous to Health Regulations (Box 6.1).

Equipment that has been in contact with blood and body fluids may transmit infection to those who service and repair it. Equipment should be thoroughly cleaned and disinfected prior to inspection and the processes undertaken should be documented on a decontamination certificate (NHS Management Executive 1993). Confusion surrounding the decontamination of equipment and the environment is by no means confined to hospitals. Invasive procedures are being performed more frequently in general practice surgeries and there is evidence that staff have inadequate knowledge about the use of decontamination procedures (Hoffman et al 1988, Morgan et al 1990, Finn & Crook, 1998). The British Medical Association has published a code of practice on the sterilisation of instruments that is particularly aimed at the primary healthcare team (British Medical Association 1989).

REPROCESSING OF SINGLE-USE EQUIPMENT

Equipment or devices that have been labelled by the manufacturer 'single use' or 'do not re-use' are intended to be discarded after use. Some devices can be safely re-used by the same patient, provided that they are kept clean (e.g. insulin syringes, intermittent urine catheters). There may appear to be economic benefits from reprocessing such devices and using them on another patient, but several issues should be considered. The disinfection or sterilisation processes available to the reprocessor may be inadequate; the process may damage the product (e.g. cause plastics to lose flexibility or crack) and the manufacturer's warranty for the product is likely to be voided and the person reprocessing it may therefore be liable should it cause any injury. If single-use items are going to be re-used, the decontamination must be validated to demonstrate effectiveness and safety and details of the procedure and number of times an item can be safely reprocessed should be carefully recorded (Medical Devices Agency 1995). The perceived economic advantages must therefore be weighed against the costs of performing and documenting the decontamination procedures and the potential liability should a problem related to re-use occur. A device assessment group, comprising the infection control doctor, infection control nurse, purchasing officer, sterile supplies manager and risk manager, should be convened to consider whether re-use is appropriate and possible, and what quality control checks are required to ensure effective reprocessing (Working Party of the Central Sterilising Club 1999).

SPECIAL DECONTAMINATION PROBLEMS

Inactivation of viruses

Most viruses have fairly fragile structures that are readily destroyed by temperatures of 70°C or higher, reached in washing machines, bedpan washers and dishwashers, and by higher temperatures achieved during boiling or steam-sterilisation (Ayliffe 1986). Blood-borne viruses, which present one of the greatest risks of transmission on instruments, are reliably destroyed by autoclaving.

Alkaline glutaraldehyde and chlorine-based agents (10 000 ppm available chlorine) are the most reliable chemicals for the inactivation of viruses, destroying them within a few minutes. Other disinfectants have variable activity (Wood & Payne 1998). Chemicals containing peroxygen compounds or peracetic acid are also virucidal and are useful in some situations. 70% alcohol is less effective against non-enveloped viruses than against those with a lipid envelope and is generally not a reliable method of decontamination (Hanson et al 1989). Phenolic disinfectants and quaternary ammonium compounds are not reliably effective against viruses and are not recommended for routine disinfection (Ayliffe et al 1993).

Inactivation of prions

The virus-like agents, prions, that cause Creutzfeldt–Jakob disease (CJD), bovine spongiform encephalopathy in cattle and scrapie in sheep, appear to be particularly resistant to destruction by conventional methods of decontamination. They do not appear to be inactivated by glutaraldehyde or formaldehyde but may be destroyed by prolonged exposure to hypochlorite. Instruments that have been used on someone known or suspected to be infected with CJD should be autoclaved at a high temperature of 134–136°C for 18 minutes or immersed in hypochlorite solution (20 000 ppm available chlorine) for 1 hour (Advisory Committee on Dangerous Pathogens 1998).

In the case of CJD, the prion is found in the nervous system and the main risk of transmission comes from surgical instruments used during surgical procedures involving neural tissue, e.g. neurosurgery and ophthalmic surgery.

REFERENCES

Advisory Committee on Dangerous Pathogens (1998) Transmissible spongiform encephalopathy agents: safe working and prevention of infection. *PL/CO (98)2.* Stationery Office, London.

Akamatsu, T., Tabata, K., Hironga, M. *et al.* (1996) Transmission of *Helicobacter pylori* infection via flexible fiberoptic endoscopy. *Am. J. Infect. Control*, **24**, 396–401.

Anderton, A. and Nwoguh, C.E. (1991) Re-use of enteral feeding tubes – a potential hazard to the patient? A study of the efficacy of a representative range of cleaning and disinfection procedures. *J. Hosp. Infect.*, **18**, 131–138.

Ayliffe, G.A.J. (1986) Viruses, specula and vaginal cancer. *Lancet*. **1**, 158

Ayliffe G.A.J., Babb J.R., Collins B.J. *et al.* (1974) *Pseudomonas aeruginosa* in hospital sinks. *Lancet* ii, 578–581

Ayliffe, G.A.J., Coates, D. and Hoffman, P.N. (1993) *Chemical Disinfection in Hospitals.* Public Health Laboratory Service, London.

Block, S.S. (1991) *Disinfection, Sterilisation and Preservation,* 4th edn. Lea & Febiger, Philidelphia, PA.

Bloomfield S.F., Smith-Burchnell C.A., Dalgleish A.G. (1990) Evaluation of hypochlorite-releasing disinfectants against the human immunodeficiency virus (HIV). *J. Hosp. Inf.* **15**: 273–278

British Medical Association (1989) *Code of Practice for Sterilisation of Instruments and Control of Cross Infection.* BMA, London.

British Standard 3970: Part 4 (1990) Sterilising and disinfecting equipment for medical products; specification for benchtop steam sterilisers for unwrapped instruments and utensils.

BS EN 554:1994 Sterilisation of medical devices: validation and routine control of sterilisation by moist heat.

Cefai, C., Richards, J., Gould, F.K. *et al.* (1990) An outbreak of *Acinetobacter* respiratory tract infection resulting from incomplete disinfection of ventilatory equipment. *J. Hosp. Infect.*, **15**, 177–182.

Coates, D. and Wilson, M. (1989) Use of dichloroisocyanurate granules for spills of body fluids. *J. Hosp. Infect.*, **13**, 241–252.

Collins, B.J. (1988) The hospital environment: how clean should a hospital be? *J. Hosp. Infect.*, **11**(Suppl. A), 53–56.

Department of Health (1990) Spills of urine; potential risk of misuse of chlorine releasing disinfecting agents. *Safety Action Bull.*, **(90)41**.

Department of Health (1992) Neuro and ophthalmic procedures on patients with, or suspected to have, or at risk of developing Creutzfeldt–Jakob Disease (CJD), or Gerstmann–Straussler–Scheinker Syndrome (GSS), *PL(92)CO/4.* HMSO, London.

Dowsett E.G. and Wilson P.A. (1981) An outbreak of streptococcus pyogenes infection in a maternity unit. *Communicable Diseases Report*, 81(17), 3

East, J. (1992) implementing the COSHH regulations. *Nursing Standard*, **6**(26), 33–35.

Finn, L. and Crook, S. (1998) Minor surgery in general practice – setting standards. *J. Public Health Med.*, **20**(2), 169–174.

Greaves, A. (1985) We'll just freshen you up, dear. *Nurs. Times*, **6 March** (Suppl.), 3–8.

Hanson, P.J.V., Gor, D., Jeffries, D.J. *et al.* (1989) Chemical inactivation of HIV on surfaces. *Br. Med. J.*, **298**, 862–864.

Haythorne, A. (1998) Alert to alternatives. *Nurs. Times*, **94**(37), 76.

Health and Safety Executive (1988) *Control of Substances Hazardous to Health Regulations.* HMSO, London.

Health Technical Memorandum 2010 Part 4: *Operational management*. HMSO, London.

Hoffman, P.N., Cooke, E.M., Larkin, D.P. *et al.* (1988) Control of infection in general practice: a survey and recommendations. *Br. Med. J.*, **297**, 34–36.

Kelsey, J.C. and Maurer, I.M. (1967) The choice of disinfectants for hospital use. *Month. Bull. Min. Health*, **26**, 110–114.

Langenberg, W., Rauws, E.A.J., Oudbier, J.H. *et al.* (1990) Patient-to-patient transmission of *Campylobacter pylori* infection by fiberoptic gastroduodenoscopy and biopsy. *J. Infect. Dis.*, **161**, 507–511.

Lilly, H.A., Lowbury, E.J.L. and Wilkens, M.D. (1979) Limits to progressive reduction of resident skin bacteria by disinfection. *J. Clin. Pathol.*, **32**, 382–385.

McAllister, T.A., Lucas, C.E., Mocan, H. *et al.* (1989) *Serratia marcesceus* outbreak in a paediatric oncology unit traced to contaminated chlorhexidine. *Scot. Med. J.* **34**, 525–528.

Medical Devices Agency (1995) The re-use of medical devices for single use only, *MDA DB 9501*. Department of Health, London.

Medical Devices Agency (1996) The purchase, operation and maintenance of benchtop steam sterilisers, *MDA DB 9605*. Department of Health, London.

Morgan, D.R., Lamont, T.J., Dawson, J.D. *et al.* (1990) Decontamination of instruments and control of cross-infection in general practice. *Br. Med. J.*, **300**, 1379–1380.

Neidner, R. and Schöpf, R. (1986) Inhibition of wound healing by antiseptics. *Br. J. Dermatol.*, **115**(S31), 41–44.

NHS Executive (1995) Hospital laundry arrangements for used and infected linen, *HSG(95)18*. HMSO, London.

NHS Management Executive (1993) Decontamination of equipment prior to inspection, service or repair. *HSG(93)26*. HMSO, London.

Oie, S. and Kamiya, A. (1996) Microbial contamination of antiseptics and disinfectants. *Am. J. Infect. Control*, **24**, 389–395.

Rotter, M., Koller, W. and Wewalka, G. (1980) Povidone-iodine and chlorhexidine gluconate-containing detergents for disinfection of hands. *J. Hosp. Infect.*, **1**, 149–158.

Russell, A.D. (1994) Glutaraldehyde: current status and uses. *Infect. Control Hosp. Epidemiol.*, **15**, 724–733.

Ryan, C.K. and Potter, G.D. (1995) Disinfectant colitis. Rinse as well as you wash. *J. Clin. Gastroenterol.*, **21**(1), 6–9.

Thompson, G. and Bullock, D. (1992) To clean or not to clean? *Nurs. Times*, **88**(34), 66–68.

Werry, C., Lawrence, J.M. and Sanderson, P.J. (1988) Contamination of detergent cleaning solutions during hospital cleaning. *J. Hosp. Infect.*, **11**, 44–49.

Wilson, J. (1995) *Infection Control in Clinical Practice*. Baillière Tindall, London.

Wood, A. and Payne, D. (1998) The action of three antiseptics/disinfectants against enveloped and non-enveloped viruses. *J. Hosp. Infect.*, **38**(4), 283–296.

Working Party of the Central Sterilising Club (1999) Reprocessing of single use medical devices in hospital. *Zentr. Steril.*, **7**, 37–47.

FURTHER READING

APIC (1996) Guideline for selection and use of disinfectants. *Am. J. Infect. Control*, **24**(4), 313–342.

Ayliffe, G.A.J., Babb, J.R. and Bradley, C.R. (1992) Sterilisation of arthroscopes and laparoscopes. *J. Hosp. Infect.*, **22**(4), 265–269.

Ayliffe, G.A.J., Lowbury, E.J.L., Geddes, A.M. and Williams, J.D. (1992) *Control of Hospital Infection – A Practical Handbook*, 3rd edn. Chapman & Hall, London.

British Thoracic Society Research Committee (1989) Bronchoscope and infection control. *Lancet*, **ii**, 270–271.

Coates, D. (1988) Household bleaches and HIV. *J. Hosp. Infect.*, **11**, 95–96.

Cowan, T. (1997) Sterilising solutions for heat-sensitive instruments. *Prof. Nurse*, **13**(1), 55–58.

Department of Health (1994) Instruments and appliances used in the vagina and cervix; recommended methods for decontamination. *Safety Action Bulletin SAB(94)22*. HMSO, London.

Department of Health (1993) *Sterilisation, Disinfection and Cleaning of Medical Equipment*. Guidance from the Microbiological Advisory Committee to the Medical Devices Directorate. HMSO, London.

Earnshaw J.J., Clark A.W., Thom B.T. (1985) Outbreak of *Pseudomonas aeruginosa* following endoscopic retrograde cholangiopancreatography. *J. Hosp. Inf.* **6**, 95–97.

Health and Safety Executive (1998) Chemical hazard alert notice – Glutaraldehyde. *CHAN 7* (revised). Stationery Office, London.

Medical Devices Agency (1996) Decontamination of endoscopes. *Bulletin DB 9607*. HMSO, London.

Medical Devices Agency (1996) Decontamination of blood gas analysers – safety notice. *MDA SN 9612*. HMSO, London.

Russell A.D., Hugo W.B., Ayliffe G.A.J. Eds. (1992) *Principles and practice of disinfection, preservation and sterilisation*. Blackwell Scientific Publications. Oxford.

7

The microbiology laboratory

INTRODUCTION

A diagnosis of infection in a patient is based on the interpretation of clinical symptoms and signs such as fever or inflammation, together with epidemiological evidence that may point to the cause, e.g. travel abroad or contact with infection. While the symptoms and signs may indicate infection and its focus, confirmation of the causative microorganism and the most appropriate form of antibiotic treatment usually requires the expertise of the microbiology laboratory.

The function of the microbiology laboratory in the diagnosis of infection is concerned with:

- the aetiological diagnosis of infection by
  - the isolation and identification of the causative microorganism
  - the detection of antibodies in the patient's blood, formed in response to an infecting microorganism and interpretation of their significance
- advising on the most appropriate antimicrobial treatment.

Selection of the most appropriate tests and correct interpretation of the results depends on the provision of properly collected specimens, accompanied by detailed, relevant information about the patient and his/her symptoms and signs. If the specimen is of poor quality, e.g. stored inappropriately for prolonged periods, then the results of tests may be unreliable.

Ideally, specimens should be taken before antimicrobial therapy is commenced; the presence of antimicrobial agents can reduce the number of microorganisms present at the site of an infection or destroy them in the specimen during transport to the laboratory, thus affecting the microbiological tests.

Viruses are a common cause of infection and are frequently implicated in outbreaks of infection in hospital, e.g. outbreaks of gastroenteritis caused by small round structured virus (Chadwick & McCann 1994). Special laboratory techniques are required to investigate and identify viruses; not all microbiology laboratories have the appropriate facilities and virology specimens may have to be sent to a specialised laboratory elsewhere.

THE COLLECTION OF MICROBIOLOGICAL SPECIMENS

The main principles of specimen collection are to:

- collect tissue or fluid from the suspected site of infection
- preserve microorganisms present in the specimen and prevent it being contaminated by others
- identify the specimen by accurately completing the label and request form
- transport to the laboratory safely and as rapidly as possible.

Selecting specimen containers

Microbiology laboratories supply various types of sterile container for the collection of clinical specimens (Figure 7.1). Plastic pots are used to collect liquid samples such as pus, urine or sputum and those with integral spoons are designed to scoop samples of faeces. Specimens placed in pots should be stored in a designated refrigerator at 4°C until they can be taken to the laboratory. They should not be stored in a refrigerator used for food. Blood specimens are collected in special bottles, which should be incubated immediately at 37°C.

Cotton wool swab sticks are used to sample mucous membranes, wounds or other lesions on the skin. These are then inserted into a tube of soft agar, which acts as transport medium, preserving any microorganisms present for approximately 24 hours. However, for the diagnosis of viral infections, bottles of viral transport medium must first be obtained from the laboratory. Immediately

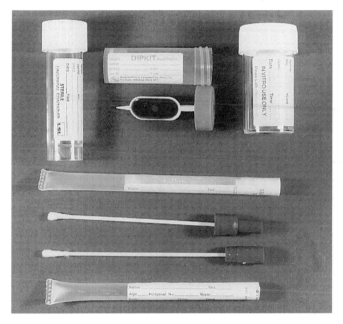

Figure 7.1 Examples of containers for specimen collection. Clockwise from top left: Universal container, e.g. for urine; Agar-coated dipslide (urine sampling); Universal container, e.g. for faeces; Wound/lesion swabs with transport medium.

after the specimen has been taken, the swab is placed in the medium and the stick is broken off. The specimen must then be sent to the laboratory without delay.

Labelling of specimens

A specimen must be correctly labelled to ensure that it can be identified and matched with its corresponding request form and that the results of the tests are related to the correct patient. The information on the request form needs to be accurate and relevant. It should identify the source of the specimen, including the specific site, for example the location of the wound where there is more than one; clinical information that may be relevant, for example, symptoms such as diarrhoea and vomiting and their duration; and current antimicrobial therapy so that the laboratory can interpret the result. An example of this is ampicillin-resistant klebsiella which is an unlikely cause of respiratory tract infection but commonly isolated in sputum of patients receiving ampicillin.

Transport of specimens

Any specimen may contain harmful microorganisms and must therefore be handled carefully to ensure that ward and laboratory staff are not exposed to risk. The container should be securely closed and any contamination on the outside removed.

The Health Services Advisory Committee (1991) has issued guidance about the safe transport of specimens, recommending that they should be sealed in plastic bags, with the request form in a separate pocket, and carried in leakproof boxes by staff trained in what to do if there is a spillage or accident. Some pathogens are considered particularly hazardous, e.g. *Mycobacterium tuberculosis*, and specimens thought to contain them need to be marked with biohazard labels (Figure 7.2; Health Services Advisory Committee 1991, Advisory Committee on Dangerous Pathogens 1990).

Nurses have a role to play in ensuring that specimens are properly labelled and sealed in the appropriate container.

TYPES OF SPECIMEN

Swabs

Nasal swabs

These are sometimes taken to investigate a purulent discharge or to detect carriage of *Staphylococcus aureus*, e.g. during an outbreak

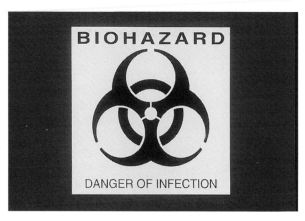

Figure 7.2   Biohazard label. Source: Wilson 1995.

of infection. The patient should be placed facing a good light source and the procedure should be explained carefully. When screening for staphylococcal carriage, the sample should be taken from the anterior nares, directing the swab upwards in the tip of the nose and rotating it gently. As the nose is normally dry, the swab should first be moistened in the transport medium.

Pernasal swabs of the nasopharynx are taken to confirm a diagnosis of whooping cough and should only be taken by a member of staff who has been appropriately trained. The swab consists of a flexible wire with cotton wool on the tip and the transport medium contains charcoal to facilitate the survival of *Bordetella pertussis*.

Throat swabs

These should be taken with the patient facing a good light source and the tongue depressed. The swab should be rubbed over the pillars of fauces and any area with visible inflammation, lesion or exudate, taking care to avoid touching the mouth or tongue.

Ear swabs

Infections of the outer ear can be sampled by carefully inserting a swab. If otitis media is suspected an aural speculum will be needed and swabbing should be carried out by medical staff.

Eye swabs

Organisms that commonly cause eye infections are delicate. They should be sampled by gently rubbing a wire loop over the conjunctiva and the lower conjunctival sac, a procedure usually performed by medical staff. 'Sticky eye' problems in babies are usually caused by staphylococci or coliforms, and a simple eye swab placed in transport medium will be adequate. If gonococcal or chlamydial infection is suspected, special transport media, obtained from the laboratory, must be used.

Vaginal or cervical swabs

A vaginal speculum is required to take these swabs, which should always be placed in transport medium. Special transport media, obtained from the laboratory, are required if infection with gonorrhoea, chlamydia or herpes simplex is suspected.

Wound swabs

The results of wound swabs can be difficult to interpret as many normal skin flora and other organisms can be present without causing infection. A diagnosis of wound infection should therefore be based on clinical signs such as inflammation, erythema, pus, swelling or unusual levels of pain rather than the identification of bacteria in a wound swab. Correct labelling of the specimen with the exact site from which it has been taken can help interpretation of the results. To maximise the chance of identifying the organisms responsible for infection, swabs should be taken from the affected part of the wound. Some authors suggest the removal of surface contamination by gentle cleaning or irrigation prior to sampling (Cooper & Lawrence, 1996). Other studies have found no difference in results if wounds are not first cleaned (Hansson et al, 1995). Pus can be sampled with a syringe and sent to the laboratory in a sterile container. If the wound or lesion is dry, the swab should first be moistened in the transport medium or sterile water, as this will improve the efficiency of sampling.

Sputum

The mouth and pharynx are colonised by various commensal flora and the particular microorganism causing the suspected respiratory tract infection may be difficult to detect among them. It is therefore important to ensure that the specimen is sputum, which will be purulent or mucopurulent, and not saliva. A physiotherapist may be able to help a patient to expectorate and a specimen is usually easier to obtain in the early morning.

Sometimes it is possible to make a preliminary identification of the microorganism causing infection of the respiratory tract by staining and microscopy. Special staining techniques are used to identify mycobacteria, including *Mycobacterium tuberculosis*, the bacterium that causes tuberculosis (p. 178). Antimicrobial treatment will be commenced if mycobacteria are found by microscopy, but the diagnosis and sensitivity to antibiotics cannot be confirmed until the organism has been cultured. These bacteria grow extremely slowly and require at least 6 weeks of incubation before colonies are visible. Since numbers of mycobacteria in the sputum may be small, a series of three sputum specimens, ideally taken on consecutive mornings, should be examined before excluding a diagnosis of tuberculosis.

Blood culture

An infection of a particular organ system, e.g. urinary or respiratory tract, may invade the bloodstream. The presence of microorganisms in the blood is called *bacteraemia* and when their presence is associated with symptoms such as high fever, chills or rigors the patient is considered to have *septicaemia*.

To detect microorganisms in the blood, samples should be taken as close to the peak of fever as possible as then the number of microorganisms circulating in the blood is likely to be greatest. Blood cultures need to be taken carefully to avoid contamination with bacteria present on the skin. The skin should first be disinfected, then blood should be withdrawn and a fresh needle used to inoculate the bottles. Usually a set of two bottles is inoculated, one to culture aerobic organisms while the other is for the culture of anaerobes.

As the number of bacteria circulating in the blood will be small, the bottles should not be refrigerated but taken to the laboratory promptly, where they will be incubated for at least a week and checked daily for signs of growth. Appropriate clinical information may assist the laboratory in identifying the microorganism, e.g. the date the symptoms started, the presence of an infection that may be the origin of the causative microorganism, and any relevant underlying, predisposing conditions such as leukaemia or HIV infection. Intravascular devices are a common source of bacteraemia and are usually associated with *Staphylococcus epidermidis*, an otherwise unusual pathogen.

Cerebrospinal fluid

These specimens are collected by medical staff, and a strict aseptic technique is required to prevent the inadvertent introduction of microorganisms and to prevent contamination of the specimen with skin microorganisms. Cerebrospinal fluid (CSF) is collected in three sterile bottles; the last bottle is less likely to contain blood cells and is therefore used to perform a cell count. In the case of suspected meningitis, it may be possible to make a rapid, provisional diagnosis by Gram-staining the specimen and detecting characteristic bacteria such as *Neisseria meningitidis* (the cause of meningococcal meningitis) under the microscope.

Urine

Urine is easily contaminated by bacteria colonising the perineum during collection of the specimen and these may confuse interpretation of the microbiological tests, rendering the result meaningless. This contamination can be reduced by asking the patient to collect a midstream specimen i.e. to pass the first part of the stream into the toilet before collecting 10–20 ml into a sterile container. Cleansing the perineum prior to collection may be of limited value in preventing contamination from the perineum (Holliday et al 1991).

If a patient has a urinary catheter, specimens of urine should be collected from the self-sealing sleeve of the drainage tube using a sterile, fine-bore needle and syringe. The sleeve should first be cleaned with alcohol and the needle inserted at an angle of 45° to avoid penetration of the far wall of the tubing. Samples should never be obtained by breaking the catheter–drainage-bag junction as this will almost certainly lead to contamination of the system. Nor should samples be taken from the drainage bag as the organisms will have multiplied in the static urine and will not represent the numbers present in the bladder (Bradley et al 1986). Catheterised patients commonly have many bacteria colonising their urine, but treatment is not usually indicated unless symptoms of infection, such as fever, are present (p. 326). The identification of white blood cells in a sample of urine viewed under the microscope is more indicative of infection than the presence of microorganisms alone.

Urine specimens should be delivered to the laboratory as soon as possible but can be refrigerated for up to 24 hours. After this time accurate assessment of the numbers and types of bacteria in the specimen may not be possible. In the community or outlying hospitals, where transit to the laboratory may be difficult, 'dip slides' may be used. These are plastic slides coated with a nutrient medium, which are dipped into a urine specimen, sealed in the container and posted to the laboratory for incubation. However, they do preclude examination of the specimen for the presence of white blood cells.

Faeces

Gastroenteritis can be caused by a range of bacteria or their toxins, viruses and parasites. Faeces contain large numbers of different bacteria and distinguishing between the commensal flora and the pathogens causing enteric infection can be difficult. Specially formulated agar media are therefore used that suppress the growth of commensal flora but allow pathogenic species to grow. Viruses in faeces are detected by electron microscopy or antigen-detection techniques, but are usually detectable only early in the course of the illness and specimens must therefore be collected as soon as an infectious cause is suspected.

Parasitic infections are identified by microscopic examination of faeces and requires a fresh specimen. An exception is for the diagnosis of threadworms. These lay their ova under the perianal skin and can be sampled by pressing sticky tape on to the skin around the anus in the morning before defecation. If amoebic dysentery is suspected, the protozoa responsible, *Entamoeba histolytica*, is more easily seen in warm faeces while it is still motile. Specimens should therefore be taken to the laboratory for examination as soon as they are passed.

VIROLOGICAL SPECIMENS

Most viruses do not survive for long outside the body. Special viral transport media (VTM) and prompt delivery to the laboratory are required for some types of specimen requiring investigation for viruses. The transport medium contains saline and protein to protect the virus together with antibiotics to prevent the growth of bacteria. Many viruses cannot be cultured in the laboratory. Serological techniques, where an increase in the level of a specific antibody in the blood is measured, are commonly used to detect them. Other viral infections are identified by electron microscopy and a few can be grown in tissue culture. Advice about the collection and transport of viral specimens can be obtained from the virology department.

The request form should clearly indicate that a viral infection is suspected, the symptoms and the date that they started. In the case of specimens of blood, information on relevant immunisations and blood products that the patient has received in the previous 6 months can assist the laboratory in assessing the significance of the results.

METHODS USED IN THE IDENTIFICATION OF BACTERIA

Methods that are used in the microbiology laboratory to identify the organisms causing infection include:

- microscopy and staining
- culture
- biochemistry testing
- sensitivity to antimicobial agents.

The appearance of the specimen itself may provide important clues for the microbiologist. It may speed diagnosis by indicating the specific tests that may be necessary; for example, foul-smelling pus suggests infection with anaerobes; and in some instances inspection may confirm a diagnosis (e.g. if segments of tapeworm are visible).

Microscopy and staining

This involves the use of a microscope to examine the specimen and identify the shape and structure of any organisms present (Figure 7.3). Bacteria occur in two main shapes; round (cocci) and rod-shaped (bacilli), although a few species are spiral-shaped and some form curved rods. Some microorganisms characteristically occur in pairs, chains or clusters of cells, while motility can also be a distinguishing feature.

Specimens can be observed directly under the microscope by preparing a 'wet film'. For this, a drop of the specimen is placed on a glass slide and covered with a thin square of glass called a coverslip. Since cells are colourless they can only be seen with difficulty in wet films. Specimens are therefore generally stained with a dye that colours the cells, prior to examination under the microscope. The most common staining method is the Gram stain; this distinguishes two main groups of bacteria (see Box 2.1), Gram-positive and Gram-negative. Another staining method, used to identify mycobacteria, is Ziehl–Neelsen (ZN) staining, which is based on the ability of these cells to retain dye despite subsequent exposure to strong acid alcohol. This explains why mycobacteria are also known as acid-alcohol-fast bacilli (AAFB).

A light microscope can be used to determine the shape and arrangement of cells but to distinguish any of the internal structures

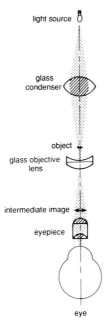

Figure 7.3   The light microscope. The compound light microscope comprises two sets of lenses: one is next to the object being viewed, the other is next to the eye. The light source is beneath the object; light travels through the object and into both lenses, which magnify the image. A standard microscope will provide an image between 100 and 1000 times larger than the actual object. Source: Wilson 1995.

of the cell or to see objects as small as 0.001 μm, such as viruses, the much more powerful electron microscope is needed. This uses a stream of electrons instead of light to magnify the object and can also provide a three-dimensional image.

Microscopy can sometimes be used to provide a rapid, provisional identification of microorganisms causing life-threatening infection. For example, examination of cerebrospinal fluid from a patient with suspected meningitis can often indicate the likely causative bacteria and enable appropriate antimicrobial therapy to be started immediately.

Culture

Microorganisms present in the specimen are identified by growing them in mixtures of sterile nutrients called culture media. The most commonly used culture media are agar plates. Nutrients are mixed with melted agar (a gel derived from seaweed), poured into flat Petri dishes and allowed to set. The specimen is inoculated on to the surface of the agar and then distributed over its surface to separate out individual bacterial cells (Figure 7.4).

Several types of media are available, since different bacteria have different nutritional needs. Specific substances can be added to the basic medium, either to promote the growth of particular organisms or to reduce the growth of non-pathogenic species present in normal flora, allowing the pathogens to grow more freely. These selective media are useful for the detection of pathogenic organisms in material such as faeces and throat secretions, which normally contain large numbers of organisms. Blood agar is used for the identification of the majority of bacteria and fungi that cause infection in humans. Chocolate agar is made of heated blood and is used to detect fastidious organisms such as *Neisseria* and *Haemophilus spp.*

Broth cultures are mixtures of nutrients without setting agents. They are used to enhance the growth of microorganisms from specimens likely to contain only a small number of organisms, such as blood. Wound swabs are usually inoculated both on to agar plates and into broth.

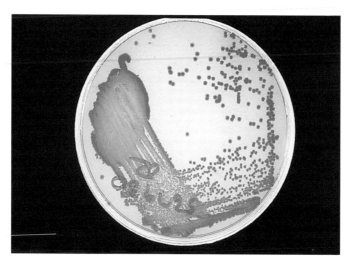

Figure 7.4 Bacterial colonies on an agar plate. Colonies of *S. marcescens* spread out on the surface of an agar plate. Source: Wilson 1995.

Once the agar or broth has been inoculated with microorganisms, they are incubated overnight, i.e. for between 18 and 24 hours. Most human pathogens grow best at body temperature and are therefore usually incubated at 37°C. If the infection may be caused by an anaerobic microorganism, which will not grow in the presence of oxygen, the cultures are incubated in special oxygen-free cabinets.

During incubation each bacterial cell will multiply many times, each multiplication occurring every 20–30 minutes in many species. After several hours, repeated division of a single cell gives rise to millions of bacteria, which are visible on the surface of the agar plate and are called colonies. The size, shape, colour and consistency of these colonies vary considerably between different species and their appearance can be used to provide clues to their identity. Some bacteria have a characteristic effect on the surrounding medium. For example, some species of streptococcus release an enzyme that breaks down blood cells in the blood agar, causing characteristic clear areas to form around each colony. Highly motile microorganisms such as proteus do not form colonies but spread over the plate in a thin film, although this can be prevented by growing them on special media lacking specific nutrients that they need for motility.

Specimens frequently contain a mixture of microorganisms, which appear as different types of colony on the agar plate. By spreading the sample out across the plate (Figure 7.5) colonies of

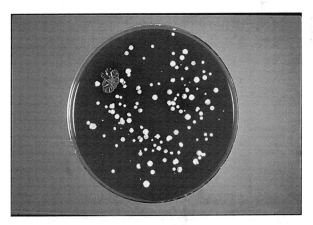

Figure 7.5 A mixed growth of several different bacteria. Specimens often contain more than one species of bacteria, which can be distinguished by the differing appearance of the colonies on the surface of the agar. Source: Wilson 1995.

different species are readily detectable. Individual colonies will be scraped off the surface of the agar and inoculated into fresh culture medium to enable further tests to be performed on each type of bacterium present in the specimen.

Analysis of biochemistry

Biochemical tests have been found to be useful for differentiating bacteria. The majority are designed to detect the presence of specific enzymes produced by organisms. For example, the different species of salmonella that cause food poisoning are morphologically and culturally identical but can be distinguished by the range of carbohydrates that they break down by the action of their enzymes. The resulting production of acid is detected by an indicator dye, which changes colour in the presence of acid. Other tests detect the breakdown of macromolecules such as gelatin or the production of particular byproducts of metabolism such as hydrogen sulphide.

A range of these standard biochemical tests can be performed in miniature plastic kits (Api Kit) (Figure 7.6) comprising a series of chambers, each containing a different carbohydrate or amino acid. Each chamber is inoculated with the test organisms, incubated overnight and a reaction determined by the subsequent change in colour. These kits enable the microorganisms to be identified quickly and accurately with the use of minimal equipment.

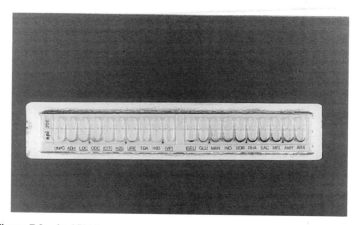

Figure 7.6   An API kit

Sensitivity to antimicrobial agents

The sensitivity of various organisms to antimicrobial agents is of major importance as a guide to appropriate therapy, but may also be of value in differentiating strains, particularly in the investigation of outbreaks of hospital-acquired infection.

The most commonly used method of antibiotic sensitivity testing is that of disc diffusion. Agar culture medium in a Petri dish is inoculated with the organisms under investigation and paper discs, each impregnated with a different antibiotic, are placed on its surface. During incubation the antibiotics diffuse out of the paper into the agar, preventing bacteria that are susceptible to the antibiotic from growing in the space around the disc. Where the bacterium is resistant to the antibiotic it grows right up to the edge of the disc (Figure 7.7).

Serological tests to identify bacteria

The cells of the immune system recognise and attack molecules on the surface of microorganisms. These molecules are referred to as antigens and can be small or large single molecules or complex proteins or carbohydrates. Specific antibodies recognise the shape of a particular antigen and bind to it. These antibodies can be

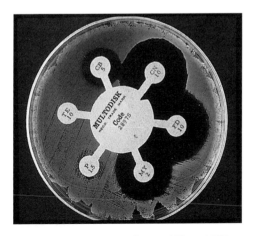

Figure 7.7 Antibiotic sensitivity testing. Source: Wilson 1995.

made into standard preparations called antisera, known to recognise and bind to antigens on specific species of bacteria. When antisera are mixed with a suspension of bacteria carrying the corresponding antigen the binding reaction results in bacterial cells becoming bound together in clumps that are clearly visible. This is called an agglutination reaction. The identity of test organisms can be confirmed by mixing them with specific antisera and observing an agglutination reaction. The use of antisera to detect antigens is widely used in the identification of pathogenic bacteria.

Some bacteria release antigenic substances into their environment; those that cause damage to the tissues of their host are called exotoxins. Bacteria that produce exotoxins are commonly identified by using specific antisera to detect the toxin, e.g. the precipitation test (Elek's procedure) used to identify toxin-producing strains of *Corynebacterium diphtheriae*.

Bacterial typing

Bacteria, like other living organisms, are classified into groups according to similarities in their structure and behaviour. Each is allocated a group name, the genus (e.g. *Escherichia*) and a specific name within the group, the species (e.g. *coli*). However, many bacteria can be further distinguished as different 'strains' within a particular species; this subdivision reflects slightly different properties of different members of the same species. This information can be useful when diagnosing a particular infection. For example, the species *Escherichia coli* is present in the normal flora of the large intestine but some strains are pathogenic through their ability to produce a range of toxins. One of these strains is verotoxigenic *E. coli* (VTEC), which has been associated with several outbreaks of haemorrhagic colitis and haemolytic uraemic syndrome, including a recent outbreak in Scotland (p. 164).

The process of distinguishing strains of bacteria is called typing and involves various techniques, depending on the species under investigation. Typing the organism by strain is an important part of the investigation of outbreaks of infection, since it can help to indicate whether several cases of the same infection are related and to determine if and how cross-infection may have occurred. Many of these tests are performed in specialised laboratories within the Public Health Laboratory Service (p. 258).

Serotyping

Some strains are identified by the presence of specific antigens on their surface or by the production of particular exotoxins. Specific antisera are used to detect each strain. This technique is commonly used to identify strains of Gram-negative bacteria such as *Escherichia coli*, *Salmonella spp.* and *Shigella spp.*

Phage typing

Like other living cells, bacteria are susceptible to infection by viruses, called bacteriophages. The phage enters the bacterial cell, takes over the mechanisms for nucleic acid and protein synthesis and, once it has replicated, lyses the cell. If an agar plate is covered with a film of bacteria, inoculated with a bacteriophage and incubated overnight, the viral infection can be detected by clear circular areas, called plaques, which appear where bacterial cells have been lysed. Susceptibility to a range of bacteriophages is characteristic of particular strains and detecting phage susceptibility is used to distinguish strains, e.g. staphylococci (Wilson & Richardson 1997).

Bacteriocin typing

Some bacteria produce complex proteins, called bacteriocins, that attack other related species of bacteria. Sensitivity to various bacteriocins is characteristic of particular strains of bacteria and identifying the range of susceptibility is a technique used in the typing of a number of intestinal organisms, including *Shigella sonnei* and *Escherichia coli*.

DNA typing

New techniques, based on the direct analysis of DNA extracted from the microorganism, are becoming more widely used in microbiological diagnosis. Fragments of DNA called 'gene probes', known to be specific for the microorganism under test, are mixed with single strands of DNA or RNA extracted from the test organism. If the probe matches the test DNA it will hybridise with it and can be detected by a radioactive label attached to the probe. Another technique, called polymerase chain reaction (PCR), causes specific sequences of nucleic acid from the organism to be synthesised in large quantities and hence detectable by hybridisation with a corresponding gene probe. This technique provides a rapid and highly accurate test capable of detecting an organism in a sample of tissue even if it is present in very small numbers.

METHODS USED IN THE IDENTIFICATION OF VIRUSES

Viruses do not grow on culture media used for bacteria. The methods used to diagnose viral infections are:

- detection of the virus by electron microscopy
- culture on living cells
- serological techniques to detect specific antibodies formed against the virus or its antigens.

Electron microscopy

Virus particles as small as 0.0001 μm are visible under an electron microscope and this technique is particularly useful for detecting viruses in stool specimens. To improve the chance of seeing viruses, specific antibodies can be added to the specimen. These cause any virus particles present to clump together and therefore become more visible.

Culture

Unlike bacteria, viruses cannot grow on artificial media since they need living cells for growth. In the laboratory, they are grown using a technique called tissue culture. This uses standard lines of cells, usually derived from mammalian fetal or neoplastic tissues. Sheets of tissue one cell thick, called *monolayers*, are attached to a glass or plastic dish, inoculated with the virus and then bathed in nutrient fluid. Cell damage can be seen in the form of a plaque, or clear area, in the monolayer. Where a mixture of viruses is present, the monolayer can be bathed in nutrient agar instead of fluid. This then solidifies and confines the virus to a single cell, enabling the subculturing of pure virus from the resulting plaque. Some specimens, e.g. CSF, can be added directly to a tissue culture, but others, which are likely to contain bacteria from sites with a normal flora (e.g. throat swabs), have to be centrifuged first.

Different viruses may cause characteristic changes in the infected cells called cytopathic effects. These can be observed under the microscope and used to identify the virus. Other viruses are detected by testing for changes in the metabolic activity of the cells or for viral components in the fluid bathing the cells, e.g. haemagglutinins, viral enzymes that cause red blood cells to clump together.

Serological tests

The proteins that make up the structure of a virus are antigenic and are recognised by the cells of the immune system, resulting in the formation of specific antibodies (p. 59). These antibodies can be detected in the blood. A serological diagnosis of infection is commonly used in virology, since tests to detect and measure these specific antibodies are easier than isolating and identifying the virus itself.

Several methods are used to detect the antibodies; the most common is the enzyme-linked immunosorbent assay (ELISA) in which specific known viral antigens are placed in small wells on a plastic plate. Serum from the patient is added and the plates are incubated. If antibody specific to the antigen in the wells is present it will bind to it. This binding reaction is then detected by a colour-producing enzyme that recognises antibodies.

Different types of antibody appear in the blood during the course of an infection (p. 59) and their detection can be used to determine whether a patient has a current or previous infection. Viral infections diagnosed by this method include rubella and hepatitis B. In the latter, the particular type of antibody present indicates whether the patient has present or past infection, or has become a chronic carrier of the virus.

Since the presence of antibody may reflect past infection, diagnosis of a current infection requires antibody levels to be measured in two samples of blood, one taken while the patient is acutely ill, the second taken 10 days later. These are described as paired or acute and convalescent sera and the level, or titre, of antibody is assessed in both specimens at the same time. Levels of antibody significantly higher in the second specimen (usually fourfold) indicate an active, current infection. A summary of tests used in virology is given in Table 7.1.

Table 7.1   Some methods of identifying viral infections

Infection	Specimen	Test	Viruses
Respiratory tract infection	Throat swab, nasopharyngeal, washings	Culture	Influenza, parainfluenza, RSV
	Paired sera	Serology	Influenza, parainfluenza, RSV, adenovirus, mumps
Vesicular skin lesions	Fluid from lesion	Electron microscopy, culture	Herpes simplex
	Serum	Serology	Varicella-zoster
Erythematous skin rash	Paired sera	Serology	Measles, rubella
Hepatitis	Serum	Serology	Hepatitis A, B and C
Eye infections	Conjunctival scrapings	Culture	Herpes simplex, Adenovirus
Gastroenteritis	Faeces	Electron microscopy	Rotavirus, Calcivirus, small round virus

INTERPRETING LABORATORY REPORTS

The identification of microorganisms in clinical specimens can take some time. In a few cases a provisional diagnosis can be made rapidly by staining and examination under a microscope. More commonly at least 18 hours is required for the microorganisms to be grown and differential tests to be applied. Additional time may be necessary where several different organisms are present in the specimen. Where the specimen contains only a few bacteria, e.g. blood, it may take several days before they have multiplied sufficiently to be detectable. Some bacteria, notably mycobacteria, grow extremely slowly and colonies can only be seen on agar after approximately 6 weeks of incubation. Providing the laboratory with a good quality, fresh specimen and accurately completed details about the infection site and symptoms can help speed the process and facilitate interpretation of the results.

When the laboratory has identified the microorganisms present in the specimen a report is compiled and sent to the patient's doctor. The process requires the help of a clinical microbiologist, a doctor who has specialised in microbiology and who can relate the laboratory findings to the clinical symptoms and also provide advice on the most appropriate form of antimicrobial treatment. Important results are phoned to the ward before a written report is sent and these results must be recorded properly in the patient's notes.

Laboratory reports can only be interpreted with knowledge of the clinical condition of the patient. Just because a pathogen and its antibiotic sensitivities are reported does not necessarily mean that the patient should be given antimicrobial therapy.

- He/she may already be recovering from the infection
- The organism may only be colonising the site and not invading the tissues to cause infection.

Advice on how to interpret the information supplied in the report can be obtained from the clinical microbiologist in the microbiology laboratory.

The information in the laboratory report may include:

- **Macroscopic appearance** (e.g. liquid, bloody stool), which will be of clinical significance and enable the reported microorganism to be matched to the patient's symptoms.
- **Microscopy**: whether pus cells, yeasts, parasites or their ova, depending on the particular specimen, are present. This information can be used to assess the significance of any microorganism isolated. For example, the presence of pus cells in a wound swab, urine sample or sputum specimen suggests infection. If pus cells are not seen, then the microorganism identified may only be colonising rather than causing infection.
- **Culture**: the presence or absence of a particular organism as requested by the doctor, e.g. *Mycobacterium tuberculosis* or *Corynebacterium diphtheriae*. The report may give only the genus of the organism e.g. Salmonella, indicating that identification to a particular species has not been made by adding the abbreviation sp. (singular) or spp. (plural). Where identification of the species has been made, the genus may be abbreviated to the first letter, e.g. *S. enteritidis*. The growth of the organism is usually described in terms of quantity, e.g. heavy (+++), moderate (++) or light (+), or, in the case of urine, more specifically as number of bacteria per millilitre of urine. This can help to assess the significance of the microorganisms identified, particularly where more than one microorganism has been isolated from one specimen. The laboratory may also qualify the presence of a particular microorganism;

for example, diphtheroids are commonly isolated from wound swabs but are invariably skin flora and not a cause of wound infection.

• **Antibiotic sensitivity**: antibiotics to which the microorganism considered to be clinically significant is sensitive or resistant will be reported to guide treatment. The results are often abbreviated to S for sensitive and R for resistant. While the report of sensitivity to antibiotics does not imply that treatment is necessary, the laboratory will sometimes withhold information on the sensitivities if the microorganism isolated is unlikely to be the cause of infection.

Other microbiology results may report the presence or absence of a particular bacterial toxin (e.g. *Clostridium difficile* toxin), or, in the case of virology reports, the presence of diagnostic antigens, (e.g. HbSAg – hepatitis B surface antigen) or the titre of specific antibody in paired sera (e.g. rubella).

Serum assay

Some antibiotics have toxic effects if they reach too high a concentration in the blood (e.g. gentamicin, vancomycin). To ensure that the levels in the blood remain high enough for effective treatment but not so high as to cause toxicity, their levels have to be regularly checked. Blood is taken immediately before a dose is administered and exactly 1 hour afterwards, to provide trough and peak levels. If the concentration of circulating drug falls outside acceptable levels then the dosage or interval between doses will need to be adjusted. The results are telephoned directly to the clinician looking after the patient.

REFERENCES

Advisory Committee on Dangerous Pathogens (1990) *Categorisation of Pathogens According to Hazard and Categories of Containment*. HMSO, London.
Bradley, C., Babb, J., Davies, J. *et al.* (1986) Taking precautions. *Nurs. Times*, 5 March, 70–73.
Chadwick, P.R. and McCann, R. (1994) Transmission of small round structured virus by vomiting during a hospital outbreak of gastro-enteritis. *J. Hosp. Infect.*, **26**, 251–260.
Cooper, R. and Lawrence, J.C. (1996) The isolation and identification of bacteria from wounds. *J. Wound Care*, **5**(7), 335–340.

Hansson, C., Hoborn, J, Moller, A. *et al.* (1995) The microbial flora in venous leg ulcers without clinical signs of infection. *Acta Dermatol. Venereol. (Stockh.)*, **75**, 24–30.

Health Services Advisory Committee (1991) *Safe Working and Prevention of Infection in Clinical Laboratories*. HMSO, London.

Holliday, G., Strike, P.W. and Masterton, R.G. (1991) Perineal cleansing and midstream urine specimens in ambulatory women. *J. Hosp. Infect.*, **18**, 71–76.

Wilson, J. (1995) *Infection Control in Clinical Practice*. Baillière Tindall, London.

Wilson, J. and Richardson, J. (1997) Keeping MRSA in perspective. *Nurs. Times*, **92**(19), 58–60.

FURTHER READING

Ayton, M. (1982) Microbiological investigations. *Nursing*, **2**(8), 226–230.

Duerden, B.I., Reid, T.M.S. and Jewsbury, J.M. (1993) *Microbial and Parasitic Infection*. Edward Arnold, Sevenoaks.

Gilchrist, B. (1996) Wound infection 1. Sampling bacterial flora: a review of the literature. *J. Wound Care*, **5**(8), 386–387.

Health and Safety Commission (1994) *Control of Substances Hazardous to Health Regulations (COSHH)*. *Approved Codes of Practice*. HSE Books, London.

Inglis, T.J.J. (1996) *Microbiology and Infection*. Churchill Livingstone, Edinburgh.

McFarlane, A. (1989) Using the laboratory in infection control. *Prof. Nurse*, **4**(8), 393–397.

McKune, I. (1989) Catch or bag your specimen? A comparative study of the contamination rates between clean catch and bag specimens of urine in children aged two years and under. *Nurs. Times*, **85**(37), 80–82.

A guide to pathogenic bacteria

The aim of this chapter is to provide basic information about those bacteria commonly encountered in health care settings. Additional information on the routes of transmission and care of patients infected with many of these organisms can be found in the appendix to Chapter 14.

CLASSIFICATION OF BACTERIA

The first system of biological classification was developed by Linnaeus during the 18th century. Although it has since been developed, the principles are still used in the classification of all forms of life, including bacteria. Organisms are placed into different groups according to similarities in their structure and characteristics. Each organism has two names, the first, the genus, indicates the group to which it belongs, the second, the species, is a specific name within the group. Bacteria within a species may be further distinguished into different strains according to specific characteristics: for example, some may be able to produce a particular toxin or be resistant to an antibiotic. In the case of bacteria, the most important differences relate to their shape and staining properties, in particular the Gram stain (p. 20). To aid their identification they are broadly grouped as follows:

• Cocci: – Gram-positive
            – Gram-negative
• Bacilli: – Gram-positive
            – Gram-negative

Curved
Small
- Acid-fast bacilli
- Spirochaetes
- Chlamydias, rickettsias, mycoplasmas

The main pathogenic genera and species in each of these groups are discussed below.

GRAM-POSITIVE COCCI

Staphylococcus

These organisms characteristically occur in clusters (Figure 8.1) and are commonly found as commensals on the skin. The main pathogenic species is *Staphylococcus aureus*, which is characterised by its ability to produce an enzyme, coagulase.

Staphylococcus aureus

S. aureus colonises the nose and skin of healthy people, especially the axillae, groin and perineum. Approximately 20% of people have the organism in their nose most of the time and a further 60% carry it intermittently. It can establish infection if it enters

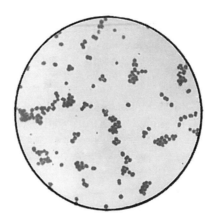

Figure 8.1 Gram-stained preparation of staphylococci, showing characteristic clusters of cells (× 1000).

damaged skin or hair follicles and is a common cause of abscesses, carbuncles and impetigo. It is also causes infection in surgical wounds and may cause more severe infections, such as osteomyelitis, septicaemia, pneumonia and endocarditis.

Some strains of *S. aureus* damage their host through the production of toxins. Toxic epidermal necrolysis (scalded skin syndrome) is caused by a particular toxin-producing strain that causes blistering skin lesions in neonates and young children and can spread rapidly through neonatal or maternity units. Toxic shock syndrome is associated with retained sanitary tampons, which support the multiplication of toxin-producing strains of *S. aureus*. The toxin causes a range of symptoms including fever, diarrhoea, scarlet-fever-type desquamative rash and hypotension. Staphylococcal enterotoxins can also cause food poisoning, characterised by vomiting and diarrhoea soon after the consumption of contaminated food.

S. aureus is a major cause of infection associated with healthcare, accounting for approximately 20% of surgical wound infections, and the second most common cause of all hospital-acquired infections (Emori & Gaynes 1993). Its presence on skin enables it to gain access easily to invasive devices, such as cannulae, and to enter wounds or skin lesions. Outbreaks of infection have been frequently reported, often associated with transmission on the hands of staff (Reybrouck 1983). Staff clothing and equipment may also be involved in transmission but, although the organism can survive in dust for prolonged periods, the environment is not considered to play an important part in transmission in most settings (Mylotte 1994). Nasal carriage is also an important risk factor for infection. The nose provides an ideal environment for the organism to multiply, and provides a source from which it can spread to other skin sites on the body. Patients who carry the organism in their nose are at increased risk of surgical wound infection, infections associated with dialysis and other device-related infections (Klutymans et al 1997). The elimination of *S. aureus* from the nose appears to reduce carriage on the skin, and the use of antistaphylococcal ointments prior to surgery has been demonstrated to reduce the rate of surgical wound infection (Klutymans et al 1996).

Methicillin-resistant strains of *S. aureus* (MRSA) cause a similar range of infections to sensitive strains and some spread easily, affecting large numbers of patients in many different hospitals

(Communicable Disease Report 1997). Patients colonised with MRSA are more likely to develop subsequent infection, especially those in intensive care with intravenous lines, pressure ulcers and surgical wounds (Coello et al 1997). MRSA is becoming an increasing problem in healthcare facilities throughout the world and special measures to limit its spread are frequently implemented in affected hospitals (p. 84).

The antibiotic of choice for the treatment of *S. aureus* infection is flucloxacillin, or erythromycin if the patient is allergic to penicillin. Methicillin-resistant strains of *S. aureus* (MRSA) are resistant to flucloxacillin and often to a range of other antibiotics, limiting treatment to vancomycin and teicoplanin.

Coagulase-negative staphylococci

Coagulase-negative species are generally considered to be non-pathogenic or of low pathogenicity; however, some, such as *Staphylococcus epidermidis*, are increasingly recognised as a cause of infection in hospitals. Their pathogenicity relates to the production of a polysaccharide referred to as slime, which enables them to adhere to and multiply on foreign materials such as catheters and artificial implants. *S. epidermidis* is a frequent cause of septicaemia in patients with central intravascular devices, particularly in immunocompromised patients, and of infection in prosthetic orthopaedic joints, cardiac valves and vascular grafts. It also causes infection in patients with cerebrospinal shunts, peritoneal dialysis catheters and urinary catheters (Hamory & Parisi 1987). *S. epidermidis* is intrinsically much more resistant to antibiotics than *S. aureus* and vancomycin is the antibiotic usually used to treat infections.

Streptococcus

In a Gram-stain preparation these cocci are characteristically seen in pairs or chains (Figure 8.2). Many species are able to rupture red blood cells, causing an area of haemolysis around colonies on blood agar plates. Those that cause complete haemolysis of red blood cells are called β-haemolytic. They are divided into Lancefield groups and many are pathogenic. Other species use partial haemolysis and are called α-haemolytic.

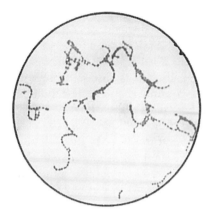

Figure 8.2 Gram-stained preparation of streptococci, showing characteristic arrangement of cells in chains (× 1000).

Lancefield group A streptococci *(Streptococcus pyogenes)*

This is an important pathogenic species, causing a range of infections, often severe, including streptococcal sore throat, erysipelas, traumatic or surgical wound infection, puerperal fever and septicaemia. Infections should be treated promptly with penicillin, to which they respond rapidly; erythromycin is a useful alternative antibiotic if the patient is allergic to penicillin. Some strains produce an erythrogenic toxin, which causes the rash of scarlet fever. Rheumatic fever and glomerulonephritis, due to a hypersensitivity reaction to the microorganism (p. 70), sometimes complicate a case of acute group A streptococcal infection. Outbreaks of streptococcal infection among hospital patients have been reported (Dowsett & Wilson 1981, Takahashi et al 1998). Necrotising fasciitis is caused by particularly virulent strains of group A streptococcus.

Lancefield groups C and G streptococci

These organisms commonly colonise the skin and mucous membranes and cause a similar range of infections to the group A streptococci, but occur less frequently. They are also associated with outbreaks of infection in hospital.

Lancefield group B streptococci *(Streptococcus agalactiae)*

These streptococci are carried asymptomatically in the vagina of a proportion of women; as a result vertical transmission to the neonate may occur either in utero or during delivery and may cause meningitis, septicaemia and pneumonia in the neonate. Infection of the neonate is more likely to occur where there is premature labour or prolonged rupture of membranes and, although early recognition and improved treatment has reduced mortality, the fatality rate is high among low-birth-weight babies. Endometritis, caesarean wound infection and septicaemia may also occur in women following delivery.

Viridans *streptococci*

This group of streptococci are α-or non-haemolytic. Species within the group form a large proportion of the normal flora of the mouth and are also found in the intestinal tract or genital tract. They are generally considered to be of low pathogenicity but are involved in the formation of dental caries and are a common cause of bacterial endocarditis. *S. mutans* adheres to tooth enamel and produces acetic and lactic acids as a byproduct of the fermentation of sugar. These acids erode the tooth enamel to cause caries. A variety of viridans streptococci, in particular *S. mitior, S. sanguis* and *S. milleri,* cause endocarditis in people with abnormal or prosthetic heart valves. The infection occurs following dental treatment, when oral streptococci may be released into the bloodstream and subsequently adhere to the heart valve.

Streptococcus pneumoniae

This is a α-haemolytic streptococcus that characteristically occurs in pairs. Pathogenic species produce complex polysaccharides, which form a capsule around the cell. *S. pneumoniae* frequently colonises the upper respiratory tract asymptomatically, but is also the commonest cause of bacterial pneumonia, often complicating a viral respiratory infection. The mortality rate of pneumococcal pneumonia is around 5%, but it is higher in the elderly and in those who develop bacteraemia. *S. pneumoniae* may also cause meningitis, otitis media and sinusitis. The treatment of choice for pneumococcal infection is penicillin G, with erythromycin recommended for patients allergic to penicillin. Resistance to penicillin was first reported in pneumococcus in the 1960s and the number of reports has gradually increased since. In the UK the level of resistance is still relatively low but increasing, with 2.9% of isolates from the most severe infections resistant to penicillin and more than 10% resistant to erythromycin (Laurichesse et al 1998). In other parts of the world, notably southern Europe and the USA, up to 50% of isolates are resistant. There appears to be a strong association between general antimicrobial usage and nasal carriage of penicillin-resistant pneumooccci in children (Avason et al 1996).

Enterococci

These bacteria, previously known as group D non-haemolytic streptococci, have recently been re-classified into a separate genus. The most common species, *E. faecalis* and *E. faecium*, are part of the normal flora of the lower intestine but can cause infections of the urinary tract, surgical wounds and soft tissues, endocarditis and septicaemia, particularly in the seriously ill or immunocompromised patients. They are intrinsically resistant to a number of antibiotics, and strains with acquired resistance to other drugs are particularly difficult to treat (Murray 1990). Vancomycin-resistant enterococcus (VRE) is resistant to the glycopeptide antibiotics that are usually used for the treatment of serious enterococcal infections. The first outbreak of hospital-acquired infection caused by VRE occurred in London in the late 1980s. Since then the number of hospitals reporting outbreaks of VRE infection has increased and some strains appear to have a propensity to spread both within and between hospitals (Johnson 1998). Immunocompromised patients are particularly vulnerable to infection and outbreaks are most likely to occur in bone-marrow transplant, intensive care, renal and liver units (Morrison et al 1996). The organism is carried between patients on the hands of staff, but equipment and the accumulation of the organism in the environment have also been implicated in transmission (Weber & Rutala 1997).

Glycopeptide-resistant strains of enterococcus may develop in the gut of the patient following antimicrobial therapy. However, there is evidence that patients may already be colonised with resistant strains before admission to hospitals and that the use of glycopeptides in animal feed additives may have encouraged their emergence in some countries (Bates et al 1994).

GRAM-POSITIVE BACILLI
Clostridium

This large group of organisms only grow under strict anaerobic conditions, can form spores under adverse environmental conditions and produce a variety of toxins. They are present in soil and animals, and occur in large numbers as commensals in the human gastrointestinal and female genital tract. A few species are major human pathogens.

Clostridium perfringens

This species is a common member of the faecal flora, but is also responsible for serious infections.

Food poisoning. C. perfringens spores commonly contaminate raw meat and poultry and the anaerobic nature of the organism enables it to multiply in internal cavities. The spores vary in their ability to resist cooking temperatures and may survive the procedure. While cooked foods are slowly cooling the spores germinate and multiply. Re-heating food before serving it will not kill all the bacteria and on ingestion they form spores and a toxin; the latter is responsible for poisoning. A large number of microorganisms need to be ingested to cause symptoms, which are characterised by abdominal pain and watery diarrhoea. C. perfringens is a common cause of outbreaks of food poisoning in the UK (Cowden et al 1995).

Skin and soft tissue infection. C. perfringens is frequently recovered from wounds without evidence of clinical infection, and often in combination with other species. Gas gangrene can complicate perforation of the bowel, septic abortion, amputation or foot ulcers. The infection develops rapidly in 1–3 days and characteristically involves destruction of muscle, release of gas into tissues and systemic toxaemia. Infection results from contamination of wounds with soil or street dust or is derived from skin contaminated with intestinal organisms. The most notorious form of clostridial infection, it was previously associated with wartime, when rapid surgical management of grossly contaminated wounds was not possible. However, cases are now associated with road traffic accidents, crush injuries or where there is underlying vascular disease. Impairment of the blood supply, the presence of dead tissue and blood clots provide anaerobic conditions that favour the growth of the organism. There is no risk of transmission to others. It can also cause a less severe infection called anaerobic fasciitis without muscle necrosis, which occasionally may spread to cause cellulitis and overwhelming toxaemia.

Clostridium difficile

This species is a common commensal in the intestine. Antibiotic therapy, in particular clindamycin, ampicillin and cephalosporins (Nye 1993), disrupts the microbial flora of the intestine, allowing C. difficile to multiply in the absence of competition from other species. Toxins released by certain strains of the organism cause necrosis of the intestinal mucosa. The condition, called pseudomembranous colitis, is characterised by severe, often bloody diarrhoea, which in some cases may be fatal. In addition to this endogenous infection, cross-infection may occur as the organism may be shed in large numbers from an affected patient and the spores can survive for prolonged periods in the environment (Hoffman 1993). A number of outbreaks of infection, particularly amongst elderly patients, have been reported (Department of Health, Public Health Laboratory Service 1994).

Clostridium tetani

This species is a common commensal of human and animal gastrointestinal tracts and its spores are abundant in soil, especially in environments animals inhabit (Figure 8.3). Spores are introduced into puncture wounds, cuts or other lesions and germinate. Germination is aided by necrotic tissue, calcium salts and the presence of other organisms that produce anaerobic conditions. As the bacteria multiply in the tissue they produce a toxin, which reaches the central nervous system, causing widespread muscle spasm. C. tetani is not an invasive organism and infection remains at the site of entry. Treatment involves managing the effects of the toxin through assisted ventilation and intensive nursing care. Associated mortality is around 30%, higher in the elderly. The immunisation of infants against C. tetani and administration of booster doses following traumatic injury has virtually eliminated cases of the disease, with less than 100 cases reported annually in the UK (Shanson 1989).

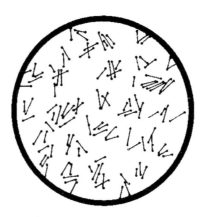

Figure 8.3 Diagram of *Clostridium tetani*, showing characteristic round terminal spores (× 1200).

Clostridium botulinum

The spores of this species are widely distributed in soil. It produces a highly potent neurotoxin, which, if ingested even in minute amounts, is sufficient to cause progressive paralysis and death from respiratory paralysis or cardiac arrest. Intensive respiratory support and the use of antitoxin have reduced the case fatality to 10%, but recovery may take months. Toxin production does not occur in an acidic environment; therefore alkaline food products are more susceptible to contamination. The toxin is readily destroyed by heat (10 minutes at 100°C), although some spores are not. Poisoning is usually associated with fruit or vegetables inadequately heated during canning and not cooked prior to consumption, and often following home preservation (Communicable Disease Report 1998). An outbreak involving 27 people in the UK was traced to hazelnut puree in yoghurt (Acheson, 1989). In infants, botulism occurs following ingestion of spores e.g. in honey which frequently contains botulinum spores, which germinate in the gut and then produce toxin (Benenson, 1995).

Corynebacterium

Several species form part of the normal flora of skin and mucous membranes. Most are commensals referred to as diphtheroids or coryneform bacilli, but some can be pathogenic. The principal human pathogen of the genus is *C. diphtheriae*.

Corynebacterium diphtheriae

This species causes diphtheria, a localised infection of the throat and a generalised toxaemia. Infection is characterised by sore throat and the formation of a tough, adherent membrane of necrotic mucosa and fibrin, which may lead to suffocation. The neck lymph glands enlarge and powerful exotoxins cause distant nerve damage, resulting in paralysis of the soft palate, eye muscles and extremities and affecting the muscle of the heart, causing myocarditis, conduction-defects and ultimately heart failure. These effects are reversible with appropriate treatment.

The infection is transmitted by respiratory droplets or items contaminated with secretions. The organism can be carried asymptomatically in the nose and throat, from where it can be transmitted to others, although not all strains are toxogenic. Patients with the disease remain infectious for several weeks after the symptoms have resolved.

In the past diphtheria was a common disease causing many deaths, particularly among young children. Since the introduction of routine immunisation in 1940, the incidence in the UK has dramatically declined and now only a handful of cases are reported each year (Department of Health 1996). However, a recent increase in cases in the former USSR, where immunisation programmes have not been maintained, illustrates the importance of such control measures. A cutaneous form of diphtheria occurs chiefly in the tropics and is an important reservoir in the transmission of the respiratory disease.

Bacillus

These aerobic organisms form spores and are widely distributed throughout the environment. A few species may cause infection.

Bacillus anthracis

This species causes anthrax, a disease of animals, particularly hoofed animals, in which it causes a fatal septicaemia; it can cause outbreaks of infection amongst farm animals. After the death of the animal, the spores remain in the soil for decades. Humans can become infected by close contact with infected animals or carcasses. Usually the infection is acquired by inoculation through the skin and causes local skin lesions; if spores are inhaled or ingested, pneumonia or gastroenteritis may follow. Infection may also be complicated by septicaemia. The use of protective clothing and decontamination procedures for hides and other animal products has reduced the incidence of the disease and it is rarely encountered in the UK.

Bacillus cereus

This species is found in dust and soil and frequently contaminates cereals and beans. Some toxin-producing strains cause food poisoning, often associated with rice. The spores on the rice survive cooking and, if left at room temperature, may germinate, multiply and release toxin. The toxin is heat-stable, not destroyed during subsequent re-heating and, when ingested, causes acute vomiting within hours. Some strains found in meat produce different toxins, which cause a rapid onset of diarrhoea. Rarely, *B. cereus* has been associated with wound infection related to contaminated linen (Barrie et al 1992) or incontinence pads (Stansfield & Caudle 1997).

Listeria

There are several species in this genus but the main human pathogen is *Listeria monocytogenes*, which is present in the faeces of a wide range of animals, in soil and in sewage. It is ingested by humans on contaminated food or is passed congenitally from mother to baby during pregnancy. Infection has been associated with soft cheeses, patés and preprepared, chilled meat meals, and outbreaks have been caused by failure of milk pasteurisation and by raw vegetables (e.g. cabbage in coleslaw) contaminated by sewage (Jones 1990). Its ability to grow at normal refrigeration temperatures of less than 10°C enables listeria to grow in chilled foods and it is also able to survive temperatures of up to 60°C.

In congenital infection, the fetus is exposed to the organism following gastrointestinal or genital colonisation in the mother. Exposure during early pregnancy usually results in the death of the fetus. If infected later, the neonate may be born with a range of serious conditions, including meningitis, pneumonitis and hepatosplenomegaly. Neonates may also be infected during delivery, by organisms colonising the vagina, and subsequently develop meningitis and bacteraemia. Infection can be transmitted to others from affected mothers or babies (Schlech 1991).

Listeria monocytogenes can infect healthy adults and children, but usually causes a mild, subclinical infection that passes unnoticed. Occasionally, clinical infection of meningitis and bacteraemia occurs, especially in the immunocompromised; however the incidence of infection in the UK is low (Newton et al 1992). To reduce the incidence of the infection, the Department of Health issued guidance recommending that pregnant and immunocompromised individuals should avoid eating foods likely to contain high numbers of the organisms, such as soft, ripened cheeses and paté, and that cook-chilled meals and ready-to-eat poultry should be re-heated prior to consumption (Department of Health 1988).

GRAM-NEGATIVE COCCI
Neisseriaceae

These cocci usually occur in pairs and many species are common commensals of the upper respiratory tract. There are two pathogenic species in the genus neisseria: *N. meningitidis*, the cause of meningococcal meningitis, and *N. gonorrhoeae*, which causes gonorrhoea.

Neisseria meningitidis

This species colonises the upper respiratory tract of approximately 10% of healthy people but can cause meningitis, septicaemia or both infections. Meningitis usually begins suddenly with intense headache, vomiting, stiff neck, photophobia, progressing to coma within a few hours. Presentation varies and includes muscle pain, drowsiness, headache and photophobia. In children, fever and vomiting are often the only sign of infection prior to loss of consciousness. Some cases develop a characteristic petechial rash, which does not blanch under gentle pressure and may be evident under pressure points such as elastic on underwear. Microscopy of cerebrospinal fluid is often helpful in making a rapid diagnosis (Figure 8.4). Overall mortality from the disease is around 8%, but is highest when septicaemia is present.

Outbreaks of infection frequently occur in the winter months, probably related to the seasonal increase in the incidence of influenza. Groups A, B and C are most commonly associated with

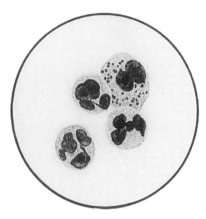

Figure 8.4 Cerebrospinal fluid from a case of meningococcal meningitis showing *Neisseria meningitidis* inside pus cells (× 475).

disease. Group B strains account for two-thirds of cases in the UK and mostly affect young children, but group C has recently increased in incidence and caused infections amongst older children and young adults. Group A strains rarely cause infection in the UK but are common in other parts of the world (Department of Health, 1996).

Meningococci are transmitted from carriers or those in the early stages of infection by respiratory droplets or direct contact, although the rate of transmission is low even within families. High carriage rates may occur in groups of young people living in crowded conditions, such as schools, universities or military camps. Carriage may persist asymptomatically for many months and eventually probably confers immunity, but in a small number of individuals the organism invades the nasopharynx and causes disease.

Early treatment of cases with benzylpenicillin is usually effective. In outbreaks of infection, where two or more cases occur within a particular community, close contacts of the cases may be given prophylactic antibiotic therapy and, if the infection is due to a group A or C strain, a meningococcal vaccine is also available. Other contacts may be screened to detect carriage of the organism. Since the overall risk of meningitis is very low routine immunisation against A and C strains is not recommended (Department of Health, 1996).

Neisseria gonorrhoeae

This organism causes gonorrhoea, a disease of the genital tract transmitted by sexual intercourse. In men it infects the urethra, producing a purulent discharge; it may extend to the prostate, seminal vesicles and epididymis or invade the periurethral tissue, producing an abscess and subsequent urethral stricture. In women the urethra and cervix are infected and the infection may spread to the lining of the uterus and fallopian tubes (salpingitis). Bacteraemia and a rash may result from primary infection and arthritis is a complication. Infants may acquire the infection from their mothers during delivery, presenting as ophthalmia neonatorum, a severe conjunctivitis that develops within 2 or 3 days of delivery. In the past, treatment with penicillin has been widely effective, but penicillin-resistant strains are now becoming common, particularly in Africa and Asia, where other antimicrobial agents may have to be used, e.g. ciprofloxacin.

Moraxella catarrhalis

A common nasopharyngeal commensal, this organism sometimes causes otitis media and low-grade infection of the respiratory tract, particularly in immunocompromised patients, although it has been associated with laryngitis, meningitis and prolonged cough in children. It may also be associated with lower respiratory tract infections in patients receiving assisted ventilation.

GRAM-NEGATIVE BACILLI

Enterobacteriaceae

This family of bacteria consists of several genera characterised by their ability to behave as anaerobes if necessary (facultative anaerobes) and to ferment carbohydrates. Many are commensals in the gastrointestinal tract of humans and animals and some are pathogens, either in the gastrointestinal tract or other sites. They are commonly referred to as enterobacteria or coliforms.

Escherichia coli

This species is a normal inhabitant of the gut, but some strains can cause gastroenteritis. Enteropathogenic strains cause gastroenteritis in young children; enterotoxin-producing strains affect both adults and children. The most notable of these strains, serotype O157, produces a verotoxin, which can cause symptoms ranging from mild diarrhoea to haemorrhagic colitis and severe abdominal pain. The illness is usually self-limiting, but in up to 10% of cases a haemolytic uraemic syndrome (HUS) develops, which can seriously impair renal function and is fatal in between 3% and 17% of those affected. Children are particularly susceptible to HUS.

E. *coli* O157 has been responsible for a number of outbreaks, often associated with undercooked minced beef, including a recent outbreak in Scotland that affected nearly 500 people, 18 of whom died (Cowden 1997). Cattle are the main reservoir of the bacterium and other vehicles of infection include unpasteurised milk, yoghurt and faecally contaminated raw vegetables. It can also be transmitted from person to person and through direct contact with animals (Communicable Disease Report, 1995a)

Coliforms are a common cause of urinary tract infection, with E. *coli* accounting for at least one-quarter of hospital-acquired urinary tract infections (Glynn et al 1997; Figure 8.5). It also causes wound infections, intra-abdominal abscesses and septicaemia and is a leading cause of meningitis in infants.

Klebsiella

Like E. *coli*, these organisms are normal inhabitants of the gastrointestinal tract, but can cause septicaemia and infect the urinary

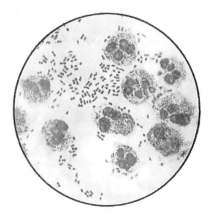

Figure 8.5 *Escherichia coli* in urine, with large pus cells also visible (× 1000).

tract and wounds. The cells are surrounded by a polysaccharide capsule, which is an important determinant of virulence and is used in the typing of different strains. The main pathogenic species is *K. pneumoniae*, a common cause of hospital-acquired infection, particularly in association with invasive devices, and frequently resistant to many antibiotics (Gormon et al 1993). In patients who have received antibiotics, *K. pneumoniae* may take advantage of the destruction of the normal flora and can be recovered in large quantities in sputum. In this situation, their presence is often not significant and therapy is unnecessary. In the community, *K. pneumoniae* sometimes causes pneumonia but usually in debilitated compromised hosts such as alcoholic patients.

Other enterobacteria

Other genera in this family include serratia, enterobacter and citrobacter. They are often resistant to many antibiotics and are increasingly recognised as hospital pathogens, responsible for septicaemia, wound and urinary tract infections in seriously ill patients. *Proteus* spp. are part of the normal flora of the gut and are a common cause of urinary tract infections. They may be present in wounds, but often without causing clinical infection; many are resistant to antibiotics and will survive when other species are destroyed by antimicrobial therapy.

Salmonella

There are more than 2000 species of salmonella; *S. typhi* and *S. paratyphi* cause enteric fever and are exclusively human pathogens, the others are present in the intestines of many animals and cause food poisoning in humans. The most commonly reported species in the UK are *S. typhimurium* and *S. enteritidis*.

Salmonella typhi and Salmonella paratyphi

These organisms cause typhoid and paratyphoid enteric fevers. The route of infection is the ingestion of food or water contaminated by faeces of a human carrier; thus they are not commonly acquired in the UK, but are in countries with untreated drinking water or poor sanitation. The severe illness is characterised by a gradual onset of constipation, dry cough and fever, followed by the emergence of a rose-spot rash and diarrhoea. The organisms reach the bone marrow via the bloodstream and multiply in the reticuloendothelial system. Subsequently, they are excreted in faeces and urine at various times during the illness and the gall bladder is frequently colonised. A proportion of those infected become carriers and continue to excrete organisms in their faeces, and less often their urine, intermittently for many years, acting as a source of infection to others.

Other salmonellas

These organisms are primarily of animal origin but cause food poisoning in humans following ingestion. Symptoms usually develop after 18 or 24 hours, beginning with nausea and vomiting and followed by diarrhoea. In the UK, infection is usually associated with poultry, since a significant proportion (up to 60%) of chickens and both egg-white and shells are likely to be contaminated with salmonella (De Louvois 1993). Transmission occurs as a result of one or more of the following: incomplete defrosting (bacteria protected from destruction by heat during cooking); cooking at too low a temperature (bacteria able to survive); cooling at room temperature (surviving bacteria multiply to a harmful level). Previously cooked food can also be contaminated by raw meat during storage. Infection may be spread from person to person, although this can be prevented by applying simple infection control measures such as handwashing after using the toilet and before preparing foods. Antibiotic therapy is not indicated, except in the very young, very old or septicaemic patient, and the main focus of treatment is rehydration.

Major outbreaks of salmonella infection in hospitals, related to poor food hygiene, have been reported and, where elderly patients are involved, fatalities are likely. In one serious outbreak in 1984, hundreds of patients at the Stanley Royd psychiatric hospital were affected and 19 died (Department of Health and Social Security 1986).

Shigella

These organisms are responsible for bacillary dysentery. The infection is acquired by direct contact with faeces or indirectly through contaminated food or water. The organisms invade the wall of the large intestine, releasing toxins that disrupt water absorption and cause ulceration of the mucosa. Infection is characterised by bloody diarrhoea. Most infections in the UK affect children and are caused by *S. sonnei*; secondary spread from person to person is common. Outbreaks of infection occasionally occur in children's nurseries, schools and residential homes for people with learning difficulties where hand-washing practices may be less than satisfactory (Communicable Disease Report 1995b).

Pseudomonas

These organisms are similar to enterobacter but are strictly aerobic and do not ferment carbohydrates. Many produce fluorescent pigments. There are many different species, which are widely distributed in nature but, except for *P. aeruginosa*, most are rarely pathogenic. They thrive in moist environments such as washbasins, although those recovered from environmental sources are rarely implicated in infection (Levin et al 1984). Recently, an outbreak of infection related to whirlpool baths was reported. The highly aerobic conditions and extensive pipework favour colonisation by pseudomonas and cross-infection is a risk when such baths are used by patients with open wounds (Hollyoak et al 1995). Of greater significance is hospital equipment contaminated by pseudomonas that has been poorly cleaned and dried and introduces infection when used on subsequent patients (Weems 1993, Humar et al 1996).

Pseudomonas aeruginosa

This species is commonly found colonising the gut. It can grow in the presence of very limited nutrients, producing a characteristic blue/green pigment. It tends to take advantage of breaches in the normal defences of the body, causing urinary tract infection in patients with urine catheters and respiratory tract infections associated with assisted ventilation or cystic fibrosis. It commonly colonises chronic open wounds, taking advantage of the moist environment and sometimes causing infection. Extensive burns are particularly vulnerable to colonisation and septicaemia may develop as a result (Weber et al 1997). It is intrinsically resistant to many antibiotics but strains resistant to drugs, such as aminoglycosides, usually used to treat infection, can cause problems in hospitals, especially in critically ill patients (Tassios et al 1997).

Yersinia

The most significant pathogen in this genus is *Y. pestis*, the cause of plague. It is carried by fleas on rats or other rodents and transferred to humans when they are bitten by the rodent fleas. Although uncommon in Europe, sporadic cases and outbreaks of plague occur in America and the tropics, where humans live in close association with rats or other rodents. The disease is characterised by high fever, enlarged, discharging lymph nodes (buboes) and in some cases pneumonitis. Those who develop respiratory infection are particularly infectious. Early treatment with antibiotics is usually effective.

Other species, notably *Y. enterocolitica*, are associated with gastroenteritis, causing diarrhoea and abdominal pain. Transmission occurs through the consumption of contaminated food, particularly undercooked pork.

Other aerobic non-fermenters

Other pathogenic Gram-negative organisms which occasionally cause infection include aeromonas, xanthomonas and acinetobacter. *Acinetobacter* is widely found in nature and is the only Gram-negative organism that is a normal commensal of human skin and as a result sometimes contaminates blood cultures. It is an unusual cause of infection but is increasingly recognised as an opportunistic pathogen in burns and intensive care patients. Outbreaks of infection have been reported, particularly in intensive care units and in association with respiratory therapy equipment (Dealler 1998). Some strains may be highly resistant to antibiotics, making treatment difficult (Musa et al 1990, Humphreys & Towner 1997).

CURVED GRAM-NEGATIVE BACILLI
Vibrio

These organisms are widely distributed in nature. The main pathogenic species is *V. cholerae*, although *V. parahaemolyticus* can cause food poisoning associated with contaminated shellfish.

Vibrio cholerae

This species causes cholera, an illness of sudden onset characterised by profuse, watery diarrhoea and abdominal cramps, and associated with the ingestion of contaminated food or water. The symptoms are caused by the release of an enterotoxin, which stimulates hypersecretion of water and chloride in all parts of the small intestine. There are two distinct biotypes of *V. cholerae*. The 'classic' variety causes a severe disease and used to be responsible for most cases. Since the 1960s, most outbreaks of infection have been caused by the 'El Tor' biotype, which is associated with a milder disease but spreads very rapidly. Cholera is endemic in some parts of the world, including south-east Asia and parts of Africa; in the UK cases are invariably acquired abroad.

Campylobacter

These microorganisms live in the intestines of many animals, especially poultry and cattle (Figure 8.6). Methods of culture and identification were not developed until the 1970s, but the organism is now recognised as a major cause of food poisoning in the UK (Wall et al 1996). Infection is commonly associated with undercooked poultry, and outbreaks related to consumption of raw or inadequately pasteurised milk or water contaminated with animal or bird faeces have also been reported (Communicable Disease Report 1995b, Cowden et al 1995). The number of bacteria required to cause infection is very low as they multiply within the gastrointestinal tract; cross-contamination from raw poultry to cooked food is therefore a significant route of transmission (Eley 1992). The organism is not associated with prolonged excretion in the faeces and person-to-person transmission is rare. After an incubation period of 3–4 days there is an acute onset of fever and headache, followed by watery, sometimes bloody, diarrhoea and very severe abdominal pain. If abdominal pain is the predominant symptom suspected appendicitis may be diagnosed.

Helicobacter

These spiral-shaped organisms were originally classified as campylobacter, but are now considered a distinct genus. The species *H. pylori* had been seen in tissue taken from the stomach of people with peptic ulcer disease but it was not until 1984, when it was realised that it required long incubation in low-level oxygen, that the organism was finally cultured (Marshall & Warren 1984). It is now recognised as a significant cause of gastritis, duodenal

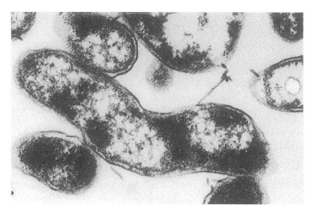

Figure 8.6 Long, curved rods of *Campylobacter* (electron micrograph).

and gastric ulcers and has also been associated with gastric cancer and heart disease (Cottrill 1996). After ingestion, helicobacter burrows into the mucous layer lining the stomach. It produces an enzyme, urease, that converts urea to ammonia, providing a microenvironment around the cell protecting it from the high acidity of the stomach. Most people infected with *H. pylori* have no symptoms, but a proportion develop a chronic gastritis that can result in damage to the mucosal surface and ulceration. 95% of patients with duodenal ulcers and 70% of those with gastric ulcers are infected with *H. pylori* and the use of antimicrobial therapy to eliminate it from the stomach can provide an effective cure in most cases. Infection is acquired through ingestion of contaminated water or contact with faeces, with the risk of infection increasing in conditions of poor hygiene and overcrowding. In developing countries a large proportion of the population become infected as children. In developed countries improved sanitation has resulted in a low incidence of infection in children; peptic ulcer disease in adults probably reflects acquisition during childhood.

SMALL GRAM-NEGATIVE BACILLI

Haemophilus

These organisms are common commensals of the respiratory tract but some strains can cause infection. The principal pathogenic species, *H. influenzae*, is commonly carried in the nasopharynx of healthy people. Some strains have capsules (capsulate), others do not (non-capsulate). Non-capsulate strains are a major cause of acute exacerbation of chronic bronchitis or bronchiectasis and of otitis media. The capsulated strain serotype b is responsible for most of the invasive infections in young children. The most common of these is meningitis, often accompanied by bacteraemia; other infections are acute epiglottitis, septicaemia, septic arthritis, osteomyelitis and pneumonia. Immunity to *H. influenzae* develops as a result of carriage of the organism, hence the occurrence of serious infection among young children. A vaccine against serotype b (Hib) is now administered to children at 2, 3 and 4 months of age; since its introduction the incidence of infection has fallen dramatically (Figure 8.7; Department of Health, 1996).

Pasteurella

These small bacilli are found in the respiratory tract of many animals. They sometimes cause infection in humans following animal bites, particularly from dogs and cats. Infected wounds are often slow to heal and may be accompanied by lymphangitis and cellulitis.

Legionella

These strictly aerobic bacteria are difficult to grow except on special media. They are commonly found in environmental water sources,

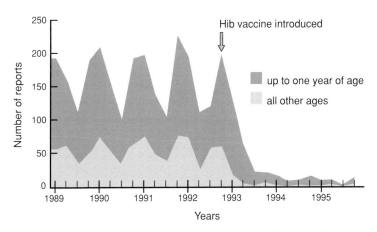

Figure 8.7 Effect of Hib immunisation on the incidence of *Haemophilus influenzae* infections in children. Source. Department of Health, 1996.

including air-conditioning systems and domestic water supplies, particularly in association with blue-green algae. The main pathogenic species in humans is *L. pneumophila*.

Legionella pneumophila

This pathogen was recognised (and named) after an outbreak of severe atypical pneumonia affecting members attending a convention of the Pennsylvania branch of the American Legion in Philadelphia in 1976. It has since been recognised in many countries as a cause of sporadic or epidemic, atypical pneumonia called legionellosis or legionnaires' disease generally affecting elderly and mildly immunocompromised people. The highest incidence is in men over 55 years and other risk factors include smoking, chronic bronchitis, emphysema, steroid or other immunosuppressive treatment and diabetes. It can also cause a similar, but milder, disease in young people, called Pontiac fever. Very few cases are reported in the UK but they are associated with a case fatality rate of 10%. Conventional antibiotic treatment for pneumonia is not effective and the disease is frequently not recognised until a late stage.

Infection is acquired by inhaling aerosols of contaminated water generated from water-cooled air-conditioning systems in large buildings such as hotels, office blocks or hospitals. Infection has also been associated with fountains, shower outlets and whirlpool spas (Hutchinson 1990). The organism can grow in temperatures between 20 and 50°C and is therefore able to survive in hot water supplies. To prevent infection, water-cooled air-conditioning systems need to be properly cleaned and maintained and water supplied at temperatures that do not favour the growth of legionella (Department of Health, 1994).

Bordetella

The species *B. pertussis* causes whooping cough, a highly communicable infection of the respiratory tract characterised by paroxysmal coughing. After an incubation period of about 2 weeks, a mild cough and sneezing develops, followed by the paroxysmal stage. During episodes of coughing, inspiration ceases and large amounts of mucus accumulate in the upper airways. When the paroxysm ends, it is followed by a stridulous inspiration or characteristic 'whoop'. Coughing may persist for 2–3 weeks and may cause cyanosis and intracranial or conjunctival haemorrhage. Brain damage is the usual cause of infant mortality. Pernasal swabs are required for sampling and *B. pertussis* is difficult to grow.

Vaccination against the infection was introduced in the 1950s and has dramatically reduced the incidence of the disease (Figure 8.8). Reductions in the rate of vaccination, related to concerns about adverse reactions, have been associated with marked increases in the number of cases (Department of Health, 1996).

Brucella

Primarily animal pathogens, these bacteria cause brucellosis, or undulant fever, in humans. *B. abortus* is the main pathogenic species in the UK; it causes spontaneous abortion in cattle and can be acquired by humans through the consumption of unpasteurised milk or contact with infected animal material. It is an occupational disease of farmers and veterinary surgeons. The disease in humans is characterised by high fever, which may re-occur over several weeks (hence 'undulant fever'), lymphadenopathy and splenomegaly. Joints and bones also sometimes become infected and the acute phase is followed by a chronic stage, which may last for years.

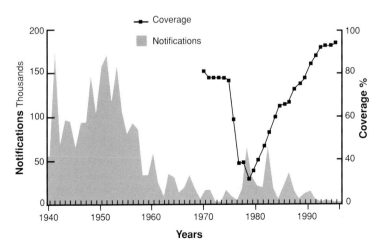

Figure 8.8 Pertussis notifications (1940–1995) and the effect of immunisation uptake (Department of Health, 1996).

ANAEROBIC GRAM-NEGATIVE BACILLI

Bacteroides

These are a large group of anaerobic bacilli, vast numbers of which are found colonising the intestinal tract, mouth and female genital tract. They can cause wound infection, abdominal or pelvic abscesses following intestinal or gynaecological surgery, often in association with other bacteria such as *E. coli*. They are usually the predominant pathogen with other anaerobic bacteria in brain abscesses and empyema. Infections can result in considerable tissue damage, characteristically produce foul-smelling pus and if untreated can spread to other sites via the bloodstream.

ACID-FAST BACILLI

Mycobacterium

Although Gram-positive, these bacteria have a cell wall with a high lipid content, making them difficult to stain; but once stained with carbol fuchsin they resist decolorisation by strong acid or alcohol, hence the term acid-alcohol-fast bacilli or AFB (Figure 8.9). They are strictly aerobic, need special culture media to meet their exacting nutritional requirements and grow extremely slowly so that the colonies are only visible after several weeks of incubation. This means that information about the species and its antibiotic sensitivities cannot be obtained for some time, although in some cases a provisional diagnosis may have been made by staining samples from the site of infection. There are more than 85 species of mycobacteria, but most are environmental bacteria, living in soil and water. A few are obligate pathogens in humans, the most important of which is *M. tuberculosis*.

Mycobacterium tuberculosis

This microorganism usually infects the lungs, causing pulmonary tuberculosis. The infection begins with a small area of inflammation surrounded by a dense granuloma. This primary infection may then resolve and calcify or may progress into active disease. In active disease affecting the lung, the granuloma extends and necrotic tissue formed as a result is removed by coughing, leaving

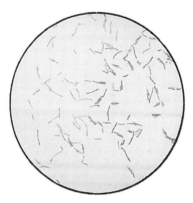

Figure 8.9   Mycobacterium tuberculosis (× 1500), showing characteristic, slightly curved, delicate bacilli.

cavities in the lung tissue. The lesions contain large numbers of mycobacteria which are released during coughing. More generalised infection may result from the spread through the bloodstream or bronchi, leading to miliary tuberculosis in the lung with lesions in other organs, e.g. lymph nodes, meninges, pericardium, peritoneum and kidney. Active disease may occur as a result of re-activation of a primary infection after many years.

Lung infection is usually manifest by a dry cough, fever, night sweats and weight loss. Samples for microbiological culture are often difficult to obtain as the organism may be present in the sputum only intermittently. Best results are obtained from early morning specimens on three consecutive days.

Pulmonary tuberculosis is transmitted from person to person through inhalation of mycobacteria carried on minute droplets expelled from the respiratory tract of a person with active disease. Although highly infectious, prolonged contact is usually required for transmission to occur. However, susceptibility is increased in those who are immunosuppressed; individuals with acquired immune deficiency syndrome have become infected after as little as 24 hours of exposure to someone with active tuberculosis (Breathnach et al 1998). Non-pulmonary forms of the disease are not readily transmissible. Patients can usually be treated at home but, if admission to hospital is necessary, the patient should be segregated in a single room, ideally with a mechanical air extraction system to filter air or direct it outside the building (Joint

Tuberculosis Committee of the British Thoracic Society 1994). Tuberculosis is a notifiable disease. The process of notification triggers the tracing and screening of close contacts and is an important part of tuberculosis control.

Prolonged chemotherapy with a combination of antituberculosis drugs is required to treat the infection (p. 96). Mycobacteria are rapidly removed from the sputum and, once effective chemotherapy has commenced, the patient will usually become non-infectious after 2 weeks (Joint Tuberculosis Committee, 1994). Chemotherapy should be supervised by a respiratory specialist to ensure that the correct treatment is prescribed. Inadequate compliance with treatment is the main cause of relapse of the disease and encourages the emergence of antibiotic-resistant strains (Mitchison 1998). Tuberculosis health visitors and clinic nurses play an important role in both monitoring compliance with treatment and tracing contacts who may have acquired the infection and require treatment. Although the incidence of multi-drug-resistant tuberculosis (MDRTB) is currently low in the UK, an outbreak among HIV-positive patients in a London hospital has been reported recently (Breathnach et al 1998). In some parts of the world, in particular in the developing world but also the USA, difficulties in maintaining compliance with therapy has led to a high incidence of MDRTB, which in some cases has been untreatable and associated with a high mortality (Morse 1996).

The Bacillus Calmette–Guérin (BCG) vaccine, a live attenuated strain derived from *M. bovis*, is used to immunise children against tuberculosis between the ages of 10 and 14. Some people exposed to the infection acquire immunity without developing active disease. Groups of people who are likely to encounter tuberculosis in their work, for example healthcare workers, veterinary surgeons, prison staff and close contacts of people with active pulmonary tuberculosis, should be tested for immunity to tuberculosis and offered vaccination if not immune (Department of Health 1996). Tuberculin skin testing (Mantoux or Heaf test) is used to determine the level of immunity to infection prior to vaccination. In these tests, a small amount of purified tuberculin protein is injected under the skin and the degree of subsequent inflammatory reaction is used to assess whether the individual is immune, non-immune or has active disease.

Other mycobacteria

Other species of mycobacterium can occasionally cause disease in humans. The primary host of *M. bovis* is cattle but it is associated with infection in humans if the disease is not controlled in cattle and milk is not pasteurised prior to consumption. *M. xenopi* and *M. kansasii* cause similar lesions in the lung to *M. tuberculosis* but as opportunistic pathogens they usually infect individuals who have abnormal lower respiratory tracts, e.g. chronic obstructive airways disease. *M. avium–intracellulare* (MAI) is a group or complex of mycobacteria that causes infection in people who have an underlying immunodeficiency, e.g. AIDS. It is acquired through the gastrointestinal tract and causes severe disseminated infection in the lung and gastrointestinal tract. Effective treatment is difficult as MAI is frequently resistant to conventional antituberculosis therapy.

Some species, e.g. *M. ulcerans* and *M. marinum*, are skin pathogens only.

Mycobacterium leprae

This species causes leprosy, a disease of the skin, nerves and mucosa, which is spread by close contact, usually among families. It is not particularly infectious, except where the nasal mucosa are affected. The damage to nerves supplying the limbs can result in severe deformities. Leprosy is a disease of tropical countries, in which around 10 million people are affected. As with tuberculosis, prolonged multiple-drug therapy is required to treat the infection and prevent resistance emerging.

SPIROCHAETACEAE

These organisms have a unique spiral structure and move by using a whip-like or corkscrew mechanism. Most species are non-pathogenic; the three genera that include pathogenic species are treponema, leptospira and borrelia.

Treponema

Treponema palladium is exclusively a parasite of humans and is the cause of syphilis. It is transmitted by sexual intercourse, probably penetrating intact mucous membranes or minor skin lesions of the genital tract, or transplacentally to the fetus. The infection starts with a local lesion or *chancre* in the genital tract. This primary lesion always heals spontaneously, but 2–8 weeks later secondary lesions appear. These include a maculopapular rash, papules in the anogenital region, axillae and mouth and, less commonly, syphilitic meningitis, chorioretinitis or periostitis. If left untreated, a latent asymptomatic state follows, which 10–25 years later develops into tertiary syphilis, with lesions affecting many systems of the body, causing dementia, osteomyelitis and cardiac abnormalities. *T. pallidum* can cross the placenta, especially in the secondary stage. Infection results in premature delivery, fetal death or congenital syphilis.

The delicate organisms die rapidly outside the body and cannot be cultured in the laboratory (Figure 8.10). In primary and secondary lesions it may be possible to find and identify *T. pallidum* by dark-field microscopy carried out in 'special clinics' (Weston 1998). Serological testing is used to diagnose secondary, latent and tertiary syphilis, as well as response to treatment.

Leptospira

These are very tightly coiled, vigorously motile spirals. The single species has many strains, which are widely distributed throughout the environment, particularly in water. Some types are saprophytic, others are parasitic and potential pathogens of humans and animals, e.g. rats, mice, dogs, cattle, pigs. Infected animals

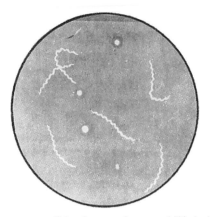

Figure 8.10   *Treponema pallidum* from a primary syphilitic lesion (× 1000).

may be diseased but commonly act as chronic healthy carriers, excreting leptospira in their urine that may remain viable in stagnant water for several weeks and enter new hosts through abrasions on the skin or mucous membranes. In the UK, infection is most commonly seen in people who work with cattle, although it may also be acquired by people swimming or canoeing in contaminated water. Leptospirosis causes symptoms similar to influenza, sometimes associated with jaundice and meningitis.

Borrelia

These are large, spiral organisms. There are several pathogenic species, although the predominant species in temperate climates is *B. burgdorferi*, which causes Lyme disease. It is transmitted from animals, particularly small rodents and deer, to humans by the bite of ticks. A characteristic rash develops around the tick bite and a subsequent inflammatory disorder can result in recurrent attacks of arthritis. In the UK, infection is most likely to occur after exposure to forest or parkland where ticks live in the vegetation. Other species of borrelia, also carried by ticks or lice, predominate in tropical climates, where they cause relapsing fever.

ATYPICAL BACTERIA

Mycoplasma

These bacteria are very small, have no cell wall and are therefore of indefinite size and shape. They are difficult to grow and require very rich media. Many species can be found in soil and elsewhere in the environment. They can also be isolated from the respiratory and urinary tract of humans. The main human pathogen is *M. pneumoniae*, which causes atypical pneumonia, a respiratory infection that unlike bacterial pneumonia, does not respond to treatment with penicillin and depends on serological techniques for diagnosis. Outbreaks of this infection occur every few years (Public Health Laboratory Service 1990). Other species, such as *M. hominis* and *Ureoplasma urealyticum*, colonise the genital tract and may be associated with sexually transmitted disease.

Rickettsia

These are very small microorganisms, which are similar in size to viruses but resemble Gram-negative bacteria. They are unable to replicate independently and therefore exist as intracellular parasites. With the exception of *R. prowazeki* they follow a cycle of transmission between arthropod (ticks, mites, fleas) and vertebrate (small wild mammals) hosts, and humans are infected accidentally. They cause two types of disease: typhus (a severe febrile illness) and spotted fevers, characterised by fever and a rash. Endemic typhus is caused by *R. typhi* and is transmitted by rat fleas and lice. It occurs in urban areas where there is a high rat population. Spotted fevers are transmitted by ticks carried by horses, dogs and rodents. For example, Rocky Mountain spotted fever, which occurs in North and South America, is caused by *R. Rickettsii* carried by dog ticks.

R. prowazeki causes epidemic typhus and is transmitted by the human body louse. The infection occurs where the risk of louse infection is high, i.e. in overcrowded and unhygienic conditions, most commonly associated with war or famine. Infection is controlled by eliminating the body louse and the conditions that enable it to survive.

Coxiella

C. burneti causes Q fever, an influenza-type illness. It is transmitted between animals (sheep, goats, cattle) by ticks, but humans are infected by handling infected meat, ingesting contaminated milk or inhaling contaminated dust. Endocarditis may occur and requires prolonged antibiotic treatment and replacement of the affected valves. Q fever is rarely seen in the UK, although a recent outbreak in east Birmingham involved over 100 people and was thought to have been spread by contaminated dust (Smith 1989).

Chlamydia

These tiny organisms are closely related to Gram-negative bacteria but do not have a cell wall and, as they cannot replicate independently, are intracellular parasites like rickettsia. They can be cultured in the laboratory but clinical samples require special transport media. The main human pathogens are *C. trachomatis*, *C. psittaci* and *C. pneumoniae*.

C. trachomatis

Most strains of this organism can only grow in columnar epithelial cells, found in the conjunctiva, cervix, urethra, respiratory and gastrointestinal tracts. C. trachomatis infection of the genital tract is the most common sexually transmitted disease in females and the cause of non-gonococcal urethritis in males. Neonatal pneumonia occurs when the organism is acquired from the birth canal during delivery. Trachoma, a common cause of blindness in southeast Asia, Africa and the Middle East, is caused by C. trachomatis infection of the conjunctiva and is spread by eye-to-eye contact.

C. psittaci

This organism infects birds, in particular psittacine birds such as parrots. It is transmitted to humans by inhalation of dust containing dried faeces of infected birds and causes psittacosis. The symptoms can range from a mild influenza-type illness to severe pneumonia. Other strains of C. psittaci can cause arthritis and abortion in animals such as sheep and cattle. Infection can be transmitted to humans who handle infected animals.

C. pneumoniae

This causes mild pneumonia in humans, who appear to be its only hosts. Outbreaks may occur in schools or other crowded institutions.

REFERENCES

Acheson, E.D. (1989) Botulism and hazelnut yoghurt. *Health Trends*, **21**, 66.
Avason, V.A., Kristinsson, K.G., Sigurdson, J.A. *et al.* (1996) Do antimicrobials increase the carriage rate of penicillin resistant pneumococci in children? Cross sectional prevalence study. *Br. Med. J.*, **313**, 387–391.
Barrie, D., Wilson, J., Hoffman, P.N. and Kramer, J. (1992) *Bacillus cereus* meningitis in two neurosurgical patients: an investigation into the source of the organism. *J. Infect.*, **25**, 291–297.
Bates, J., Jordens, J.Z. and Griffiths, D.T. (1994) Farm animals as a putative reservoir for vancomycin-resistant enterococcal infection in man. *J. Antimicrob. Chemother.*, **34**, 507–514.
Benenson, A.S. (ed.) (1995) *Control of Communicable Diseases Manual*. American Public Health Association, Washington, DC.
Breathnach, A.S., de Ruiter, A., Holdsworth, G.M.C. *et al.* (1998) An outbreak of multi-drug resistant tuberculosis in a London teaching hospital. *J. Hosp. Infect.*, **39**(2), 111–118.

Coello, R., Glynn, J.R., Gaspar, C. *et al.* (1997) Risk factors for developing clinical infection with methicillin resistant *Staphylococcus aureus* (MRSA) amongst hospital patients initially only colonised with MRSA. *J. Hosp. Infect.*, **37**, 39–46.

Communicable Disease Report (1995a) Interim guidelines for the control of infections with Vero cytotoxin producing *Escherichia coli* (VTEC). *CDR Rev.*, **5**(6), R77–R80.

Communicable Disease Report (1995b) The prevention of human transmission of gastrointestinal infections, infestations and bacterial intoxications. A guide for public health physicians and environmental health officers in England and Wales. *CDR Rev.*, **5**(11), R157–R172.

Communicable Disease Report (1997) Epidemic methicillin resistant *Staphylococcus aureus*. *CDR Weekly*, **7**(22), 191.

Communicable Disease Report (1998) Botulism associated with home-preserved mushrooms. *CDR Weekly*, **8**(18), 159.

Cottrill, M.R.B. (1996) *Helicobacter pylori*. *Prof. Nurse*, **12**(1), 46–48.

Cowden, J.M. (1997) Scottish outbreak of *Escherichia coli* O157 November–December 1996. *Euro Surveillance*, **2**(1), 1–2.

Cowden, J.M., Wall, P.G., Adak, G. *et al.* (1995) Outbreaks of foodborne infectious intestinal disease in England and Wales: 1992 and 1993. *CDR Rev.*, **5**(8), R109–R117.

Dealler, S (1998) Nosocomial outbreak of multi-resistant *Acinetobacter* sp. on an intensive care unit: possible association with ventilation equipment. *J. Hosp. Infect.*, **38**(2), 147–148.

De Louvois, J. (1993) Salmonella contamination of eggs. *Lancet*, **342**, 366–367.

Department of Health (1988) ML/CMO (89)3 and Press release 89/369 – statements of advice on listeria and food.

Department of Health (1994) The control of legionellae in healthcare premises – a code of practice. *HTM 2040*. HMSO, London.

Department of Health (1996) *Immunisation Against Infectious Disease*. HMSO, London.

Department of Health and Public Health (1994) *Clostridium Difficile* Infection Prevention and Management Joint Working Group Report. *PL (94)CO/4*. BAPS Health Publications Unit.

Department of Health and Social Security (1986) *The Report of the Committee of Enquiry into an Outbreak of Food Poisoning at Stanley Royd Hospital*. HMSO, London.

Dowsett, E.G. and Wilson, P.A. (1981) An outbreak of *Streptococcus pyogenes* infection in a maternity unit. *Commun. Dis. Rep.*, **81**(17), 3.

Eley, A.R. (ed.) (1992) *Microbial Food Poisoning*. Chapman & Hall, London.

Emori, T.G. and Gaynes R.P. (1993) An overview of nosocomial infection, including the role of the microbiology laboratory. *Clin. Microbiol. Rev.*, **6**, 87–107.

Glynn, A., Ward, V., Wilson, J. *et al.* (1997) *Hospital Acquired Infection: Surveillance, Policies and Practice*. Public Health Laboratory Service, London.

Gormon, L.J. Sanai, L., Notman, W. *et al.* (1993) Cross-infection in an intensive care unit by *Klebsiella pneumoniae* from ventilator condensate. *J. Hosp. Inf.*, **23**, 17–26.

Hamory, B.H. and Parisi, J.T. (1987) *Staphylococcus epidermidis*: a significant nosocomial pathogen. *J. Infect. Control.*, **15**, 59–74.

Hoffman, P.N. (1993) *Clostridium difficile* and the hospital environment. *PHLS Microbiol. Digest*, **10**(2), 91–92.

Hollyoak, V., Allison, D. and Summers, J. (1995) *Pseudomonas aeruginosa* wound infection associated with a nursing home's whirlpool bath. *Communicable Dis. Rep.*, **5**(7), R100–R102.

Holmes, S. (1989) Careful food handling reduces the risk of listeria. *Prof. Nurse*, **4**(7), 322–324.

Humar, A., Oxley, C., Lu Sample, M. *et al.* (1996) Elimination of an outbreak of Gram-negative bacteraemia in a hemodialysis unit. *Am. J. Infect. Control*, **24**, 359–363

Humphreys, H. and Towner, K.J. (1997) Impact of *Acinetobacter* spp. in intensive care units in Great Britain and Ireland. *J. Hosp. Infect.*, **37**(4), 281–286.

Hutchinson, D.N. (1990) Nosocomial legionellosis. *Rev. Med. Microbiol.*, **1**, 108–115.

Johnson, A.P. (1998) Antibiotic resistance among clinically important Gram positive bacteria in the UK. *J. Hosp. Infect.*, **40**, 17–26.

Joint Tuberculosis Committee of the British Thoracic Society (1994) Control and prevention of tuberculosis in the United Kingdom: Code of Practice 1994. *Thorax*, **49**, 1193–1200.

Jones, D. (1990) Foodborne listeriosis. *Lancet*, **336**, 1171–1174.

Klutymans, J., Van Belkum, A. and Verbrugh, H. (1997) Nasal carriage of *S. aureus*: epidemiology, underlying mechanisms and associated risks. *Clin. Microbiol. Rev.*, **10**, 505–520.

Klutymans, J.A., Mouton, J.W., Vanden Bergh, M.F.Q. *et al.* (1996) Reduction in surgical site infection in cardiothroacic surgery by elimination of nasal carriage of *S. aureus*. *Infect. Control. Hosp. Epidemiol.*, **17**, 780–785.

Laurichesse, H., Grimaud, O., Wraight, P. *et al.* (1998) Pneumococcal bacteraemia and meningitis in England and Wales: 1993 to 1995. *Commun. Dis. Public Health*, **1**(1), 22–27.

Levin, M.H., Olsen, B., Nathan, C. *et al.* (1984) Pseudomonas in the sinks in an intensive care unit: relation to patients. *J. Clin. Pathol.*, **37**, 424–427.

Marshall, B.J. and Warren, J.R. (1984) Unidentified curved bacilli in the stomachs of people with gastritis and peptic ulceration. *Lancet*, **i**, 1311–1315.

Mitchison, D.A. (1998) How drug resistance emerges as a result of poor compliance during short course chemotherapy for tuberculosis. *Int. J. Lung Dis*, **2**(1), 10–15.

Morrison, D., Woodford, N. and Cookson, B.D. (1996) Epidemic vancomycin-resistant *Enterococcus faecium* in the UK. *Clin. Microbiol. Rev.*, **1**(2), 146.

Morse, D.I. (1996) Directly observed therapy for tuberculosis. *Br. Med. J.*, **312**, 719–720.

Muhlemann, M.F. and Wright, D.J.M. (1987) Emerging pattern of Lyme disease in the United Kingdom and Irish republic. *Lancet*, **i**, 260–262.

Murray, B.A. (1990) The life and times of the enterococcus. *Microbiol. Rev.*, **3**(1), 46–65.

Musa, E.K., Desai, N. and Casewell, M.V. (1990) The survival of *Acinetobacter calcoaceticus* inoculated on fingertips and on formica. *J. Hosp. Infect.*, **15**(3), 219–227.

Mylotte, J.M. (1994) Control of methicillin-resistant *Staphylococcus aureus*: the ambivalence persists. *Infect. Control Hosp. Epidemiol.* **15**, 73–77.

Newton, L., Hall, S.M., Pelevin, M. *et al.* (1992) Listeriosis surveillance: 1991. *Communicable Dis. Rev.*, **2**(12), R142–R144.

Nye, F.J. (1993) Clinical features and treatment of *Clostridium difficile* diarrhoea. *PHLS Microbiol. Digest*, **10**(2), 77–78

Public Health Laboratory Service (1990) *Mycoplasma pneumoniae* infections in England and Wales. *Communicable Dis. Rep.* **18**, 1.

Reybrouck, G. (1983) Role of hands in the spread of nosocomial infection: 1. *J. Hosp. Infect* **4**, 103–110.

Schlech, W.F. (1991) Listeriosis: epidemiology, virulence and the significance of contaminated foodstuffs. *J. Hosp. Infect.* **19**(4), 211–224.

Shanson, D.C. (1989) *Microbiology in Clinical Practice*, 2nd edn, John Wright, Bristol.

Smith, G. (1989) Q fever outbreak in Birmingham UK. *Lancet*, **ii**, 557.

Stansfield, R. and Caudle, S. (1997) *Bacillus cereus* and orthopaedic surgical wound infection associated with incontinence pads manufactured from virgin wood pulp. *J. Hosp. Infect.*, **37**(4), 336–337.

Takashashi, S., Yomoda, S., Tanimoto, K. *et al.* (1998) *Streptococcus pyogenes* hospital-acquired infection within a dermatological ward. *J. Hosp. Infect.*, **40**, 135–140.

Tassios, P.T., Gennimata, V., Spaliara-kalogeropoulou, L. *et al.* (1997) Multiresistant *Pseudomonas aeruginosa* serogroup O:11 outbreak in an intensive care unit. *Clin. Microbiol. Infect.*, **3**(6), 621–628.

Taylor, D. and Littlewood, S. (1998) Respiratory System: part 2. *Tuberculosis Nurs. Times*, **94**(11), 50–53.

Wall, P.G., de Louvois, J., Gilbert, R.J. and Rowe, B. (1996) Food poisoning: notifications, laboratory reports, and outbreaks – where do the statistics come from and what do they mean? *CDR Rev.*, **6**(7), R93–R99.

Weber, J.M. Sheridan, R.L., Pasternack, M.S. *et al.* (1997) Nosocomial infections in pediatric patients with burns. *Am. J. Infect. Control.*, **25**, 195–201.

Weber, D.J. and Rutala, W.A. (1997) Role of environmental contamination in the transmission of vancomycin-resistant enterococci. *Infect. Control Hosp. Epidemiol*, **18**, 306–309.

Weems, J.J. (1993) Nosocomial outbreak of *Pseudomonas cepacia* associated with contamination of reusable electronic ventilator temperature probes. *Infect. Control Hosp. Epidemiol.*, **14**(10), 583–586.

Weston, A. (1998) Striking back at syphilis. *Nurs. Times*, **94**(3), 30–32.

FURTHER READING

Albino, J.A. and Reichman, L.B. (1997) Multidrug-resistant tuberculosis. *Curr. Opin. Infect. Dis.*, **10**, 116–122.

Bannister, B.A., Begg, N.T. and Gillespie, S.H. (1996) *Infectious disease.* Blackwell Science, Oxford.

Beaumont, G. (1998) Resistant movement (enterococcus). *Nurs. Times*, **94**(37), 69–75.

Casewell, M.W. (1998) The nose: an underestimated source of *Staphylococcus aureus* causing wound infection. *J. Hosp. Infect.*, **40**(Suppl. B), S3–S12.

Davies, A. (1998) Chlamydia: the most common sexually transmitted infection. *Nurs. Times*, **94**(5), 56–58.

Doyle, M.P. (1990) Pathogenic *Escherichia coli*, *Yersinia enterocolitica* and *Vibrio parahaemolyticus*. *Lancet*, **336**, 1111–1115.

Duerden, B.I., Reid, T.M.S. and Jewsbury, J.M. (1993) *Microbial and Parasitic Infection*, 7th Edn. Edward Arnold, London.

Hospital Infection Control Practice Advisory Committee (HICPAC) (1995) Recommendations for preventing the spread of vancomycin resistance. *Am. J. Infect. Control*, **23**, 87–94.

Williams, P. and Ellison, J. (1998) Food fears. *Nurs. Times*, **94**(28), 72–73.

9

A guide to viruses

INTRODUCTION

Viruses are intracellular parasites, which require a host cell to provide the necessary structures and materials for their replication. Most viruses replicate in specific tissue and are transmitted by inhalation, ingestion, inoculation, sexual contact or transplacentally, depending on the site or tissue affected. For example, measles viruses replicates in the respiratory tract, poliovirus in the gastrointestinal tract; and they are transmitted by secretions from these tissues.

Viral infections are usually of acute onset and self-limiting, causing symptoms for a few days or weeks until they are destroyed by the host's immune system. The effect on the host depends on the particular cells involved and their function. For example, if motor neurone cells in the central nervous system are infected by the poliovirus, they are destroyed and the muscles they supply will be paralysed. Some viruses destroy cells they invade, others only disrupt cell function, while others cause no damage at all. A few induce changes in the genetic material of cells, causing them to be transformed into malignant cells. Some complications associated with viral infection (e.g. rashes, arthritis) are due to the immune response mounted by the host against the infection. In some cases, extensive tissue damage results from the destruction of virus-infected cells by the immune defences (e.g. destruction of liver cells invaded by the hepatitis B virus).

Intact skin forms an effective barrier against invasion by viruses and a break is necessary to allow the virus to enter. Some viruses cause localised lesions (e.g. herpes simplex) and others (e.g. hepatitis B) cause a generalised infection involving several body systems. Many viruses enter at mucosal surfaces in the respiratory, gastrointestinal or genitourinary tracts. They may then replicate locally before being spread via the bloodstream to other target tissues. Some viruses (e.g. adenoviruses) can replicate inside phagocytic white cells, using them as a means to travel in the bloodstream, while being protected from attack by the immune system.

The basic structure of all viruses is very similar, consisting of a piece of nucleic acid, surrounded by a protein coat (p. 26). The use of powerful electron microscopes has allowed examination of their detailed structure and enabled a system of classifying viruses into groups to be developed. The classification is based on a number of characteristics:

- type of nucleic acid, either DNA or RNA
- symmetry of the capsid, which may be arranged as a hollow sphere (cubic), spiral (helical) or more complex structure
- presence or absence of a lipid envelope
- size.

A summary of viral classification is given in Tables 9.1 and 9.2.

This chapter considers clinically significant viruses, grouped under the following headings:

- Respiratory viruses
- Gastrointestinal viruses
- Hepatitis viruses
- Retroviruses
- Herpes viruses
- Pox viruses
- Papovaviruses
- Rhabdoviruses
- Togaviruses
- Haemorrhagic fevers
- Virus-like agents.

Chapter 2 describes the structure and replication of viruses. Additional information on their route of transmission and the care of affected patients is outlined in the appendix to Chapter 14 (p. 365).

Table 9.1 Summary of the main groups of human RNA viruses

Group	Capsid symmmetry	Size	Viruses in group	Infections
Picornaviruses	Cubic	24–35	Enteroviruses	
			• Poliovirus	Poliomyelitis
			• Coxsackie virus	Hand, foot and mouth disease
			• Echoviruses	Meningitis
			• Rhinoviruses	Common cold
			• Hepatitis A virus	Hepatitis
Togaviruses	Cubic	40–70	Alphaviruses	Encephalitis
			Flaviviruses	Yellow fever, dengue fever
			Rubella virus	Rubella
Reoviruses	Cubic	60–80	Reoviruses	
			Rotaviruses	Gastroenteritis
Retroviruses	Cubic	100	HIV	AIDS
			HTLV	Lymphoma
Orthomyxoviruses	Helical	80–120	Influenza viruses	Influenza
Paramyxoviruses	Helical	100	Parainfluenza virus	Respiratory infection
		120	Measles virus	Measles
			Mumps virus	Mumps
			Respiratory syncytial virus	Bronchiolitis
Rhabdoviruses	Helical	80–180	Rabies virus	Rabies
Coronaviruses	Helical	80–130	Coronaviruses	Common cold
Arenaviruses	Helical	110	Arenavirus	Lassa fever
Unclassified viruses			Marburg virus	Haemorrhagic fever
			Ebola virus	Haemorrhagic fever
			Calciviruses	Gastroenteritis, hepatitis E

RESPIRATORY VIRUSES

The viruses described in this section mainly affect the respiratory tract. They are spread by respiratory droplets containing the virus, which are expelled by coughs and sneezes and land on the mucous

Table 9.2 Summary of the main groups of human DNA viruses

Group	Capsid symmmetry	Size	Viruses in group	Infections
Parvoviruses	Cubic	20	Parvovirus	Erythema infectiosum
Papovaviruses	Cubic	50	Papilloma virus	Warts
Adenoviruses	Cubic	50	Adenoviruses	Respiratory infection, conjunctivitis
Herpes viruses	Cubic	120	Herpes simplex virus	Cold sores, encephalitis, genital herpes
			Varicella-zoster virus	Chickenpox, shingles
			Human herpes virus 6	Roseola infantum
			Cytomegalovirus	Infectious mononucleosis
			Epstein–Barr virus	Infectious mononucleosis
Poxviruses	Complex	230–300	Variola virus	Smallpox
			Orf virus	Skin lesions
			Molluscum contagiosum virus	Skin lesions
Unclassified		42	Hepatitis B virus	Hepatitis B

membranes of another person. Direct contact with respiratory secretions on freshly contaminated hands, handkerchiefs and eating utensils also contributes to their spread (Ansari et al 1991). Children are most vulnerable to many of these respiratory tract infections and particular care is required in paediatric wards or other areas caring for young children. Transmission can be limited by isolation of affected children and careful handwashing after any contact with respiratory secretions.

Adenoviruses

These are icosahedral viruses with characteristic antennae (see Figure 2.2). More than 40 different adenoviruses are known and they are an important cause of respiratory tract infection in young children, most of whom will have encountered the virus by the age of 10. They cause a runny nose, mild pharyngitis or tracheitis, cough and fever. The symptoms usually last between 3 and 5 days. Immunity develops after infection but is specific to the particular type of adenovirus and subsequent infection with a different serotype may occur. The virus can also become latent, remaining in the epithelial cells of the nasopharynx, replicating slowly and although not causing any symptoms of infection, available for transmission to others.

Adenoviruses can also cause conjunctivitis, often lasting for several weeks, and swimming pools have been implicated in outbreaks of infection (Piedra et al 1992). Conjunctivitis can occur in conjunction with upper respiratory tract infection or following trauma to the eye. Epidemics associated with contaminated ophthalmic solutions have also been reported (Straube et al 1983)

Orthomyxoviruses (influenza viruses)

These helical RNA viruses have a lipid envelope with spikes that enable them to penetrate mucus and attach to receptors on the host's respiratory mucous membranes. They replicate in the mucous membranes but their effect is more general, causing influenza, an illness associated with sore throat, cough, myalgia, lethargy and high fever. The incubation period is very short, only 2–3 days. Since these symptoms are associated with a number of viral infections, a diagnosis may be made by isolating the virus from nasopharyngeal specimens or demonstrating a rise in the antibody level in paired sera (p. 143). Although not usually a serious illness, influenza can cause pneumonia and myocarditis and recovery is often prolonged, particularly in the elderly. Damage to the cilia of the epithelium of the respiratory tract, an important component of the normal defences against infection, enables subsequent secondary infection by bacteria, in particular *Staphylococcus aureus*, which can cause a severe, often fatal, pneumonia. The virus is readily transmitted by respiratory droplets and epidemics and pandemics are common, with the elderly being particularly vulnerable (Communicable Disease Report, 1998a).

There are three types of influenza virus: A, B and C. Type A causes most epidemics and also infects a variety of birds and animals as well as humans. Immunity to influenza depends on the recognition by the host of antigenic proteins on the surface of the virus. These antigens are complex and unstable, making it difficult for the immune system to recognise and respond to them. Minor changes to the antigens occur through mutation of the nucleic acids that encode them; these changes are termed *antigenic drift*. Larger changes, called *antigenic shift*, occur when a completely new combination of antigens emerges. Immunity to a previously encountered strain will not be protective against the strain with a new combination of antigens. The antigenic types of prevalent influenza viruses are carefully monitored to predict those likely to cause epidemics and enable appropriate vaccines to be prepared. Once a particular strain has caused an epidemic, a large proportion of the population will develop immunity. The strain may then circulate within the bird and animal populations for many years until it is introduced into and infects a new, susceptible population.

Influenza virus vaccines

These are prepared every year to protect against the strain considered most likely to be prevalent in the coming winter. In 80% of cases they protect against infection and, where infection does occur following vaccination, the risk of serious complication such as a secondary bacterial pneumonia is considerably reduced. Influenza epidemics can cause considerable mortality. During the winter of 1989–90, 26 000 people died in the UK of influenza A or from secondary infections (Reilly, 1990). Annual immunisation is therefore recommended for people who are most at risk of developing serious illness should they acquire influenza, e.g. those with chronic respiratory or heart disease, diabetes or immunosuppression. Elderly people living in nursing homes should also be vaccinated as infection can spread rapidly in these settings (Department of Health, 1996).

Reye's syndrome

This is an acute encephalopathy that occurs as a rare complication of influenza B and some other viral infections in children. It has a high mortality and is thought to be associated with the use of aspirin during the infection (Committee on Infectious Diseases 1982).

Paramyxoviruses

These are enveloped RNA viruses, which cause a variety of respiratory illnesses. The main human pathogens in the group are measles, mumps, parainfluenza viruses and respiratory syncytial virus.

Measles

This virus causes an acute respiratory illness with fever, cough, running nose and conjunctivitis. Raised red spots with white centres like grains of sand (Koplik's spots) form on the buccal mucosa. After about 7 days a characteristic rash appears, first on the face and then spreading over the whole body; this is caused by the cell-mediated immune response to the infection (p. 62). Secondary infections of bronchopneumonia and otitis media are common; encephalitis occurs more rarely. These complications are most likely to occur in poorly nourished or clinically ill children and the associated mortality is high in children under 1 year of age (Benenson 1995). Subacute sclerosing panencephalitis (SSPE) is a rare, but fatal, complication of measles infection, usually associated with acquisition of the virus before 1 year of age.

Infection is spread by respiratory droplets. The incubation period is usually 10 days and infectivity lasts for 2 days before the onset of symptoms and approximately 4 days after the rash has appeared. Measles is a notifiable disease (p. 260) and routine immunisation of young children is recommended, using the combined live vaccine measles, mumps and rubella (MMR). Prior to the introduction of a measles vaccine in 1968 epidemics of the infection, affecting up to 800 000 people, occurred in 2-year cycles. MMR was introduced in 1988 and immunisation levels in children in excess of 90% were achieved; this has dramatically reduced the incidence of the infection (Department of Health 1996). Since October 1996 it has been recommended that children should receive two doses, one after the first birthday and another before school entry. Concerns about a relationship between vaccination and Crohn's disease or autism have been expressed but no clear association has been demonstrated (Communicable Disease Report 1998b). If susceptible patients in hospital are exposed to the virus, they can be protected from developing the infection by specific immunoglobulin.

Mumps

This virus causes an acute inflammatory swelling of the salivary glands, usually the parotid glands, and prior to the introduction of the vaccine was a common cause of meningitis in children under 15. About 20% of males develop orchitis if they acquire the infection after puberty. Many infections are subclinical but still induce lifelong immunity. The virus is transmitted by airborne droplets, it has an incubation period of about 3 weeks and those affected are infectious for a week before and after the appearance of symptoms. Mumps is a notifiable disease. Vaccination is recommended for children and the vaccine is included in the MMR vaccine.

Respiratory syncytial virus (RSV)

This virus is a major cause of viral respiratory illness in young children, particularly those under two. It starts like a common cold but within 24 hours the infant is acutely ill with cyanosis and respiratory distress. It mainly causes bronchiolitis, but can also cause pneumonia, croup, otitis media and other febrile respiratory tract infections. Adults may also acquire the infection, which tends to be mild, except in the elderly or those with chronic lung or heart conditions. It is transmitted by infected respiratory secretions and by contamination of hands. Outbreaks of infection tend to occur most commonly in the autumn or winter and infected people can continue to shed the virus for several weeks after symptoms have resolved. Children admitted to hospital with RSV infection should be isolated while symptomatic to reduce the risk of transmission (Madge at al 1992). Infection induces short-term immunity, so that subsequent infections occur but are usually milder.

Parainfluenza viruses

These viruses cause a variety of mild respiratory infections, including croup and bronchiolitis, particularly in children under 5.

Rhinoviruses

There are over 100 different types of RNA virus, which cause the common cold. However, there are many other virus groups that cause colds, including coxsackie and coronaviruses. Immunity to the particular type and strain of virus develops after each exposure, but the large number of types and their relative importance and distribution during outbreaks makes complete immunity to all of them unlikely.

Rubella (German measles)

This virus causes a mild febrile illness with a macular rash that starts on the face and spreads to the trunk and limbs. The incubation period is between 2 and 3 weeks and the period of infectivity is from 1 week before symptoms until 4 days after the onset of the rash. In non-immunised populations it mostly occurs in young children and young men are also commonly affected. The most significant morbidity associated with the virus occurs if a non-immune women acquires the infection during the first 4 months of pregnancy. It may then cause severe congenital defects in the fetus, including heart abnormalities, microcephaly and hepatosplenomegaly. A third of infants born with congenital rubella die within the first few months. Infection in adults is sometimes associated with joint pains and arthritis, especially in women. Rubella is a notifiable disease. In the UK, rubella vaccine is given routinely to children as part of the combined live MMR vaccine, and postpartum vaccination should be offered to women shown by serological tests to be non-immune during pregnancy.

Parvoviruses

These are small, round DNA viruses. There are a number of types and B19 is most often implicated in human infections. It causes erythema infectiosum (slapped cheek syndrome or fifth disease), a common childhood infection consisting of a mild febrile illness lasting 2–3 days, followed by a typical rash on the cheeks. The virus is spread by respiratory secretions but patients are no longer infectious by the time the rash has appeared. In adults the infection can be associated with arthralgia, which can range from very mild to full arthritis. In individuals with a chronic haemolytic anaemia (e.g. sickle cell anaemia or thalassaemia) infection may precipitate an aplastic crisis resulting in a very low haemoglobin. Infection during the first or second trimester of pregnancy can result in severe fetal abnormalities or spontaneous abortion, although in most cases the virus does not cross the placenta and the baby is unaffected.

GASTROINTESTINAL VIRUSES

These are viruses whose point of entry or primary site of infection is the gastrointestinal tract, from which they are often shed in faeces in extremely large numbers. They are transmitted through contact with faeces, either directly on hands or indirectly from contaminated food and water. Some viruses (e.g. small round structured virus, rotavirus) may also be transmitted through contact with vomit. Outbreaks of infection in hospitals and nursing homes, where person-to-person spread can occur easily, have frequently been reported (Mitchell et al 1989, Green et al 1998). They are also associated with outbreaks of food-borne infection from a variety of food sources or infected food handlers (Luthi et al 1996).

Picornaviruses

These are small, icosahedral RNA viruses and include several important groups of viruses, in particular the enteroviruses.

Enteroviruses

This large genus is associated with a wide spectrum of diseases. They are excreted in faeces and transmitted through contaminated food or water, or by contaminated hands, but are rarely associated with disease of the gastrointestinal tract. They establish infection in the lymphoid tissue of the gut or pharynx and from there spread in the bloodstream to other parts of the body. There are several subgroups: poliovirus, coxsackie virus, echovirus and hepatitis A virus.

Poliovirus. 95% of infections are subclinical; some patients experience headache, gastrointestinal disturbance, malaise and stiffness of neck and back. In one in 1000 cases, the virus spreads to the anterior horn of the spinal cord or brain stem, where the resulting destruction of motor neurones causes paralysis, which may be permanent or result in death. In some developing countries poliovirus is widespread, causing epidemics of infection with transmission occurring through contact with faeces or respiratory secretions. In the UK, since the introduction of routine immunisation in the 1950s, the number of cases has declined to two or three a year, although immunisation levels of at least 90% must be maintained to ensure that the virus is unable to spread through the population (p. 69). However, people who travel abroad may be at risk of acquiring infection and should ensure that they are fully protected by immunisation if appropriate. There are three types of poliovirus and all of them are contained in the live, attenuated vaccine used for immunisation in the UK. Three doses of vaccine are recommended to ensure that immunity develops to each type. Vaccine virus is excreted in the faeces for several weeks and may be acquired by non-immunised contacts; hands should therefore be carefully washed after contact with faeces. Infection with the vaccine virus occurs very rarely in recipients of the vaccine or their contacts, with an average of only one or two cases a year, none paralytic cases. Inactivated, rather than live, polio virus vaccine is available for protection of the immunocompromised, who may be more vulnerable to infection with virus in the live vaccine (Department of Health, 1996).

Coxsackie viruses. There are many different types of these viruses, which cause a wide range of syndromes, notably: hand, foot and mouth disease, a stomatitis associated with lesions on the palms, fingers and soles; herpangina, a pharyngitis with vesicular lesions; common colds; less commonly myocarditis, especially in neonates; epidemic myalgia, an acute pain in the chest and abdomen with fever and headache, which resolves after about a week; and meningitis and paralysis mimicking poliomyelitis, most of which recover completely. Coxsackie viruses are spread through contact with both faeces and respiratory secretions.

Echoviruses. These viruses cause acute, febrile illnesses, diarrhoea and mild upper respiratory tract infections, and may also cause meningitis.

Hepatitis A. This virus first replicates in the gastrointestinal tract and then spreads to the liver. It is transmitted by contact with faeces and causes dull abdominal pain and fever and, in some people, acute hepatitis, which is followed by jaundice. The virus cannot be cultured in the laboratory and diagnosis is therefore made by serological tests. Unlike hepatitis B virus, hepatitis A is not transmitted in blood, infection is not complicated by a carrier state and it does not cause chronic hepatitis. Outbreaks of hepatitis A infection commonly occur among groups of children and young adults, e.g. in schools, nurseries and colleges. The infection has a long incubation period of about 30 days and patients are infectious for 7–10 days before the symptoms develop and for a few days afterwards. The transmission of infection can be prevented by handwashing after contact with faeces. Food-borne infection may also occur and sewage-contaminated shellfish have been responsible for several outbreaks (O'Mahony et al 1983), as have raspberries (Reid & Robinson, 1987). A vaccine against hepatitis A infection is now available and recommended for travellers where there is a risk of contracting infection. Individuals over 50 years of age and those born in areas where hepatitis A is prevalent who have a past history of jaundice may already be immune. Haemophiliacs, some laboratory workers and homosexual males should be offered the vaccine. Passive immunisation with immunoglobulin is offered to contacts of cases of hepatitis A infection and may be a useful means of protecting contacts in the event of an outbreak.

Rotavirus

This is an RNA virus that has a two-layered capsid, giving it a characteristic wheel-shaped appearance (Figure 9.1). It is difficult to grow in cell cultures but can be detected in the faeces by enzyme-linked immunoassay (ELISA) or electron microscopy. It causes severe gastroenteritis characterised by fever, vomiting and watery diarrhoea. Hospitalisation may be required to treat dehydration. Children are particularly susceptible from the age of 6 months, when protection from maternal antibodies has declined. By 6 years of age, most children will have been exposed to the infection and

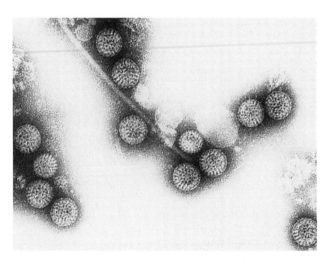

Figure 9.1   Rotavirus particles in a faecal suspension (electron micrograph).

have developed sufficient antibodies to protect against or moderate the symptoms of subsequent infections. Adults therefore usually have a mild illness, although the elderly are more vulnerable to serious illness.

The incubation period for the infection is short, between 24 and 72 hours. Large numbers of viruses are excreted in the faeces during the acute phase of the illness and transmission to others through contact with faeces, and possibly respiratory secretions, occurs readily. Outbreaks of infection in paediatric wards, children's homes or wards and homes for the elderly are especially likely to occur during the winter when the incidence of rotavirus infection reaches its peak.

Other viral causes of gastroenteritis

Many other viruses cause gastrointestinal infection, usually characterised by diarrhoea. Astroviruses and caliciviruses e.g. Norwalk virus, small round structured viruses (SRSVs) and small round viruses (SRVs) cause outbreaks of infection similar to that of rotavirus. They may be food- or water-borne and are readily spread from person to person through contact with faeces or vomit (Chadwick & McCann 1994). The incubation period is short, usually 1–2 days. They cannot yet be propagated in cell cultures; identification by electron microscopy is easiest in the first 48 hours of illness and can be important in determining the source and extent of spread of an outbreak of infection. Preventing transmission requires handwashing after any contact with faeces or vomit, careful disposal of excreta and preferably single-room care, especially in paediatric, care of the elderly or neonatal wards (Dowsett, 1988).

Hepatitis E is a calicivirus. It causes an infection similar to hepatitis A, is rarely seen in Europe but is endemic in parts of south-east Asia, the former Soviet Union and north Africa, causing large outbreaks of hepatitis. Infection is usually associated with poor sanitation, particularly sewage-contaminated water. It is also spread from person to person by contact with faeces. Young adults are most likely to become infected and, although it generally causes a mild illness, infection during pregnancy can disrupt blood coagulation and has a high mortality (Zuckerman, 1990). The incubation period is 2–6 weeks and, although chronic carriage does not occur, the virus may be excreted in the faeces for several days after the onset of jaundice.

Enteric adenoviruses are a common cause of gastroenteritis in young children, with similar symptoms to rotavirus but a longer incubation of approximately 10 days.

Many of these gastrointestinal infections only confer short-term immunity in most people so that re-infection is likely to occur on subsequent exposure.

HEPATITIS VIRUSES (BLOOD-BORNE)

At least five viruses are known to primarily infect liver cells, causing viral hepatitis, associated with inflammation and liver damage. Two of these viruses are transmitted by the faecal–oral route, hepatitis A (a picornavirus) and hepatitis E (a calicivirus); they are discussed in the section on gastrointestinal viruses above. The remaining viruses, hepatitis B, hepatitis C and hepatitis D, are transmitted by the inoculation of infected blood or body fluids and are described below. Other viruses cause hepatitis as part of a generalised infection, e.g. Epstein–Barr, cytomegalovirus, congenital rubella.

Hepatitis B

This is a small, enveloped DNA virus, with a double-shelled, spherical capsid and an inner core containing the nucleic acid (Figure 9.2). The hepatitis usually has an insidious onset with anorexia, nausea and vomiting, mild fever and jaundice. The incubation period may vary, according to the mode of transmission and dose of virus received, from 1–6 months (Benenson 1995). About 60% of infections are asymptomatic but a small proportion are very severe, causing extensive liver damage and liver failure.

The virus is transmitted by blood and other serum-derived body fluids (e.g. semen and vaginal secretions). For transmission to occur the infectious fluid must have contact with a mucosal surface or damaged skin, or be inoculated through the skin. Saliva has been found to contain low concentrations of the virus, but has been shown to transmit infection only when inoculated through the skin by a bite (Cancio-Bello et al 1982). Infection can also be transmitted by sexual intercourse and from mother to baby during delivery or perinatally; subsequent transmission to household contacts may also occur.

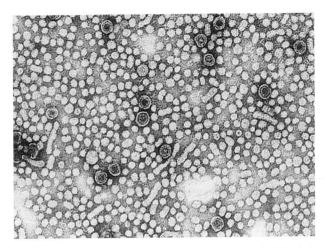

Figure 9.2 Hepatitis surface antigen (HBsAg) purified from the blood of a carrier. The large particles with an inner core are complete infectious virions (electron micrograph).

Between 2% and 10% of those infected as adults become chronic carriers of the virus. About a quarter of those who become chronic hepatitis B carriers develop progressive hepatitis, which can ultimately lead to cirrhosis and liver carcinoma. The risk of becoming a carrier is highest when the infection is acquired as a child, and increases to 90% where it is acquired perinatally (Department of Health, 1996). In countries with a high prevalence, such as south-east Asia, Africa and parts of North and South America, perinatal transmission is common and up to 20% of the population may be carriers of hepatitis B.

In most European countries, the prevalence of hepatitis B is less than 2% and transmission is more likely to occur as a result of sexual contact, sharing contaminated needles, needlestick injuries or human bites. Intravenous drug-users, haemophiliacs, residents of institutions for people with severe learning difficulties, renal dialysis patients, homosexuals and family contacts of carriers are more at risk of infection. All blood and blood products donated for transfusion are screened for hepatitis B antigens.

Serological markers of hepatitis B infection

Laboratory diagnosis of hepatitis B is made by serological tests. The presence or absence of hepatitis antigens and antibodies can be detected and used to indicate the progress of infection and the emergence of a chronic carrier state (Table 9.3). People whose blood contain HBeAg are most infectious, but if antibody to this antigen (antiHBe) is detected, infectivity is usually low.

Healthcare workers infected with Hepatitis B

Healthcare workers are at risk of acquiring infection as a result of contact with blood and other body fluids, particularly following injury with contaminated needles or other sharp instruments. A third of healthcare workers exposed to hepatitis B by a needle-stick injury with HBeAg-positive blood acquire the infection (Royal College of Pathologists 1992). The risk of acquiring infection in clinical settings can be minimised by the routine use of blood and body fluid precautions which are described in Chapter 12. The

Table 9.3 Summary of Hepatitis B serology

Blood marker	Interpretation
HBsAg	Surface antigen, a polypeptide that makes up the viral envelope, is present in acute and chronic infections and in carriers
HBeAg	Derivative of the core antigen. Its presence indicates active viral replication and a high level of infectivity. It appears early in the course of infection and is usually eliminated by the production of anti-HBe
HBcAg	Viral nucleic acid or core antigen. It is found in the liver and is not readily detectable, but the corresponding antibody can be
Anti-HBs	Antibody formed against the surface antigen. The last antibody to be produced, its presence indicates that the infection has resolved and immunity has been established. It is measured after a course of Hepatitis B vaccine and indicates immunity as it protects against re-infection
Anti-HBe	Antibody formed against the HBe antigen, which appears during the first 3 weeks of infection. It usually indicates a low level of infectivity. If HBe antibodies are not produced, the virus is not eliminated, chronic carriage is established and the blood remains very infectious
Anti-HBc	Antibody formed against the core antigen. It appears early in the infection, initially as IgM and then as IgG. It persists in the blood indefinitely and is a useful marker of recovery from previous infection

Advisory Committee on Dangerous Pathogens (1995) has made recommendations on preventing exposure to blood-borne viruses in the workplace, with particular reference to health and safety legislation. More specific guidance on preventing the transmission of hepatitis B and blood-borne viruses in clinical settings is also available (Department of Health 1993, UK Health Departments 1998).

A healthcare worker who becomes a chronic carrier of the virus may also transmit infection to patients during invasive procedures, where there is a risk that a small injury to the healthcare worker can result in blood entering the tissues of the patient. Several outbreaks of infection among patients operated on by infected surgeons have been reported (Heptonstall 1991). These are usually associated with surgeons who are HBeAg-positive; however, transmission is still possible even if the healthcare worker is HBeAg-negative (Sundkvist et al 1998). Healthcare workers who are HBeAg-positive should not perform procedures where there is a risk that injury to the worker may cause the patient's open tissues to be exposed to the worker's blood. These include surgical, dental and obstetric procedures, where the hands may be in a confined anatomical space and in contact with sharp instruments, bones or teeth (Department of Health 1993).

Vaccination against Hepatitis B

Hepatitis B vaccine is genetically engineered and yeasts are used for its production. Vaccination is recommended for people whose occupation or lifestyle increases their risk of acquiring infection, babies born to mothers who are chronic carriers of the virus, and healthcare workers whose work brings them into direct contact with blood, body fluids or tissues. A full course of three injections over a 6 month period confers immunity in 90% of individuals, although a good immune response is less likely in those over the age of 40. Immunity should be confirmed by a blood test after the full course of vaccination has been given.

A specific hepatitis B immunoglobulin is also available and can be used to provide short-term, passive immunity to non-immune people exposed to infection. Healthcare workers who have a needle-stick injury should be assessed and managed by the Occupational Health Department to ensure that the risk of acquiring hepatitis B is minimised (UK Health Departments 1998).

Hepatitis D

This is a defective virus, which cannot replicate without hepatitis B virus. Co-infection with the two viruses often results in a serious and chronic illness. Hepatitis D virus is found wherever hepatitis B is endemic, but it is most prevalent in South America, parts of Russia and the Mediterranean. Hepatitis D is transmitted in the same way as hepatitis B and, since it is dependent on the latter, vaccination and infection control precautions against hepatitis B will also protect against hepatitis D.

Hepatitis C

This RNA virus has never been isolated but its antigens have been identified and serological tests are now available. It has been known for many years that a blood-borne virus that was neither hepatitis A nor B caused viral hepatitis following blood transfusion. In the USA, 90% of transfusion-associated hepatitis is now recognised to be caused by hepatitis C virus (Choo et al 1990), although the introduction of routine testing of donated blood means that this is now an unlikely route of transmission. Like hepatitis B, the virus can be transmitted by contaminated needles, but it is less likely to be acquired through sexual contact or transmitted from mother to baby. The prevalence of infection in developed countries, indicated by the presence of hepatitis C antibodies in the blood, is between 1% and 2% of the population, but it is higher in parts of Africa and eastern Europe, and in Egypt 15% of the population have the antibody.

Many cases of acute infection are asymptomatic and only a minority develop jaundice. However chronic infection develops in about 85% of those infected and as many as 20% develop cirrhosis 10–20 years after infection. Liver failure due to hepatitis C infection is a major reason for liver transplantation and morbidity related to the infection is predicted to increase (Di Bisceglie 1998).

In the UK blood transfusions have been tested for antibodies to hepatitis C since 1991 and the incidence of infection is generally low, with less than 1 in 1000 donors found to carry the virus (Neal et al 1997), However, some intravenous-drug-using populations have a high incidence of infection and the long-term disease related to chronic hepatitis is likely to present considerable health-care problems (Goldberg et al 1998). There is no vaccine or specific immunoglobulin available. The infection control precautions recommended for hepatitis B apply to hepatitis C also (UK Health Departments 1998).

RETROVIRUSES

These viruses have an RNA genome but use an enzyme called reverse transcriptase to make a corresponding strand of DNA, which is then integrated into the chromosome of the host cell. Retroviruses cause sarcomas and leukaemia in many animals. There are four retroviruses that infect humans: two human T-cell lymphotrophic viruses (HTLV-1 and -2) and two human immunodeficiency viruses (HIV-1 and -2). Retroviruses have envelopes, and are transmitted by sexual contact or inoculation of blood and body fluids through the skin. They infect cells that have CD4 receptors on their surface, notably the T4 lymphocytes of the immune system.

Human T-cell lymphotrophic virus (HTLV)

HTLV-1 infects T4 lymphocytes, inducing them to proliferate and cause leukaemia and lymphomas. It can also induce a myelopathy similar to multiple sclerosis. The infection is endemic in Japan, the Caribbean, central Africa and South America. HTLV-2 is associated with hairy cell leukaemia.

Human immunodeficiency virus (HIV)

HIV causes acquired immune deficiency syndrome (AIDS). Its primary target is the T4 lymphocytes, which have an important role in the co-ordination of the cellular immune system (p. 62). They are gradually depleted during the course of the disease, with a subsequent impairment of the immune response (Greene 1993).

Individuals with AIDS are therefore susceptible to infection by a range of microorganisms, which can invade human cells but which are normally kept in check by T lymphocytes. These include protozoa (e.g. Cryptosporidium and *Pneumocystis carinii*), fungi (e.g. Cryptococcus), viruses (e.g. Cytomegalovirus and herpes simplex) and intracellular bacterial infections (e.g. with mycobacteria). These microorganisms are usually unable to establish infection or cause only mild symptoms in immunocompetent people, but they cause serious, disseminated infection in those whose immune response has been impaired by HIV.

HIV is acquired through sexual contact, inoculation of blood or body fluids through the skin by contaminated needles or other sharp items, and exposure of mucous membranes. It is also transmitted transplacentally from mother to baby. The virus is present in blood, semen, vaginal secretions, cerebrospinal fluid, amniotic fluid and synovial fluid. It is also probably transmitted in breast milk (Mok 1993). The amount of virus found in saliva is not sufficient to enable transmission (Centers for Disease Control 1988).

HIV infection is diagnosed by serological tests that detect antibodies to the virus, although detection of viral antigens (p. 141) and nucleic acid sequences is now also possible. Antibodies to HIV are detectable in the bloodstream 1–3 months after infection, but the virus remains latent within T cells and up to 10 years can elapse before symptoms of infection develop. The trigger that eventually switches on replication of the virus is unknown, but may be related to acquisition of other infections, to drugs or environmental factors. Once HIV infection has progressed to AIDS the prognosis is poor and survival is unlikely. Early treatment with antiviral drugs is not able to cure the infection but appears to prolong survival. If given to pregnant women treatment may reduce the risk of transplacental transmission to the fetus (Rutter 1998).

HIV infection has now spread throughout the world, with an estimated 30 million people infected. All countries have been affected, but about 63% of infected people live in sub-Saharan Africa, where HIV is endemic in some countries (World Health Organization, 1997).

HIV-2 is very similar to HIV-1 but has only been identified in people from west Africa.

In the UK, approximately 2000 new cases of AIDS are reported each year. The prevalence of HIV is estimated to be at 0.09% of those aged between 15 and 49 but varies between regions (Communicable Disease Report, 1998c). It is highest in London and the south-east, with three-quarters of patients with AIDS living in the Thames regions. Approximately 60% of infections have been acquired through homosexual partners, 30% through heterosexual partners and 10% from IV drug use. Transmission between homosexual men appeared to decline in the 1980s, but recently the number of cases has been increasing and the concurrent increase in incidence of other sexually transmitted diseases in this group suggests that the trend towards safer sexual practice has been reversed. Nearly 80% of people infected with HIV heterosexually acquired the infection abroad, and most of the remainder had been exposed to infection through sexual contact with partners at high risk of HIV infection (Communicable Disease Review 1997). The transmission of HIV among intravenous drug users has declined since the mid-1980s, probably as a result of successful needle exchange programmes (Madden et al 1997).

Healthcare workers are at risk of acquiring infection through exposure to blood and body fluids, particularly following needlestick injury. Worldwide, at least 95 healthcare workers have acquired the virus through occupational exposure, although the risk is much lower than Hepatitis B (Communicable Disease Report 1998d, Heptonstall et al 1993). Currently there is no vaccine against the virus. Treatment with zidovudine, lamivudine and indinavir is recommended for healthcare workers who have been exposed to blood known or strongly suspected to be infected with HIV, but must be given soon after exposure and its protective effects are uncertain (UK Health Departments 1997). Risk exposures include needlestick injuries and contamination of broken skin, eyes or mouth with blood or body fluids. All employers should have a written policy on the management of exposure to bloodborne viruses and should have a designated doctor (usually in Occupational Health) able to assess the risk of exposure and be responsible for postexposure prophylaxis and follow-up (UK Health Departments 1998).

Preventing the transmission of HIV depends on education to discourage high-risk behaviour such as unprotected sexual contact and sharing used needles to inject drugs. In clinical settings, the routine use of blood and body fluid precautions is recommended to prevent transmission; these are discussed in Chapter 12. The Advisory Committee on Dangerous Pathogens (1995) has made recommendations on preventing transmission in the workplace, with particular reference to health and safety legislation, and additional guidance on preventing transmission in clinical settings has been provided by the UK Health Departments (1998).

The risk of transmission from healthcare workers infected with HIV to patients in most healthcare settings is remote. Healthcare workers infected with HIV must seek appropriate medical and occupational health advice and should not perform exposure-prone procedures (where there is a risk that injury to the worker results in blood entering the open tissues of the patient; NHS Management Executive, 1994).

HERPES VIRUSES

These are enveloped DNA viruses characterised by their ability to cause latent infections that may subsequently become reactivated. The group includes the herpes simplex viruses (1 and 2), varicella-zoster virus (chickenpox and shingles), cytomegalovirus, Epstein–Barr virus and human herpes virus 6.

Herpes simplex virus

There are two types of herpes simplex virus. Although each type is usually associated with specific sites in the body, type 1 affecting the lips, nose and oropharynx (less often the skin or eye) and type 2 the genital tract, infections of the genital tract may be caused by either type.

Type 1 herpes virus (HSV-1) is commonly acquired in childhood and is often asymptomatic, but may present with vesicles then ulcers on the gums and oral mucosa. The primary infection, usually acquired in childhood, is sometimes associated with a febrile illness, stomatitis and meningoencephalitis. Meningoencephalitis is a serious infection with a high mortality for which the only effective treatment is the early use of acyclovir. HSV-1 can also cause herpetic whitlow, an infection of the finger in healthcare workers following accidental inoculation from herpes lesions.

After the primary infection the virus persists in a latent state in local nerve cells, periodically re-emerging to cause a cluster of vesicles at the margin of the lip called cold sores, often triggered by other infections, physical stimuli, such as sun, or menstrual periods. Meningoencephalitis sometimes occurs in association with a reactivation, and more severe disease may occur in those who are immunosuppressed. Herpes simplex infection of the eye can result in ulceration and scarring of the cornea, which may seriously impair vision; recurrent infections are common. Individuals with eczema are prone to skin infection with HSV called eczema herpeticum, which can be fatal.

Herpes virus type 2 (HSV-2) mainly occurs in adults and is usually transmitted by sexual contact. It causes lesions on the genital tract, including the cervix, vulva, glans penis, prepuce, perineal skin, anus, buttocks and mouth. The primary infection resolves in approximately 1 week and the virus remains in nerves supplying the area. Recurrent lesions occur when the virus is reactivated by hormone fluctuations, changes in the immune system or infection. The infection cannot be cured but symptoms can be alleviated by acyclovir. Babies born to mothers with active genital herpes are at risk of disseminated infection and encephalitis. The virus can also be transmitted congenitally if the mother acquires a primary infection while pregnant. Infection in neonates has a high mortality, although early treatment with acyclovir is effective in many cases. Particular care must be taken to avoid transmission from mothers with active lesions or affected babies. Staff should wear aprons and gloves for contact with vaginal discharges and the mother should be reminded to wash her hands carefully before handling her baby (Valenti 1998).

Transmission of HSV occurs by direct contact with the lesions, although the virus can survive for many hours on items such as cutlery or towels. Gloves should be worn for all direct contact with lesions and hands should be washed after their removal (see routine blood and body fluid precautions, Chapter 12). Staff with active herpes simplex lesions should not care for immunocompromised patients or newborn babies, and those with herpetic whitlows should not have any patient contact.

The characteristic lesions do not usually require confirmation of the diagnosis by laboratory tests; however the virus can be detected in vesicle fluid by electron microscopy and tissue culture. In suspected meningoencephalitis, tests to detect herpes simplex DNA or antibodies in cerebrospinal fluid or serum can be useful in establishing an early diagnosis.

Varicella-zoster virus (VZV)

Varicella is the term used to describe chickenpox, the primary infection caused by this virus. It spreads by inhalation of respiratory droplets or by direct contact with lesions and respiratory secretions, is common among children and, since it is highly infectious, 90% of adults in the UK are immune (Department of Health 1996). It causes a mild fever and vesicular rash, which usually starts on the face and trunk, followed, often sparsely, by the limbs. Diagnosis can be confirmed by identifying the virus in vesicle fluid by electron microscopy or tissue culture (Figure 9.3). Primary infection

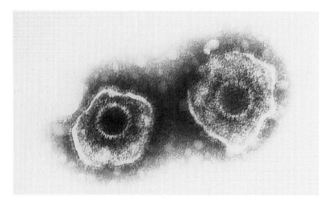

Figure 9.3 Two Herpesvirus particles from a vesicle of a patient with chickenpox (electron micrograph).

in adults can be serious and may be complicated by severe pneumonia. Children or adults with impaired immunity are also vulnerable to disseminated infection, which is frequently fatal. If chickenpox is acquired during the first 3 months of pregnancy it may cause fetal abnormalities and a mother who acquires the infection a few days before delivery may transmit the infection to the newborn infant. In this situation, specific immunoglobulin should be given to the baby to prevent severe disease developing (Craddock-Watson 1990).

The incidence of infection varies throughout the year, with a peak occurring between March and May. The incubation period is 2–3 weeks and the infectious period begins a few days before the rash appears and continues for a further 5 days. Infection confers lifelong immunity and secondary infections are rare.

Controlling the spread of chickenpox in a hospital setting can present considerable problems, particularly where immunocompromised patients may be at risk of acquiring the infection (Stover & Bratcher 1998). Patients with chickenpox should be nursed in single rooms and gloves and aprons should be worn for contact with lesions or respiratory secretions. Since the risk of transmission is high, only those known to be immune should care for affected patients. If they cannot give a history of having had chickenpox their immune status can be established by serological tests. This is necessary when staff are in contact with immunocompromised patients, who are particularly vulnerable to serious disease should they acquire the infection.

Herpes zoster, or shingles, is the infection caused by reactivation of varicella-zoster virus. Following chickenpox infection, the virus remains latent in sensory nerve ganglia. Reactivation causes the virus to travel along the nerves and erupt in the skin, causing vesicles, severe pain in the affected area, fever and malaise. The site of the lesions depends on the root nerve responsible but they commonly occur on the torso or face. The effects may be severe in the immunocompromised and prolonged neuralgia may continue after the lesions have healed, especially in the elderly. VZV may be transmitted from zoster lesions to non-immune individuals, in whom it causes the primary infection, chickenpox. Shingles is not activated through exposure to chickenpox, since it only occurs as a reactivation of the primary infection.

Cytomegalovirus (CMV)

This is a very common infection, which in most cases is asymptomatic but can cause an infectious-mononucleosis-like illness. 80% of the population have had the infection by the time they reach adulthood (Tookey & Peckham 1991). Following the primary infection, the virus remains latent in the body and can cause recurrent infections. During an acute infection CMV is excreted in urine, saliva, breast milk and vaginal secretions, and excretions of the virus may persist periodically for many years. Natural transmission is by saliva or sexual contact; transfused blood and organ transplant may also transmit CMV.

The most severe form of the disease occurs in neonates who acquire the infection as a result of primary or reactivated maternal infection, from cervical secretions during delivery or postnatally from breast milk. It causes a severe generalised infection involving the central nervous system and liver; intrauterine death may occur and the fatality rate is high. Those who survive often have mental retardation, motor disabilities, hearing loss and chronic liver disease. In later life, serious generalised disease may also occur in individuals who are immunodeficient.

Epstein–Barr virus (EBV)

This virus is responsible for most cases of infectious mononucleosis (glandular fever). It infects B lymphocytes, and the viral antigens that appear on the surface of affected B lymphocytes induce the production of characteristic, abnormal, mononuclear T lymphocytes. The initial site of infection is the salivary glands and virus is shed in saliva throughout the course of the infection. Approximately 20% of those infected retain EBV in their salivary glands and continue to excrete the virus long after the infection has resolved. The virus is transmitted by contact with saliva, particularly by kissing, and occurs most commonly among young adults. The main symptoms are fever, sore throat and lymphadenopathy. Some cases develop an enlarged spleen and mild hepatitis; however, most infections are asymptomatic.

The incubation period is between 4 and 6 weeks and, although it resolves eventually, the symptoms can persist for long periods. Serological tests to detect antibodies to the virus are used to confirm the diagnosis.

In Africa and Papua New Guinea, Epstein–Barr virus is associated with a tumour of B lymphocytes called Burkitt's lymphoma. There is evidence that, in these countries, malaria is an important co-factor in its development, the primary infection occurring early in life and the lymphoma emerging 2–12 years later. The same lymphoma sometimes occurs in immunosuppressed people, e.g. those with AIDS. More recently, evidence has been emerging that a reactivation of EBV is responsible for Hodgkin's disease, a tumour of the lymphatic system (Benenson 1995). Nasopharyngeal carcinoma has also been associated with EBV and is prevalent in China, North Africa and among Inuits, but not elsewhere.

Human herpes virus 6

This virus causes an acute febrile illness called roseola infantum in young children. Most infections are mild, with a high fever that lasts for 3–4 days and is followed by a rash.

POX VIRUSES

These are large enveloped viruses with a brick-like shape and complex structure. The viruses in this group are responsible for smallpox (variola), cowpox, orf and molluscum contagiosum.

Smallpox (Variola virus)

This virus was responsible for the deaths of millions of people in previous centuries. The World Health Organization began a world-wide eradication programme that by 1980 had resulted in the eradication of the disease. The virus is now stored only in two laboratories in the world, one in Atlanta, Georgia, USA and one in Moscow. Cowpox virus (Vaccinia virus) resembles smallpox, but causes a mild disease in cattle that can be transmitted to humans. Edward Jenner used cowpox virus to develop the first vaccine against smallpox infection.

Vaccinia virus continued to be used to immunise against small-pox. Originally it was either pure smallpox or cowpox virus but, following passage through animals, it has been altered so that when used for vaccination it usually produces only a few local pox lesions, while still conferring immunity to smallpox.

Orf

This is a pustular mouth infection of sheep and goats, which can be transmitted to farmers, shepherds and veterinarians. Lesions developing into ulcers appear on the hands, arms and face and enlarge into blisters before crusting over. They take several weeks to heal. A vaccine is available to prevent the infection in sheep.

Molluscum contagiosum

This is a mild, localised infection of the epidermal skin cells, which causes small raised nodules to develop. Transmission occurs by direct contact, including sexual contact. (Baxby 1990).

PAPOVAVIRUSES

These are DNA viruses (Figure 9.4). They include the human papilloma viruses (HPV) and wart viruses. There are many different types of HPV, most of which cause benign genital warts. Genital warts are among the most common sexually transmitted diseases treated in STD clinics in England and Wales (Wright 1998). Types 16, 18, 31 and 33 are strongly associated with cervical cancer; types 6 and 11, which account for about 95% of genital warts, are rarely associated with cancers but are associated with low-grade cervical invasive neoplasm (Etherington & Shafi 1996).

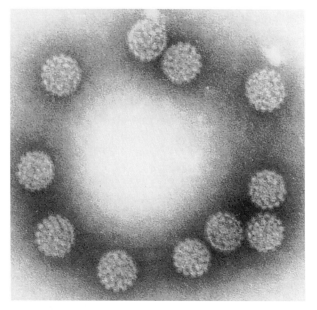

Figure 9.4 Papovavirus from a plantar wart (electron micrograph).

RHABDOVIRUS

This RNA virus is shaped like a bullet and is enveloped. It causes a form of viral encephalitis called rabies, which has an insidious onset with paraesthesia around the site of the wound, fever and headache followed by severe throat spasms on swallowing (hence a fear of drinking water), delirium, convulsion and death from respiratory paralysis. From the point at which the virus enters the body, it travels along the nerves to the brain. The incubation period ranges from a few days to several months depending on how far the virus must travel to reach the brain. Once established, the infection inevitably results in death. The virus is able to infect all mammals and is transmitted by being bitten or by contact of open skin sites with saliva of affected animals.

Although many thousands of people worldwide die of rabies each year, the infection is uncommon in developed countries. The disease has been virtually eradicated in many western European countries following an immunisation programme among foxes, the major reservoir of the infection.

The risk of acquiring rabies after being bitten, licked or scratched by dogs or other animals can be reduced by washing the wound as soon as possible with soap and running water for several minutes. Local doctors will know if rabies is likely in that area; in the case of patients seeking advice on their return to the UK, specialist advice must be sought. Postexposure prophylaxis with rabies vaccine and specific immunoglobulin will depend on the degree of risk.

TOGAVIRUSES

This is a large group of over 300 RNA viruses, most of which are transmitted by arthropods. The most important are the flaviviruses and bunyaviruses, which cause a variety of diseases in tropical and subtropical regions.

Flaviviruses

Diseases caused by these viruses include dengue and yellow fever. Dengue is a febrile illness with joint and muscle pain and gastrointestinal bleeding. It is transmitted by mosquitoes and is very common in Asia, Africa and Central and South America. As there are several serotypes of the virus, exposure confers immunity, but only to the particular type: subsequent infection with other types is possible.

Yellow fever ranges from non-specific symptoms to an acute illness with fever, vomiting and prostration. 20–50% develop hepatic and renal damage, leading to jaundice and death (Benenson 1995). The virus is transmitted by mosquitoes and is found in South America and Africa. Infection is followed by lifelong immunity. Yellow fever vaccine is available and in urban areas control of mosquito populations can prevent transmission of the disease.

Bunyaviruses

The main human pathogens in this group are sandfly fever virus and hantavirus. Sandfly fever is a mild febrile illness that occurs in the Mediterranean, Africa, India and China. It is transmitted by sandflies. Hantaviruses cause a haemorrhagic fever, which in Europe is usually mild but in Japan, Korea and parts of Russia can be very severe, with kidney failure, hypotension and shock.

Another form of the virus has been identified as causing respiratory distress syndrome, which was first recognised in 1993 when an epidemic occurred in south-west America. Hantaviruses are carried by rodents and transmitted by direct contact with the animals or by inhalation of dust containing their excreta.

HAEMORRHAGIC FEVERS

Lassa fever virus

This arenavirus causes an acute haemorrhagic disease, which has a mortality rate of about 25%. The infection is characterised by the gradual onset of malaise, fever, sore throat, vomiting, diarrhoea, chest and abdominal pain, with an intermittent spiking fever. Severe cases result in hypotension, haemorrhage, encephalopathy and shock. Plasma from previously infected patients has been used as treatment, as has the antiviral agent ribovirin. Outbreaks and sporadic cases occur in west Africa following direct contact with the excreta of a particular species of rat that carries the virus. Transmission from person to person may occur through direct contact with the blood, pharyngeal secretions or urine of an infected person.

Current advice from the Department of Health is that all acute hospitals should have policies on the safe management of patients with pyrexia of unknown origin. Where there is a strong suspicion of a viral haemorrhagic fever (VHF) the patients should be transferred to a high-security isolation unit. Where there is a slight or moderate suspicion of a VHF, standard blood and body fluid precautions are sufficient until a diagnosis has been confirmed; in 95% of cases, malaria will be found to be responsible for the symptoms (Advisory Committee on Dangerous Pathogens 1997).

Marburg and Ebola viruses

These RNA viruses have caused outbreaks of viral haemorrhagic fever, with a high rate of mortality. Infection is probably transmitted from monkeys (Jahrling et al 1990). The first outbreak of Marburg virus occurred in 1967, when seven German laboratory workers died after handling tissue from Ugandan monkeys. Person-to-person transmission can occur via infected blood, and special isolation facilities are recommended for the care of affected patients (see Lassa fever; Advisory Committee on Dangerous Pathogens 1997).

VIRUS-LIKE AGENTS: PRIONS

Prions are abnormal proteins that do not have their own nucleic acids; instead they appear to replicate by using the genome of their host. They are highly resistant to inactivation by heat and chemicals, withstanding both standard autoclaving and most chemical disinfectants.

Prion proteins have been found in association with a number of rare animal and human diseases that have long incubation periods and cause progressive, and ultimately fatal, damage to the nervous system. Creutzfeldt–Jakob disease (CJD) is a spongiform encephalopathy that causes softening and destruction of brain tissue, leading to presenile dementia. It appears to be related to a similar encephalopathy in sheep called scrapie and to bovine spongiform encephalopathy (BSE) in cattle. Kuru is another prion disease of humans reported only in cannibalistic tribes in New Guinea.

The route of transmission of prions has not been clearly established. Some cases are acquired genetically, and iatrogenic transmission on surgical instruments used in neurosurgical procedures and in preparations of human growth hormone derived from pituitary glands and corneal implants has been reported (Brown et al 1992). The epidemic of BSE in cattle appears to be related to the consumption of bone-meal-derived animal carcasses, including other cattle, and associated with a change in processing practices, which meant that meal was no longer treated with organic solvents and heated to high temperatures. The processes may have reduced the amount of prion present (Haywood 1997).

The incidence of CJD in the UK has increased, but remains very low at around 50 deaths annually. The largest increase has occurred in people over 70 years of age and probably reflects improved diagnosis of the disease. A small number of people under 30 have developed a variant form of CJD that are likely to be linked to exposure to BSE, but a link has yet to be proved (Cousens et al 1997).

The main risk of transmission of CJD in clinical settings is through contact with tissues from the brain, spinal cord or eye. Body excretions and secretions have not been implicated in the transmission of infection and the use of routine infection control procedures (Chapter 12) is recommended for most aspects of care of patients known or suspected to be infected with CJD. Surgical procedures involving contact with brain, spinal cord or eye tissues should be carried out with the minimum number of staff present, using liquid repellent gowns, gloves, masks and visors. Instruments used during these procedures must be destroyed by incineration after use. Instruments used in other surgical or clinical procedures and exposed to blood or other tissues can be re-used but must receive high-level decontamination processes, either sodium hypochlorite at a concentration of 20 000 ppm for 1 hour or sterilisation in a porous-load autoclave at 134–138°C for 18 minutes (Advisory Committee on Dangerous Pathogens 1998).

REFERENCES

Advisory Committee on Dangerous Pathogens (1995) *Protection Against Blood-borne Infections in the Workplace: HIV and Hepatitis.* HMSO, London.

Advisory Committee on Dangerous Pathogens (1997) Management and control of viral haemorrhagic fevers. *PL(97)1.* Stationery Office, London.

Advisory Committee on Dangerous Pathogens (1998) Transmissible spongiform encephalopathy agents; safe working and the prevention of infection. *PL/CO(98)2.* Stationery Office, London.

Ansari, S.A. Springthorpe, S. Sattar, S.A. *et al.* (1991) Potential role of hands in the spread of viral infections; studies with human parainfluenza virus 3 and rhinovirus 14. *J. Clin. Microbiol.,* **29**, 2115–2119.

Baxby, D. (1990) Poxviruses. In: *Principles and Practice of Clinical Virology* (eds Zuckerman, A.J. *et al.*), 2nd edn. John Wiley, Chichester.

Benenson, A.S. (1995) *Control of Communicable Disease in Man,* 16th edn. American Public Health Association, Washington, DC.

Brown, P., Preece, M.A. and Will, R.G. (1992) 'Friendly fire' in medicines: hormones, homografts and Creutzfeldt–Jakob disease. *Lancet,* **340**, 24–27.

Cancio-Bello, T.P., de Medina, M., Shorey, J. *et al.* (1982) An institutional outbreak of hepatitis B related to a human biting carrier. *J. Infect. Dis.,* **146**(5), 652–656.

Centers for Disease Control (1988) Update: universal precautions for prevention of HIV transmission in health care settings. *MMWR,* **36**(2S), 3S–18S.

Chadwick, P.R. and McCann, R. (1994) Transmission of a small round structured virus by vomiting during a hospital outbreak of gastro-enteritis. *J. Hosp. Infect.,* **26**, 251–259.

Choo, Q.L., Weiner, A.J., Overby, L.R. *et al.* (1990) Hepatitis C virus: the major causative agent of viral non-A non-B hepatitis. *Br. Med. Bull.,* **46**(2), 423–441.

Collee, J.G. (1990) Foodborne illness: bovine spongiform encephalopathy. *Lancet,* **336**, 1300–1303.

Committee on Infectious Diseases (1982) Special report: Aspirin and Reye's syndrome. *Paediatrics* **69**, 810.

Communicable Disease Review (1997) The epidemiology of HIV infection and AIDS. *Commun. Dis. Rev.,* **7**(9), 118–136.

Communicable Disease Report (1998a) An outbreak of influenza in four nursing homes in Sheffield. *Commun. Dis. Rep.,* **8**(16), 139.

Communicable Disease Report (1998b) MMR vaccine is not linked to Crohn's disease or autism. *Commun. Dis. Rep.,* **8**(13), 113.

Communicable Disease Report (1998c) The global HIV epidemic. *Commun. Dis. Rep.,* **8**(26), 227.

Communicable Disease Report (1998d) Occupational transmission of HIV infection. *Commun. Dis. Rep.*, **8**(22), 193.

Cousens, S.N., Zeidler, M., Esmonde, T.F. *et al.* (1997) Sporadic Creuzfeldt–Jakob disease in the United Kingdom: analysis of epidemiological surveillance data for 1970–96. *Br. Med. J.*, **315**, 389–395.

Craddock-Watson, J.E. (1990) Varicella-zoster virus infection during pregnancy. In: *Current Topics in Clinical Virology*, (ed. Morgan-Capner, P.) Public Health Laboratory Service, London, pp. 1–28.

Department of Health (1993) *Protecting Healthcare Workers and Patients from Hepatitis B. Recommendations of the Advisory Group on Hepatitis.* HMSO, London.

Department of Health (Welsh Office, Scottish Office Department of Health, DHSS (Northern Ireland)) (1996) *Immunisation against Infectious Disease.* HMSO, London.

Di Bisceglie, A.M. (1998) Hepatitis C. *Lancet*, **351**, 351–355.

Dowsett, E.G. (1988) Human enteroviral infections. *J. Hosp. Infect.*, **11**, 103–115.

Etherington, I. and Shafi, M. (1996) Human papilloma viruses and cervical screening. *Genitour. Med.*, **72**(3), 153–154.

Goldberg, D., Cameron, S. and McMenamin, J. (1998) Hepatitis C virus antibody prevalence among injecting drug users in Glasgow has fallen but remains high. *Commun. Dis. Public Health*, **1**(2), 95–97.

Green, J., Wright, P.A., Gallimore, C.I. *et al* (1998) The role of environmental contamination with small round structured viruses in a hospital outbreak investigated by reverse – transcriptase polymerase chain reaction assay. *J. Hosp. Inf.* **39**(1), 39–46.

Greene, W.C. (1993) AIDS and the immune system. *Sci. Am.*, **Sept.**, 20–110.

Haywood, A.M. (1997) Transmissible spongiform encephalopathies. *New Engl. J. Med.*, **337**, 1821–1828.

Heptonstall, J. (1991) Outbreaks of hepatitis B virus infection associated with infected surgical staff. *Commun. Dis. Rev.*, **1**, R81–R85.

Heptonstall, J., Gill, O.N., Porter, K. *et al.* (1993) Health care workers and HIV: surveillance of occupationally acquired infections in the United Kingdom. *Commun. Dis. Rev.*, **3**(11), 147–153.

Jahrling, P.B., Geisbert, T., Dalgard, D. *et al* (1990) Preliminary report: isolation of Ebola virus from monkeys imported to USA. *Lancet*, **335**, 502–505.

Luthi, T.M., Wall, P.G., Evans, H.S. *et al.* (1996) Outbreaks of foodborne viral gastro-enteritis in England and Wales: 1992 to 1994. *Commun. Dis. Rev.*, **6**(10), R131–R135.

Madden, P.B., Lamagni, T., Hope, V. *et al.* (1997) The HIV epidemic in injecting drug users. *Commun. Dis. Rev.*, **7**(9), R128–R130.

Madge, P., Payton, J.Y., McColl, J.H. *et al.* (1992) Prospective controlled study of four infection control procedures to prevent nosocomial infection with respiratory syncytial virus. *Lancet*, **340**, 1079–1083.

Mitchell, E., O'Mahony, M., McKeith, I. *et al.* (1989) An outbreak of viral gastro-enteritis in a psychiatric hospital. *J. Hosp. Infect.*, **14**(1), 1–8.

Mok, J. (1993) Breast milk and HIV-1 transmission. *Lancet*, **341**, 930–931.

Neal, K.R., Dornan, J. and Irving, W.L. (1997) Prevalence of hepatitis C antibodies among health care workers of two teaching hospitals. Who is at risk? *Br. Med. J.*, **314**, 179–180.

NHS Management Executive (1994) AIDS-HIV infected health care workers: guidance on the management of infected health care workers. *HSG(94)16.* HMSO. London.

O'Mahony, M.C., Gooch, C.D., Smyth, D.A. *et al.* (1983) Epidemic hepatitis A from cockles. *Lancet*, **i**, 518–520.

Patterson, W.J., Painter, M.J. (1999) Bovine spongiform encephalopathy and new variant Creutzfeldt-Jakob disease: an overview. *Commun. Dis. Public Health*, **2**: 5–13.

Piedra, P.A., Kasal, J.A., Norton, J.H. *et al.* (1992) Description of an adenovirus type 8 outbreak in hospitalised neonates born prematurely. *Paediatr. Infect. Dis. J.*, **11**(8), 460–465.

Reid, T.M.S. and Robinson, H.G. (1987) Frozen raspberries and hepatitis A. *Epidemiol. Infect.*, **98**, 109–112.

Reilly, H. (1990) High risk groups are not getting their flu vaccine. *Gen. Practit.*, **28 Sept.**, 26.

Royal College of Pathologists (1992) *HIV Infection: Hazards of Transmission to Patients and Health Care Workers During Invasive Procedures. Report of a Working Party.* Royal College of Pathologists, London.

Rutter, T. (1998) Short course of zidovudine cuts transmission of HIV. *Br. Med. J.*, **316**, 645.

Stover, B.H. and Bratcher, D.F. (1998) Varicella-zoster virus: infection, control and prevention. *Am. J. Infect. Control.*, **26**, 369–384.

Straube, R.C., Thompson, M.A., Van Dyke, R.B. *et al.* (1983) Adenovirus type 7b in a children's hospital. *J. Infect. Dis.*, **147**(5), 814–819.

Sundkvist, T., Hamilton, G.R., Rimmer, D. *et al.* (1998) Fatal outcome of transmission of hepatitis B from an e antigen negative surgeon. *Commun. Dis. Public Health*, **1**(1), 48–50.

Tookey, P. and Peckham, C.S. (1991) Does cytomegalovirus present an occupational risk? *Arch. Dis. Childh.*, **66**, 1009–1010.

UK Health Departments (1997) Guidelines on post-exposure prophylaxis for health care workers occupationally exposed to HIV. *PL/CO(97)1.* Stationery Office, London.

UK Health Departments (1998) Guidance for clinical health care workers: protections against infection with blood-borne viruses. Recommendation of the Expert Advisory Group on AIDS and the Advisory Group on Hepatitis. Stationery Office, London.

Valenti, W.M. (1998) Selected viruses of nosocomial importance. In: *Hospital Infections*, 4th edn. (eds Bennett, J.V. and Brachman, P.S.). Little, Brown & Co., Boston, MA.

World Health Organization (1997) *The World Health Report 1997.* WHO, Geneva.

Wright, T. (1998) Genital warts: their etiology and treatment. *Nurs. Times*, **94**(7), 52–54.

Zuckerman, A.J. (1990) Hepatitis E virus. *Br. Med. J.*, **300**, 1475–1476.

FURTHER READING

Communicable Disease Review (1997) The epidemiology of HIV infection and AIDS. *Commun. Dis. Rev.*, **7**(9), R118–R136.

Dolan, M. and Hughes, N. (1997) Hepatitis C: a bloody business. *Nurs. Times*, **93**(45), 71–74.

Duerdin, B.I., Reid, T.M.S. and Jewsbury, J.M. (1993) *Microbial and Parasitic Infections.* Edward Arnold, London.

Fagan, E.A. (1992) Hepatitis A to G and beyond. *Br. J. Hosp. Med.*, **47**(2), 127–131.

Teo, C.G. (1992) The virology and serology of hepatitis: an overview. *Commun. Dis. Rev.*, **2**(10), R109–113.

10

A guide to fungi, protozoa, helminths and ectoparasites

FUNGI

Fungal infections are an increasingly common cause of serious hospital-acquired infection, particularly in association with intensive therapy, multiple courses of antibiotics and intravascular catheters (Flanagan & Barnes 1998). Systemic fungal infections in leukaemic patients are now associated with almost as many deaths as bacterial infections (Bodey 1988). Broad-spectrum or combinations of antibiotics given to prevent or treat bacterial infections eradicate the normal bacterial population, thus enabling fungi, which are unaffected by the commonly used antibiotics, to establish themselves and cause opportunistic infections. However, a proportion of infections are caused by contaminated equipment or transmitted on the hands of staff (Strasbaugh et al 1994).

Infections caused by fungi, called *mycoses*, can be superficial, affecting body surfaces (e.g. skin, hair, nails), or deep, invading tissues and causing systemic infections in people with damaged immune responses. The main forms of fungal infection that affect humans are summarised in Table 10.1.

Aspergillus

This genus of saprophytic moulds is widely distributed in the environment. In immunocompetent individuals they are a rare cause of infection but are occasionally associated with chronic superficial ear infections and can infect burns and other wounds. Some people who regularly inhale dust, e.g. farm workers, can develop an allergy to the fungus.

Systemic infection, usually caused by *Aspergillus fumigatus*, can occur in the severely immunocompromised and the incidence of

Table 10.1   Summary of human mycoses

Fungus	Disease	Site of infection
Superficial mycoses		
Candida	Thrush	Mucous membranes of the mouth and vagina, skin flexures
	Peritonitis	Following bowel surgery or CAPD
	Enteritis	Following treatment with broad-spectrum antibiotics
Dermatophytes	Ringworm (scalp, body, nails), athelete's foot	Keratinised layers of skin, hair and nails
Deep mycoses in the immunocompromised		
Aspergillus	Invasive aspergillosis	Lung and other tissues
	Aspergilloma	Grows in body cavity
Cryptococcus	Cryptococcosis (chronic meningitis)	Begins as a local infection but develops into a systemic infection
Pneumocystis carinii	Pneumonia	Lung
Candida	Systemic candidiasis	Can establish infection, via the bloodstream, in kidneys or brain, or cause endocarditis

these infections has increased as more aggressive chemotherapy treatments and organ transplant programmes are introduced (Manuel & Kibbler 1998). Aspergillosis is a serious infection, which involves the lung and other tissues and is frequently fatal.

Patients most at risk of invasive aspergillosis are those on long-term immunosuppressive therapy, who have had an organ or bone-marrow transplant or who have AIDS. Infections are commonly acquired endogenously but outbreaks have been reported, particularly in association with high numbers of airborne aspergillus spores in the air such as may occur during building construction (Humphries et al 1991). Water sources (e.g. ice-machines, nebulisers), dressing materials, contaminated kitchen surfaces and food (e.g. tea, coffee, pepper, cereals, powdered milk) have also been associated with outbreaks (Loudon et al 1996, Manuel & Kibbler 1998). The use of air filtration to protect vulnerable, immunocompromised patients has been recommended and regular cleaning of surfaces to remove dust is also an important control measure (Barnes & Rogers 1989, Manuel & Kibbler 1998).

Candida

85% of all fungal infections in the critically ill are caused by candida spp. and most of these are caused by the species *Candida albicans* (Beck-Sague & Jarvis 1993, Lipman & Saadia 1997). This yeast commonly colonises mucous membranes in the respiratory, gastrointestinal and female genital tract. Under certain circumstances it proliferates and causes superficial infections at these sites, e.g. thrush of the mouth or vagina, nappy rash in infants and skin infection of warm moist areas such as the groins, axillae and breasts. Chronic infection of the nail beds can occur in people whose hands are regularly in water. Predisposing factors to infection include diabetes mellitus, general debility, immunosuppression, indwelling urinary or intravenous catheters, antibiotics that disrupt the normal flora and steroid therapy. In women, oral contraception and pregnancy are also predisposing factors for vaginal thrush (Greer 1998).

People who are immunosuppressed are particularly susceptible to candida infection. Superficial infection of the mouth may spread to the oesophagus, stomach and other parts of the gastrointestinal tract. Systemic candida infections can also cause septicaemia, endocarditis and abscess formation in the kidneys and brain. The critically ill are particularly susceptible to serious candida infection; predisposing factors include the use of broad-spectrum antibiotics, total parenteral nutrition and invasive monitoring with urinary or intravascular catheters. Invasive infections can be difficult both to diagnose and to treat (Flanagan & Barnes 1998).

Although candida infection is normally acquired endogenously (p. 37), cross-infection may occur (Burnie et al 1985, Fowler et al 1998). To minimise the risk of transmission, gloves should be worn for contact with the mucous membranes of all patients (e.g. oral hygiene) and hands should be washed after these procedures.

Cryptococcus

This yeast is found in high numbers in pigeon droppings in many parts of the world. Cryptococcosis is usually an opportunistic infection. If cryptococcus is inhaled by a person with a compromised immune system, it can lead to chronic meningitis, which is fatal if not treated. The infection is seen in people with AIDS and has also been associated with outbreaks of infection in people who have had kidney transplants (Brooks & Remington 1986). Diagnosis is made by microscopic examination and culture of cerebrospinal fluid.

Dermatophytes

These are filamentous fungi and include several genera that cause superficial infections of the keratin found in skin, hair and nails, called *ringworm* or *tinea*. Infections are readily transmitted from person to person. They are distinguished by the site of infection. Tinea pedis (athelete's foot) causes scaling, cracking or blistering of the skin between the toes. It is spread by direct contact with the lesions or with contaminated floors or surfaces in showers or swimming pools. Tinea capitis (scalp ringworm) causes scaly patches on the scalp. Hairs in affected areas become brittle and break off, causing patches of baldness. It is spread by direct contact and by combs, clothing or other articles contaminated with affected hair. Outbreaks of infection, possibly transmitted in schools, have been reported and can be difficult to control as 6–12 weeks of treatment are required to eliminate the infection and asymptomatic carriers may be missed (Communicable Disease Report 1995). Tinea corporis (body ringworm) causes reddish, vesicular ring-shaped lesions on the skin. They are transmitted through direct contact with skin and contaminated items. Tinea unguium causes nail ring-worm, where the nail thickens, becomes brittle and disintegrates. It does not appear to spread from person to person very easily.

Some species are found in animals, such as dogs, cats and cattle, but can also be transmitted to humans.

Histoplasma capsulatum

This fungus can exist as a single cell (yeast) or a filament. It can be recovered from soil contaminated by bird or bat excreta in North and South America, Africa, Asia and Australia. Inhalation of the spores can cause histoplasmosis, a lung infection, which is often asymptomatic but which may cause severe pneumonia and disseminated infection in the immunocompromised. In AIDS sufferers, infection may be reactivated and cause serious generalised infection.

Pneumocystis carinii

This organism has generally been considered to be a protozoon but recent genetic studies suggest that it is more like a fungus. It can be isolated from the lungs of healthy people, in whom it causes no symptoms, and antibody to the organism has been demonstrated in a large proportion of the adult population. However, in the malnourished or immunocompromised it causes a serious interstitial pneumonia, possibly as a result of reactivation of previous infection. Confirmation of the diagnosis of pneumocystis pneumonia requires sampling of the bronchi, usually by bronchoscopy. The widespread use of prophylactic antibiotics against the organism in people with AIDS has reduced the incidence of infection in this vulnerable group.

PROTOZOA

These are unicellular members of the animal kingdom. Only a few species are parasitic in humans, but their ability to multiply very rapidly by asexual reproduction can enable them to cause major infections. Some protozoa have complex life cycles requiring stages of development in different hosts such as animals and insects.

Protozoal infections are unusual in the UK but as foreign travel is now much more common they are increasingly seen in people returning from visits abroad. The protozoal infections discussed in this chapter are summarised in Table 10.2.

Plasmodium

The four species of this organism cause malaria. Malignant malaria, caused by *Plasmodium falciparum*, has the highest mortality. *P. vivax, P. ovale* and *P. malariae* cause a milder illness called benign malaria. The plasmodia share their life cycle between humans and mosquitoes, are transmitted by the bite of the female insect and are not transmitted from person to person, except possibly by the transfusion of infected blood products. Although not occurring naturally in the UK, malaria is an important imported disease, affecting approximately 2000 people returning from abroad each year. Malaria must always be considered as a possible cause of fever in a patient who has been in a tropical or subtropical

Table 10.2 Protozoal infections

Protozoon	Other hosts	Disease in humans	Site of infection
Cryptosporidium	Domestic animals	Cryptosporidiosis	Intestine, causing diarrhoea (chronic and severe in the immunocompromised)
Entamoeba histolytica	None	Amoebic dysentery	Intestine; rarely causes lung, brain or liver abscesses
Giardia lamblia	Wild and domestic animals	Giardiasis	Small intestine
Leishmania	Sandflies	Cutaneous leishmaniasis	Skin
		Visceral leishmaniasis	Reticuloendothelial cells
Plasmodium	Mosquito	Malaria	Erythrocytes
Toxoplasma	Cat, can also infect domestic animals	Toxoplasmosis	Brain abscesses in the immunocompromised; fetal abnormalities if acquired in early pregnancy
Trypanosoma	Tsetse fly	Sleeping sickness	Central nervous system
	Reduviidae bugs	Chagas' disease	Central nervous system and muscle cells

country, regardless of whether or not antimalarial prophylaxis has been taken. A person infected with *P. falciparum* is highly likely to die if not treated.

Sexual reproduction in the plasmodium life cycle occurs in the digestive tract of the mosquito and is followed by asexual reproduction and the build-up of large numbers of plasmodia in the salivary glands. These are injected into the human host when the mosquito feeds. Within an hour they penetrate the liver of the new host, where they replicate asexually many times, reaching up to 40 000 in number. After 6–10 days they are released into the blood and invade red blood cells, causing a malarial attack. They then begin another phase of asexual division, which causes the infected red cells to rupture and release new parasites. *P. falciparum* infects up to 40% of erythrocytes, affecting cells at any stage of maturity. Their subsequent destruction has serious consequences, including anaemia and tissue hypoxia, and is frequently fatal.

The cycles of erythrocytic replication are accompanied by bouts of fever, chills and sweating when red blood cells burst open and toxins and metabolites are released. The period between bouts varies from 36–72 hours, depending on the species. *P. falciparum* has an incubation period of 7–14 days and treatment with quinine is usually effective if started promptly.

P. vivax and *P. ovale* mostly infect young red blood cells and *P. malariae* old cells, so that these species do not cause the same degree of erythrocyte destruction as *P. falciparum* and are generally not life-threatening, except in the very young, very old or immunodeficient. *P. vivax* and *P. ovale* can persist in the liver, causing re-infection with bouts of fever periodically for many years.

The incidence of malaria is related to the distribution of the 60 species of anopheles mosquitoes capable of transmitting it. These are found in tropical and subtropical areas throughout the world where there is a source of stagnant water in which they can breed. In areas where *P. falciparum* is endemic, the local population is exposed to infection from early childhood. As many as 10% of those infected will die before they are 5 years old. Others gradually develop immunity, which limits the severity of the illness. Immunity is only short-term, so that repeated exposure is required if the severity of illness is to be controlled. People who leave endemic areas gradually lose their immunity and are as susceptible to infection if they return to the area as other visitors. Some genetic traits, such as sickle-cell trait, which is common in west Africa, result in defective red blood cells with a reduced susceptibility to malaria.

Prophylaxis against malaria is mandatory for travellers to endemic areas and up-to-date advice must be sought before travelling, as resistance to some drugs is common. To be effective, the prophylactic drugs must be commenced a week before the visit, taken regularly and continued for 4 weeks after returning. However, such prophylaxis does not completely protect against infection, especially as resistance to conventional antimalarial drugs is becoming increasingly widespread (Communicable Disease Report 1998). The use of physical barriers against mosquito bites is therefore most important, e.g. screened living and sleeping areas, long-sleeved clothing and insect repellents (Communicable Disease Report 1997).

Giardia lamblia

The cyst form of this protozoon may be present in large numbers in the stools of entirely asymptomatic persons. In some people the flagellate form (trophozoite) attaches to the mucosa of the small intestine, causing diarrhoea, steatorrhoea, abdominal cramps and weight loss (Figure 10.1). It occurs throughout the world, but is more common in areas with poor sanitation. It is acquired by drinking untreated or unfiltered water, or by swimming in fresh water. However, person to person transmission through contact with faeces may also occur, especially amongst young children. Cases in the UK are often acquired abroad. Giardiasis is diagnosed by observing the distinctive cysts in formed stools, or cysts and trophozoites in liquid stools. Examination of duodenal contents may be necessary to establish the diagnosis. Infection can be effectively treated with metronidazole but only symptomatic patients require treatment.

Trichomonas vaginalis

This flagellate protozoon causes trichomoniasis, a common sexually transmitted disease. It affects up to 20% of sexually active young women (Benenson 1995), in whom it causes vaginitis, an intense vulval irritation and a greenish-yellow discharge with a foul odour. In males it causes a urethritis and can persist in the prostate, seminal vesicles or urethra. The infection can be treated with metronidazole.

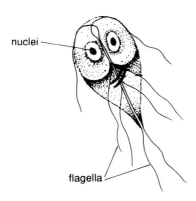

nuclei

flagella

Figure 10.1 *Giardia lamblia* trophozoite.

Entamoeba histolytica

Entamoeba histolytica causes amoebic dysentery, an infection of the large bowel. Infection is acquired through the ingestion of cysts in faecally contaminated food or water and occurs worldwide, especially in areas where sanitation is poor. Disease ranges from asymptomatic to an acute dysentery, with frequent stools containing blood and mucus and colicky abdominal pain. This may progress to an ulcerative-colitis-type disease, and rarely abscess formation in the liver, brain or lung. The amoeba exist in two forms: the trophozoite, which invades the tissues, causing intestinal disease; and the cyst, which has a hardy, protective coating, is excreted in faeces and, following ingestion by another individual, divides into new amoebæ (Figure 10.2). Infection is diagnosed by microscopic examination of stools for cysts, but considerable skill and a fresh specimen is required in order to distinguish them from other entamoebæ which are non-pathogenic. Infection can be treated with metronidazole, and diloxanide is used to eradicate cysts from asymptomatic excreters.

Toxoplasma

The cat is the primary host of *Toxoplasma gondii*. The sexual reproduction part of its life cycle takes place in the intestine of the cat and infective cysts are subsequently passed in the faeces. Cysts can remain viable in soil for up to a year and, if ingested by humans or other animals, can multiply in their tissues. Human infection is acquired by ingestion of cysts present in undercooked meat or cat faeces. Once ingested, active forms are released in the duodenum, reproduce asexually and circulate

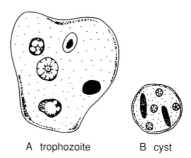

A trophozoite   B cyst

Figure 10.2 *Entamoeba histolytica*. **A.** Trophozoite. **B.** Cyst.

around the body, invading and destroying cells, particularly in muscles, brain and eye. However, immunity develops rapidly and most infections are subclinical, or cause a mononucleosis-like illness. The organism may form cysts in tissues, which usually remain dormant but can be reactivated in people who are immunosuppressed, resulting in large cerebral abscesses or retinitis.

Infection during pregnancy is more serious, causing fetal cerebral calcification, chorioretinitis, hydrocephalus, microcephalus or stillbirth. If acquired in late pregnancy, the fetal effects are mild, but it can cause a chronic retinitis.

Cryptosporidium

This protozoon attaches to the epithelial cells of the intestinal tract, causing watery diarrhoea that is mild and self-limiting, lasting 1–2 weeks, in normal people but severe and prolonged in people who are immunosuppressed (e.g. with AIDS) and is frequently a contributory factor in their death. Antibiotic treatment is unnecessary in patients with normal immunity and generally disappointing in those who are immunosuppressed.

The oocysts are transmitted in contaminated water or food, from person to person or from animal to person. Oocysts excreted in the faeces can survive in the environment for long periods and are resistant to water-treatment chemicals.

Leishmania

There are several pathogenic species of leishmania, all having animal reservoirs and all transmitted by sandflies. They are found in many parts of the world, including south-east Asia, the Middle East, Central and South America and parts of Africa and the Mediterranean area. There are two types of the disease. The cutaneous or mucocutaneous form affects the skin, causing ulcers that can persist for many months and re-occur after healing; in some cases, the nose and mouth are affected and extensive tissue damage results. The visceral form, kala-azar, is a systemic disease. The parasite spreads from the site of inoculation to multiply in reticuloendothelial cells throughout the body, particularly the spleen, liver and bone marrow. Untreated cases are usually fatal.

Trypanosoma

These flagellated protozoa are transmitted by blood-sucking insects. In Africa, two species, *Trypanosoma rhodesiense* and *T. gambiense* are spread by the tsetse fly and cause sleeping sickness. The organism is introduced by the bite of a tsetse fly, at the site of which a painful lesion develops. A febrile illness follows and in the later stages the central nervous system is involved, with typical sleeping sickness syndrome, i.e. lassitude, inability to eat, tissue wasting and unconsciousness. Without treatment the infection is ultimately fatal, although the course of the disease lasts many months. In Central and South America, a different species, *T. cruzi*, spread by a blood-sucking bug, causes Chagas' disease. The trypanosomes live in the intestines of the blood-sucking bug and are excreted in the faeces. They enter a human host when faeces are rubbed into a bite, abrasion or mucous membrane such as the eye. The parasite multiplies rapidly at the site, causing a swelling called a chagoma, and is spread in the lymphatic system. They enter and destroy nerve and muscle cells, especially in the heart. Infection in children is often fatal. The bug lives in mud walls and thatched roofs of houses and attempts to control the disease have relied on improving the standard of housing and the use of insecticides in infested buildings.

HELMINTHS

These multicellular parasites cause a variety of diseases in humans, which, although not a major problem in the UK, are a common cause of morbidity in many tropical and subtropical countries. There are three distinct groups: nematodes (roundworms), cestodes (tapeworms) and trematodes (flukes).

Nematodes

The most important pathogens in this group are *Ascaris lumbricoides*, *Toxocara canis*, threadworm (*Trichuris trichuria*), hookworm and filarial worms.

Ascaris lumbricoides

This worm infects the intestine, particularly of children. The infection is acquired by ingesting eggs from faecally contaminated soil or uncooked, contaminated food. The larvae grow and develop in the lung and return to the intestine to mature, and the eggs are excreted in the faeces. The eggs mature in the soil and are infective after 2–3 weeks. The worm occurs throughout the world but is most common in tropical countries, where sanitary conditions are poor and children contaminate the soil with faeces. The infection is usually mild, but can aggravate nutritional deficiencies and may cause bowel obstruction and pneumonitis.

Toxocara

The usual reservoir of this worm is dogs (although one species is carried by cats). It is acquired by humans through contact with soil contaminated with dog faeces, or by eating contaminated, unwashed, raw vegetables. The eggs take a few weeks to mature in the soil, but then remain infective for many months. After ingestion, the eggs hatch in the intestine and migrate to the liver, lungs and eye. The symptoms of infection are usually mild, with a raised white cell count and hepatomegaly. Lesions in the eye may result in loss of vision several years after infection. The infection probably exists worldwide, but only about 300 new cases of toxocariasis are recognised annually in the UK (Wright 1990).

Threadworm *(Enterobius vermicularis)*

This worm is only about 1 cm in length and commonly infects the large intestine, particularly of young children (Figure 10.3). The main symptoms are perianal itching and sometimes secondary infection where the skin has been scratched. Adult female worms come out of the anus while their host is asleep and lay thousands of eggs on the skin. The eggs are then distributed directly on the hands as the irritation is scratched, or indirectly on clothes, towels or bedding. The eggs survive outside the body for about 2 weeks.

The infection can be diagnosed by applying transparent sticky tape to the perianal area. Eggs adhere to the tape and can be seen under the microscope. It is probably the most common helminth infestation seen in the UK, and causes great anxiety and distress. Children between 5 and 12 years of age, and their parents, are most commonly affected (Willis 1990). Treatment with mebendazole or piperazine is effective if coupled with simple hygiene precautions and treatment of the whole family.

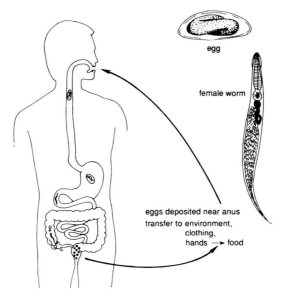

egg

female worm

eggs deposited near anus
transfer to environment,
clothing,
hands ⟶ food

Figure 10.3 Life cycle of the threadworm.

Cestodes (tapeworms)

These are flatworms that are composed of a head (the scolex) and a series of segments; they can vary in length from a few centimetres to several metres, depending on the species. There are two species of tapeworm that commonly infect humans: *Taenia solium* has a larval stage in pigs and *T. saginata* has a larval stage in cows. Humans are infected by ingesting undercooked meat containing larval cysts. The scolex emerges from the cyst and attaches to the wall of the intestine. The segments of the body are formed at the head; they gradually mature so that those at the end of the worm are full of eggs, drop off and are released in the faeces. Eggs ingested by the appropriate animal hatch in its gut and migrate into the muscles, where they form larval cysts containing the scolex.

The adult worms usually cause only gastrointestinal disturbance but the larvae of *T. solium* can invade the muscle and establish cysts in humans. These can have serious effects where they occur in the heart, eye or brain. Infection with cestodes is very rare in the UK but more common in South America, Africa, south-east Asia and eastern Europe. Only eight cases of cerebral cystercosis were reported in the UK between 1981 and 1990 (Public Health Laboratory Service 1990).

Echinococcus

The adult worm is only 5–8 mm in length and lives in the intestine of dogs, which are the definitive host. Eggs are excreted in faeces and contaminate grass, which is then eaten by sheep, the intermediate host (although it can also infect cows, goats or horses). The larvae travel to the liver, less often to the lungs, where they form cysts (hydatid cysts), which contain thousands of heads of immature worms. Humans may be infected by ingesting eggs picked up from the dog's coat or eating contaminated, uncooked vegetables. Cysts most commonly occur in the liver, but the lung and the brain may be affected. Careful surgical removal is the usual form of treatment, but if the contents of the cyst leak there is a risk of anaphylactic shock or the development of numerous peritoneal cysts.

Trematodes (flukes)

These are small hermaphrodite helminths, which are flat, unsegmented and have complicated reproductive systems. Part of their life cycle takes place in freshwater snails. There are four types that affect humans: liver flukes, intestinal flukes, lung flukes and schistosomes.

Liver flukes (Fasciola)

These usually infect sheep and cows, but can also infect humans. Infection is acquired by eating vegetation carrying the fluke cysts, which break open in the gut to release the worm. This migrates to the liver and bile duct and passes its eggs out in the faeces. These develop into larvae in water and enter water snails, in which they develop into free-swimming forms. These are released in large numbers from the snails, attach to vegetation and form into cysts. Symptoms of infection include abnormal liver function tests, biliary colic and jaundice. Infections have been reported in South America, the Middle East, Asia, Australia and also in Europe.

Intestinal flukes (Fasciolopsis)

These infect pigs and humans in east Asia. Eggs passed in the faeces hatch in water and the larvae infect fresh water snails. After a phase of development the larvae leave the snail and form cysts on aquatic vegetation. These are ingested by humans and the fluke attaches to the intestine, causing ulceration and obstruction of the gut.

Lung flukes

Lung flukes occur in east Asia, particularly China, Africa and South America. They infect dogs, cats, pigs and wild animals as well as humans. They are acquired by eating larvae in freshwater crabs or crayfish. These penetrate the gut wall and migrate to the lungs, where they develop into a cyst. Eggs are released into the bronchioles and are either coughed out in sputum or swallowed and released in faeces. The eggs hatch in water and enter snails to undergo a development phase before emerging to infect the crustaceans. The symptoms of infection are cough, haemoptysis and chest pain. The effects can be mild and the infection can persist for many years.

Schistosomes (Bilharzia)

Schistosomes are blood flukes that live in the blood vessels of the abdominal wall. Eggs are excreted in faeces or urine, hatch into larvae in water and enter freshwater snails, where they undergo a development phase before leaving as free-living larvae. They penetrate the skin of humans working or washing in the water and are carried in the blood to the large bowel or bladder, where they mature and migrate to the blood vessels (Figure 10.4). Symptoms of large-bowel infection include abdominal pain, anaemia, diarrhoea and enlarged liver and spleen, and of bladder infection terminal haematuria and frequency. Schistosomiasis can also induce portal hypertension, hydronephrosis and intestinal or bladder cancer. The disease occurs in many parts of the world, especially in Africa, South America and Asia. Antihelminthic drugs are quite effective; however good sewerage systems, mollusicides and education about avoiding working or washing in potentially contaminated water are needed to prevent transmission of the disease.

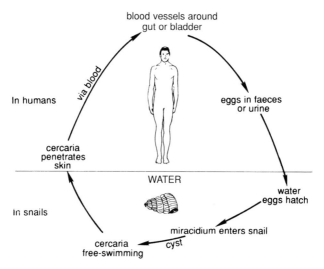

Figure 10.4 Life cycle of schistosomes.

ECTOPARASITES

A number of insects are human parasites; the most commonly encountered in the UK are lice and scabies.

Lice

There are hundreds of species of lice but only three are human parasites, and each infects a specific site on the body.

Head louse

This species lives on head and eyebrow hair and is between 1 and 4 mm long. The female louse sticks her eggs on to the base of hairs, laying about eight eggs a night. These hatch after 7–10 days and the shell of the egg, the nit, remains attached to the hair shaft. The adult louse lives for about 3 weeks, feeding off the blood of its host. It can transfer to another host when the two heads are in direct contact, enabling it to crawl across. However, as lice prefer temperatures of at least 31°C, they keep as close to the scalp as possible and prolonged, close contact is required for them to transfer to another head (Maunder 1993). Hypersensitivity to the louse saliva or faeces can cause intense irritation. Head lice are commonly found on schoolchildren and spread readily among family and friends. Conventional treatments are insecticides based on malathion (an organophosphate), carbanyl or pyrethroid. These are applied to the hair and left in contact for a period of time before washing off with shampoo. Resistance to these agents is common and health authorities may recommend the use of a single agent, changing to a different type every 3 years. Concern over the harmful effects of using chemicals, particularly the organophosphates and the difficulty of eradicating lice from children has led to the introduction of alternative methods of treatment, which many people have found to be successful (Figure 10.5).

Body louse

This louse is similar to, but larger than, the head louse. It lives in clothing rather than hair, only moving on to the body to feed. The adult louse lays its eggs in the seams of clothing, producing several hundred in its 3-week life span. The bite marks appear on the skin around the seams, in particular along the collar line or waistband, and are very itchy. These lice are destroyed when clothes are washed in hot water, and 15 minutes of hot tumble-drying will destroy both lice and eggs. As they need to feed regularly from the body they will die if the clothing is not worn for a few days. Their transmission has been associated with poor living conditions, war and overcrowding. Some infections are transmitted by lice, for example trench fever (*Bartonella quintana*), relapsing fever (*Borrelia recurrentis*) and typhus (*Rickettsia prowazeki*).

Crab (pubic) louse

Crab lice are broader and flatter than other lice and live on coarse body hair, such as pubic, axillary and chest hair. They can also live in eyebrows and facial hair. The female louse lays her eggs on the shaft of the hair. These hatch in 7–8 days and take another 2 weeks or more to mature. After 4–6 weeks the body begins to react to the louse bites and severe itching around the anus and vagina develops. Although frequently transmitted by sexual contact, they can also transfer by other forms of close physical contact,

Bug Busting is the best way to detect head lice

This is the way we BUST the bug on the thirty first in the evening!

Everyone should check using the Bug Busting method on 31 October and every fourth day for two weeks to prevent lice from circulating

Starter info for under-sevens

▼ Wash your children's hair as you normally do.

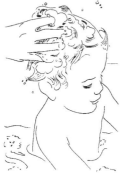

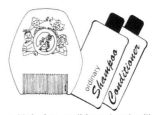

▲ **Wash, rinse, condition and comb, will leave the lice without a home!**

● Often there are very few lice on a head and no itching.
Check the whole family...

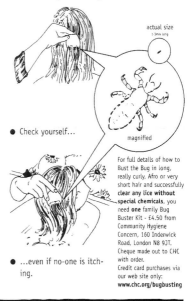

actual size
1-3mm long

magnified

● Untangle and straighten the hair using conditioner and a wide-tooth comb. Then, leaving the hair full of conditioner, comb the whole head section by section with the Bug Buster.

Slot the teeth right into the hair at the roots and draw to the tips.

Soaking-wet lice stay still; even baby lice cannot escape the Bug Buster. Check the comb for lice in the foam between each stroke and remove them.

● Check yourself...

Rinse hair thoroughly and comb again.
The wetter, the better!

For full details of how to Bust the Bug in long, really curly, Afro or very short hair and successfully **clear any lice without special chemicals,** you need **one** family Bug Buster Kit - £4.50 from Community Hygiene Concern, 160 Inderwick Road, London N8 9JT. Cheque made out to CHC with order.
Credit card purchases via our web site only:
www.chc.org/bugbusting

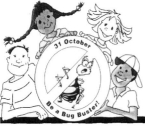

● ...even if no-one is itching.

☎ **Help Line:** 0181 341 7167
©1998 Community Hygiene Concern

Design: Aitor Ibarra • Illustration: Lisa Kershaw & Jo Lin Lee
Reg. Charity No: 801371

Figure 10.5 Alternative methods of controlling head lice.

e.g. from mother to children via axillary hair. Malathion, carbaryl and lindane can be used for treatment and should be applied to all hair on the body except the head.

Scabies

This is caused by a small mite, *Sarcoptes scabiei*, which lives in the deep epidermal layers. It burrows horizontally through the skin, the burrows appearing as tiny white lines with the mite, a brown spot, at one end.

The female mite lays two to three eggs in the burrows each day and lives for about 6 weeks. Male mites do not make burrows. The most common sites where mites live are the inner wrist and between the fingers, although they may also occur on the feet, groins, axillae and buttocks (Taplin 1986). About 4–6 weeks after infection, sensitisation to the mite causes an intense itching, not necessarily at the site of mite infection. The rash often appears on the hands, arms, legs and around the waist (Maunder 1983). A dermatologist can take scrapings from a burrow to confirm a diagnosis of scabies by detection of the eggs or female mite under the microscope. This is important to ensure adequate tracing and treatment of contacts. Treatment with lindane or malathion involves application of the solution to all parts of the skin except the head.

The mite is not easily transmitted from person to person and prolonged contact is required for it to transfer to another host. However, outbreaks may occur, e.g. in long-stay elderly care wards or units, and in the UK the incidence has increased recently (Barnet and Morse 1993).

Norwegian 'crusted' scabies

This form of scabies is seen in people with immunodeficiency, who are unable to control the mite, which subsequently multiplies rapidly, spreading all over the body. There may be as many as 2 million mites in a severe infestation, compared to an ordinary infestation, which involves only around 11 mites (Johnsen et al 1991). The skin lesions become dry and cracked and can be heavily contaminated with mites. Such individuals are very infectious and outbreaks of infection commonly spread through vulnerable populations, e.g. in AIDS units and nursing homes.

Healthy contacts with a normal immune system will develop conventional scabies (Sirera et al 1990)

REFERENCES

Barnes, R.A. and Rogers, T.R. (1989) Control of an outbreak of nosocomial aspergillosis by laminar air-flow isolation. *J. Hosp. Infect.*, **14**, 89–94.

Barnet, N.J. and Morse, D.L. (1993) The resurgence of scabies. *Commun. Dis. Rev.*, 3(2), R32–R33.

Beck-Sague, C.M. and Jarvis, W.R. (1993) National Nosocomial Infection Surveillance System. Secular trends in the epidemiology of nosocomial fungal infections in the United States, 1980–1990. *J. Infect. Dis.*, **167**, 1247–1251.

Benenson, A.S. (1990) *Control of Communicable Diseases in Man*. American Public Health Association. Washington, DC.

Bodey, G.P. (1988) The emergence of fungi as a major hospital pathogen. *J. Hospital Infection* 11(Suppl A): 411–426.

Brooks, R.G. and Remington, J.S. (1986) Transplant-related infections. In: *Hospital Infections*, 2nd edn (eds Bennett, J.V. and Brachman, P.S.) Little, Brown & Co., Boston, MA.

Burnie, J.P., Odds, F.C., Lee, W. *et al*. (1985) Outbreak of systemic *Candida albicans* in an intensive care unit caused by cross infection. *Br. J. Med.*, **290**, 746–748.

Communicable Disease Report (1995) Scalp ringworm in London. *Commun. Dis. Rep.*, **5**(38), 179.

Communicable Disease Report (1997) Guidelines for the prevention of malaria in travellers from the United Kingdom. *Commun. Dis. Rep.*, **7**(10), R138–R151.

Communicable Disease Report (1998) Rise in falciparum malaria imported from east Africa. *Commun. Dis. Rep. Wkly.*, **8**(20), 175.

Flanagan, P.G. and Barnes, R.A. (1998) Fungal infection in the intensive care unit. *J. Hosp. Infect.*, **38**(3), 163–177.

Fowler, S.L., Rhoton, B., Springer, S.C. *et al*. (1998) Evidence for person-to-person transmission of *Candida lusitaniae* in a neonatal intensive care unit. *Infect. Control. Hosp. Epidemiol.*, **19**(5), 343–345.

Greer, P. (1998) Vaginal thrush: diagnosis and treatment options. *Nurs. Times*, **94**(4), 50–52.

Humphries, H., Johnson, E.M., Warnock, D.W. *et al*. (1991) An outbreak of aspergillosis in a general ITU. *J. Hosp. Infect.*, **18**(3), 167–178.

Johnsen, C., Bellin, E., Nadal, E. *et al*. (1991) An outbreak of scabies in a New York City jail. *Am. J. Infect. Control*, **19**(3), 162–163.

Lipman, J. and Saadia, R. (1997) Fungal infections in critically ill patients. *Br. Med. J.*, **315**, 266–267.

Loudon, K.W., Coke, A.P., Burine, J.P. *et al*. (1996) Kitchens as a source of *Aspergillus niger* infection. *J. Hosp. Infect.*, **32**, 191–198.

Manuel, R.J. and Kibbler, C.C. (1998) The epidemiology and prevention of invasive aspergillosis. *J. Hosp. Infect.*, **39**, 95–109.

Maunder, J. (1983) The increase in scabies. *Postgrad. Doctor*, **6**, 198–202.

Maunder, J. (1993) An update on head lice. *Health Visitor*, **66**(9), 317–18.

Public Health Laboratory Service (1989) Toxoplasmosis. *PHLS Microbiol. Dig.*, **6**(3), 69–73.

Public Health Laboratory Service (1990) Summary of Taenia reports to CDSC.

Taplin, D. (1986) Cutaneous infestations. In *Modern Management of Skin Diseases* ed. Vickers, C.F.H. Churchill Livingstone, Edinburgh, pp. 18–25.

Sirera, G., Ruis, F., Romeu, J. *et al.* (1990) Hospital outbreak of scabies stemming from two AIDS patients with Norwegian scabies. *Lancet*, **335**, 1227.

Strausbaugh, L.J., Sewell, D.L., Ward, T.T. *et al* (1994) High frequency of yeast carriage on hands of hospital personnel. J. Clin. Micro., **32**, 2299–2300.

Willis, J. (1990) Common pests. *Nurs. Times (Community Outlook)*, **Sept.**

Wright, J. (1990) Toxocariasis – the canine threat. *Prof. Nurse*, **5**(10); 519–521.

FURTHER READING

Lane, R.P. and Crossley, R.W. (eds) (1993) *Medical Insects and Arachnids*. Chapman & Hall, London.

Manuel, R.J. and Kibbler, C.C. (1998) The epidemiology and prevention of invasive aspergillosis *J. Hosp. Infect.*, **39**(2), 95–109.

Rhame, F.S. (1991) Prevention of aspergillosis. *J. Hosp. Infect.*, **18**, 466–472.

Robinson, R. (1986) Scratching the surface. *Nurs. Times*, **34**, 71–72.

11

Infection associated with healthcare: the infection control programme

INTRODUCTION

Prior to the 19th century death from infection was commonplace and no effective treatments were available, although attempts were made to control spread through the use of quarantine. In the UK, the industrial revolution of the 1800s facilitated the spread of disease, with many people living in squalid conditions without sewerage, drainage or water supplies. At that time an infant mortality rate of 200 per 1000 births was not uncommon. By the mid-19th century, the importance of sewage disposal and clean supplies of water had been recognised and medical officers were put in place in each district to initiate and oversee measures to improve public health. Public health acts of Parliament passed in 1872 broadened the role of these medical officers to include other aspects of public health, such as food hygiene, infectious disease control, child welfare and venereal disease clinics. The effects of better living conditions, nutrition and the introduction of widespread vaccination against some of the most serious infections began to have a dramatic effect on the incidence of infectious disease. Between 1840 and 1900, the death rate in Britain fell from 25 to 15 per 1000 and life expectancy increased from 40 to 50 years.

Nowadays, the comprehensive programme of immunisation for all children in the UK has virtually eliminated many of the more serious infections that would have claimed many lives in the past. However, new threats are emerging; the Human immunodeficiency virus (HIV), first recognised in the early 1980s, will probably have infected 30–40 million people worldwide by the year 2000 (World Health Organisation 1993). The increasing tendency to travel abroad has seen many people return with tropical diseases such as malaria and has enabled antibiotic-resistant bacteria to transfer between countries and become major international problems.

The association between hospitals and infection has been recognised for thousands of years. Some of the earliest hospitals, established in Asia, Egypt, Palestine and Greece hundreds of years before the birth of Christ, used practices designed to prevent infection, such as avoiding touching wounds, the isolation of infected patients and the use of hot ovens for the sterilisation of instruments. Unfortunately, these ideas did not persist and, until the end of the 19th century, hospitals were likely to be overcrowded and to lack any measures to prevent the transmission of infection (Selwyn 1991). Mortality rates were high and patients operated on in hospitals were much more likely to die than those operated on in the community (Simpson 1869). Florence Nightingale (1863) introduced the principles of hygiene and infection control in the care of patients and gradually, as an understanding of microbiology developed, the incidence of hospital-acquired infection decreased. This was greatly facilitated by the introduction of antibiotics, the first effective treatments for infection, in the 1940s. However, the problem of hospital-acquired infection has not been eliminated. Advances in medical technology have meant that many patients who otherwise would have died can be treated, but are made more vulnerable to infection through the use of invasive devices, immunosuppressive therapy and broad-spectrum antibiotics. In addition, many types of bacteria have evolved mechanisms for resisting antimicrobial agents, causing infections that can be extremely difficult to treat.

This chapter reviews the problem of infection associated with healthcare, the reasons why hospital patients are particularly susceptible and the size and cost of the problem. It also discusses how the advisory services that implement and monitor practices intended to prevent and control infection are structured at a local level.

INFECTION ASSOCIATED WITH HEALTHCARE

Hospitals, by definition, are places to which the sick are taken for treatment. They will be in close proximity to other sick people, some of whom may have infections. They will also have frequent contact with a wide range of health care staff and equipment, which can act as both sources of infection and provide routes of transmission. All these factors help to provide the ideal environment for microorganisms to be transferred from one person to another.

Patients are especially vulnerable to infection if they have predisposing factors which increase their risk. These include the following.

- **Underlying disease.** Severe disease such as carcinoma or leukaemia, and drugs and treatments such as steroids and chemotherapy affect the ability of the immune system to respond to infection. Local factors, such as poor peripheral perfusion in diabetics, may lead to necrosis of tissue and hence increased susceptibility to infection. Poor blood supply to a wound may also be caused by pressure, vascular disease or necrosis. Effects of the disease process may increase the risk of infection at vulnerable sites; for example, faecal incontinence increases the risk of urinary tract infection.
- **Extremes of age.** The immune response is affected by extremes of age. In the neonate and young child, the immature immune system is unable to respond rapidly or effectively to invasion by microorganisms. Immunity may gradually be lost with age, making the elderly more vulnerable to infections or to reactivation of microorganisms encountered in earlier life.
- **Breaches in normal defences.** Bacteria, e.g. lactobacilli in the vagina, which normally colonise mucosal surfaces and protect them from invasion by more harmful microorganisms, may be destroyed by antibiotic therapy, allowing antibiotic-resistant microorganisms to replace them. The treatment of hospital patients frequently involves bypassing or damaging the normal body defences. The skin is breached by surgical procedures, intravenous devices or decubitus ulcers; the urinary tract by urinary catheters or other instruments; and the respiratory tract by intubation and artificial ventilation. Invasive devices are increasingly featuring in the management of patients at home. These patients are vulnerable to infection introduced either by healthcare workers or by themselves.
- **Antimicrobial resistance.** Hospital patients are highly likely to receive antibiotic therapy for treatment of infection or as pro-

phylaxis against infection prior to surgery. As a result of regular exposure to antibiotics, resistant strains of bacteria are more likely than sensitive strains to prevail in the hospital environment and, in addition, many strains have a particular capacity to spread from one person to another (Wade et al 1991).

• **Special units** often present considerable hazards. Patients in an intensive care unit are likely to be severely ill, mechanically ventilated, fed intravenously and catheterised, procedures that bypass the normal defences of the body. It is therefore not surprising to find high rates of infections among these critically ill patients (Glynn et al 1997). Premature babies in neonatal care units have immature immune systems that make them highly susceptible to infection, and the opportunity for introducing infection is increased by the need to handle them frequently.

Obviously, not all patients in hospital are exposed to factors that increase their risk of infection. To help identify those patients at particular risk of acquiring infection associated with healthcare Bowell (1992) has devised a scoring system, which takes account of those underlying diseases, invasive procedures and treatments that increase the risk of acquiring infection (List 11.1). Making an assessment of an individual's risk of infection can enable actions aimed at preventing infection to be incorporated into the care planning process (Kingsley 1992).

The boundaries between hospital and community are now much more blurred than in the past. Patients may be treated in hospital but returned rapidly to the community, receiving care as outpatients or in their own homes. Identifying and distinguishing between those infections acquired in hospital and those acquired in the community is often not possible. Patients who have invasive devices and are cared for in their own homes may be at lower risk of acquiring infection, particularly by antibiotic-resistant bacteria, from other patients, although home conditions may not be as conducive to preventing infection. The principles of infection control apply to healthcare provided at home or in hospital but may need to be adapted to cope with local circumstances.

THE SIZE OF THE PROBLEM

It is difficult to establish precisely how many infections are acquired as a result of healthcare, since accurate records are often not kept

---

List 11.1   Factors that can increase the risk of infection (Adapted from Bowell 1992)

General factors
- *Age*: very young or very old
- *Nutrition*: emaciation, obesity, dehydration
- *Mobility*: immobile or poor mobility
- *Incontinence*: urinary or faecal
- *General health*: debilitation

Local factors
- *Oedema*: pulmonary, ascites
- *Ischaemia*: necrosis, thrombus
- *Skin lesions*: wounds, burns, ulceration, device insertion sites
- *Foreign bodies*: implants, sutures

Invasive procedures
- *Intravenous cannulas*: peripheral, central
- *Surgery*: anaesthesia, wound
- *Intubation*: ventilation, suction, humidification
- *Catheterisation*: intermittent, indwelling, irrigation

Drugs
- Cytotoxics
- Antibiotics
- Steroids

Diseases
- Carcinoma
- Leukaemia
- Renal disease
- Liver disease
- Immunodeficiencies

---

and collation and analysis of information is time-consuming. Different measures can be used to define the size of the problem. The most commonly used are incidence and prevalence (p. 49). It is important to distinguish between these two measures, since a prevalence rate will appear to be much higher than an incidence rate. This is because a prevalence study counts the number of patients with infection at one point in time and as patients with infection are likely to stay in hospital for longer, they are more likely to be included in this type of survey.

Studies suggest that approximately 6% of patients admitted to hospital acquire an infection during their stay (Glenister et al 1992, Haley et al, 1985). The most common infections are of the urinary tract, lower respiratory tract and wounds; bloodstream infections are much less common, although they are likely to have more serious consequences for the patient (Figure 11.1). Data on

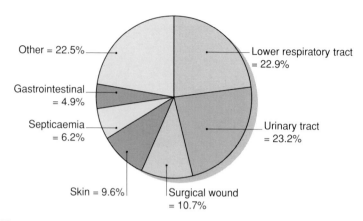

Figure 11.1 The distribution of the main types of hospital-acquired infection (Source: Emmerson et al 1996).

the occurrence of infection can be misleading. For example, the National Prevalence Studies (Box 11.1) undertaken in 1980 and 1994 suggest that the prevalence of surgical wound infection has fallen from 1.78 to 1.1 per 100 patients, but the trend towards early discharge from hospital following surgery and surgical treatment of patients as day cases means that many surgical wound infections are not be detected while the patient is still in hospital. Other infections acquired as a result of treatment in hospital may also present after discharge, e.g. respiratory tract infection following surgery and urinary tract infection following catheterisation.

The major types of infection acquired by patients in hospital are urinary tract, lower respiratory tract, surgical wound and bloodstream infections; these account for approximately 60% of hospital-acquired infection (HAI). Other important sites of HAI include non-surgical wounds such as ulcers and pressure sores, vascular lines and the gastrointestinal tract. The predisposing factors of the main HAI are summarised below and are discussed in more detail in Chapter 13.

Urinary tract infection

These are the most common infections associated with healthcare, accounting for 23% of HAI. Most are related to urethral catheter-

---

Box 11.1   The Second National Prevalence Survey of Infection in Hospitals. Source: Emmerson et al 1996.

The aims of this survey were to record the overall prevalence of infection in hospital and to assess the associated risk factors. It took place over a 15-month period, in acute specialities of 157 hospitals in the United Kingdom and Ireland. The median number of patients included in the survery by each hospital was 239. Each participating hospital would take several days to complete the survey, but where possible a whole ward would be surveyed in one session. Two people, one a doctor, entered data on all patients on the ward into a standardised questionnaire on a laptop computer. The data included the age, sex and admission type of the patients, underlying disease, specific drug therapies, presence of invasive devices, surgical or other invasive procedures and information on any infection present that met the definitions of infection developed for the survey.

The mean prevalence of HAI was 9%, but ranged from 2% to 29%. The rate of HAI was higher in teaching hospitals (11.2%) than non-teaching hospitals (8.4%). 66.5% of infections occurred in the urinary tract, surgical wounds, lower respiratory tract and skin. A further 14% of patients in hospital had community-acquired infections, particularly lower respiratory tract, urinary tract and skin infections.

---

isation. This device enables bacteria to enter the bladder, either along the outside of the tube or through its lumen. The presence of the catheter prevents microorganisms from being flushed out by the normal filling and emptying of urine, enabling them to colonise the bladder. Microorganisms may spread to the kidneys or invade the bloodstream. Urinary tract infection occurs most commonly in those groups of patients likely to be catheterised, such as those treated in urology, gynaecology and orthopaedic units (Glynn *et al.* 1997).

Lower respiratory tract infection

These account for 23% of HAI and can occur as bronchitis, tracheitis or pneumonia. Pneumonia is often a very serious infection, which results in the death of about one-third of those affected. Microorganisms are aspirated from the oropharynx or inhaled and the risk is increased by devices that bypass the normal defences (e.g. endotracheal tubes) and by reduced levels of consciousness (e.g. sedation). Nasogastric tubes increase the reflux of fluid from the stomach and facilitate colonisation of the oropharynx and subsequent aspiration of microorganisms into the lung.

Immunocompromised patients are vulnerable to pneumonia caused by opportunistic pathogens such as aspergillus, and outbreaks of respiratory viral infections sometimes occur among hospital patients, especially children.

Surgical wound infection

These account for nearly 11% of HAI, although this rate of infection is an underestimate, since many patients will have been discharged from hospital before the infection becomes apparent. The risk of infection is increased where the procedure involves a region of the body that is heavily colonised by bacteria, e.g. the bowel. Foreign material implanted in the wound, for example a joint replacement, increases the risk of infection. The skills of the surgeon are of paramount importance in preventing subsequent infection; prolonged procedures, tissue damage, necrosis and haemotoma formation are all important risk factors in the development of surgical wound infection.

Bloodstream infection

These account for approximately 6% of HAI, but are responsible for considerable morbidity and mortality. Infections caused by Gram-negative bacteria are particularly difficult to treat because these organisms produce a range of toxins, which have serious systemic effects. Some bloodstream infections develop from another focus of infection, e.g. affecting the urinary tract, respiratory tract or wound, but a significant proportion of bloodstream infections are directly related to intravenous therapy, particularly central vascular devices. Skin commensals such as *Staphylococcus epidermidis*, which are otherwise unusual causes of infection, can establish infection in the blood through the colonisation of invasive devices, particularly in immunocompromised patients.

Patients with infectious diseases

Some infections can be easily spread from person to person and present particular problems in hospitals. Other patients may be especially vulnerable to infection and the frequent movement of staff between patients facilitates the spread of microorganisms.

Isolation precautions are therefore used to prevent transmission of these microorganisms from the infected patient to other patients or staff. These are discussed in more detail in Chapter 14.

Sometimes, spread to other patients or staff does occur, and is termed an outbreak of infection. While outbreaks of infection are uncommon, considerable resources are required to control them, such as additional staff to carry out isolation procedures, supplies of protective clothing, laboratory tests and treatment for affected patients (Barness 1989).

Common causes of outbreaks of infection in hospitals are shown in List 11.2. In recent years, bacteria that are highly resistant to a wide range of antimicrobial agents have emerged. Many of them also have the capacity to spread readily between vulnerable patients in hospitals and between hospitals and nursing homes, presenting major problems to those places affected. Outbreaks of methicillin-resistant *Staphylococcus aureus* (MRSA) now affect as many as 80 hospitals at any one time in England and Wales (Communicable Disease Report 1997). Controlling outbreaks of infection caused by MRSA can involve the use of considerable resources. The ICT may spend considerable time swabbing staff and patients to detect carriage; affected patients require treatment with topical creams to eliminate carriage or expensive antibiotics to treat infection; and ward or bed closures may be required. Cox et al (1995) reported an MRSA outbreak that lasted 2 years, with the cost of control measures reaching nearly £500 000.

List 11.2   Some microorganisms commonly associated with outbreaks of infection in hospitals

Bacteria
- *Clostridium difficile*
- Antibiotic-resistant organisms eg MRSA, VRE, penicillin-resistant pneumococci
- Salmonella (food poisoning)
- Group A streptococci
- *Mycobacterium tuberculosis*

Viruses
- Chickenpox
- Gastrointestinal viruses, e.g. Rotavirus, small round structured virus, Norwalk agent
- Respiratory viruses, e.g. influenza, RSV

COSTS OF INFECTION ASSOCIATED WITH HEALTHCARE

Infections acquired as a result of healthcare cause considerable morbidity and mortality. The costs of these infections to the hospital need to be considered in terms of the costs of treatment, specialist care and extra days spent in hospital. However, many infections acquired in hospital are not detected until the patient has been discharged and the costs of treatment fall to the general practitioner and community nursing services (Elliston et al 1994). There are also costs to society in terms of loss of earnings, productivity and social security payments, which may impinge on both the patients and their carers (Plowman et al, 1997). Studies to quantify the associated costs indicate that some infections, such as respiratory tract infection and bloodstream infections, are more costly than others (Haley, 1992). Coello et al (1993) estimated that in England the costs of treatment varied from approximately £500 for a urinary tract infection to over £3000 for patients who develop multiple infections. The overall costs to the nation from HAI acquired by surgical patients was estimated at over £170 million. Outbreaks of infection can also be costly. Barness et al (1989) calculated the costs of an outbreak of *Salmonella* that affected 17 patients and two staff to be over £21 000.

Currie and Maynard (1989) estimated that, if an effective infection control programme could be implemented thoughout the UK, over £15 million could be saved. The costs of establishing and maintaining an infection control programme are considerable, but as pointed out by Daschner (1991), an infection control programme can help to eliminate costly and ineffective practices and reduce pollution of the environment.

IMPLICATIONS FOR SERVICE QUALITY

The NHS has a clear responsibility to ensure that the services provided are of high quality. The framework through which NHS organisations are accountable for safeguarding high standards of care and improving quality is described as clinical governance (Department of Health 1998). This concept requires accountability for quality at a corporate level, with clear lines of responsibility for the overall quality of care within the organisation and a range of mechanisms in place to establish and monitor the quality of services (List 11.3). In addition, healthcare professionals have an individual responsibility to maintain a high standard of practice, with support from professional development programmes and codes of professional practice, conduct and discipline. The Commission for Health Improvement (CHI) will be a statutory body responsible for policing the adoption and operation of clinical governance and providing advice and support to service providers and a National Institute of Clinical Excellence (NICE) is to be established to facilitate and promote the use of evidence-based clinical guidelines (Wilson 1998).

While it may not be possible to prevent all infections, the risk can be reduced by maintaining high standards of infection control practice (Chapters 12 and Chapter 13). Employing measures to prevent infection is therefore an essential part of quality. Infection control policies and procedures should be evidence-based and there should be systems in place for auditing practice, monitoring the occurrence of infections and using this information to identify where the quality of care may be improved. The infection control team has responsibility for advising other clinical staff and for planning and implementing a programme of activity directed at preventing and controlling infections.

List 11.3 Clinical governance (Source: Wilson 1998)

Framework for clinical governance
Corporate accountability
- Chief executive accountable
- Clear lines of responsibility

Internal mechanisms
- Individual accountability
- Professional regulation
- Professional development

External support structures
- Commission for Health Improvement (CHI)
- National Institute of Clinical Excellence (NICE)

Core principles of clinical governance
- Clinical audit
- Evidence-based practice
- Clinical effectiveness
- Risk management
- Risk reduction programmes
- Monitoring outcomes of care
- Learning lessons from complaints
- Dissemination of good practice

Risk management

A key part of clinical governance is a systematic approach to identifying events that could have adverse consequences and implementing appropriate measures to control them. This process involves identifying and investigating adverse events to ensure that the lessons learnt from them are incorporated into practice, together with identifying and controlling practices that have the potential to result in harm (Dickson 1995).

Another dimension of risk management is the financial benefits associated with minimising the exposure of NHS organisations to litigation where effective risk reduction systems are in place (Moss 1995). This has taken on increasing importance since the removal in the late 1980s and early 1990s of Crown immunity, which in the past exempted hospitals from prosecution and prevented enforcement of some legislation, e.g. food safety.

Risks could affect either staff or patients and a risk management policy will focus on the structures and policies that are in place to address these risks. Infection control has an important part to play in risk management, with the safe handling of patients, equipment and body fluids being fundamental to preventing patients or staff acquiring infection in hospital. For example, needlestick injuries to staff are known to carry a significant risk of transmission of blood-borne viruses. A clearly stated policy on the safe disposal of used needles, training of staff who handle them, the provision of sufficient, appropriate disposal containers and a system for monitoring accidental injuries are all essential parts of managing the risk associated with needlestick injury.

MANAGEMENT ARRANGEMENTS FOR THE PREVENTION AND CONTROL OF INFECTION

The significance of an effective programme to prevent HAI was demonstrated by a major American study carried out in the 1980s called the Study of the Efficacy of Nosocomial Infection Control (SENIC). It evaluated the infection control activity in 338 hospitals and, through the review of clinical records, measured how the rate of HAI changed in the 5-year period after the infection control programme was established. Those hospitals with a comprehensive infection control programme featuring all the

---

List 11.4   Components of an infection control programme
(SENIC study, cited in Haley et al, 1985)

Infection control personnel co-ordinating the programme
- Trained infection control doctor
- One infection control nurse to every 250 beds

Control activities
- Detect, investigate and control outbreaks of infection
- Produce, implement and monitor policies
- Educate staff

Surveillance activities
- Identify infections
- Analyse data
- Disseminate results

---

components described in List 11.4 were able to reduce the rate of HAI by 32%, compared to hospitals with a poor or non-existent programme, where the rate of HAI increased by 18% during the same period. The results of this study have important implications for clinical practice. They suggest that a significant proportion of HAI can be prevented and that the quality of the infection control programme makes a difference. The study also highlighted the combination of activities that were important for an effective infection control programme, identifying surveillance of HAI as a key component and the important role of specialist staff, the infection control nurse and infection control doctor.

The chief executive of the hospital is responsible for ensuring that effective arrangements for infection control are in place and a planned programme has been defined and is regularly reviewed. Planning and implementing an infection control programme requires the expertise of specialist staff and all hospitals are recommended to employ an infection control nurse and infection control doctor to take on this role (NHS Executive 1995). They work as a team, liaising regularly, providing advice on infection control to all disciplines of staff, and implementing measures required by the programme. The infection control team (ICT) report to the chief executive and are supported by an infection control committee (Figure 11.2).

In addition to providing specialist advice, the ICT has several functions:

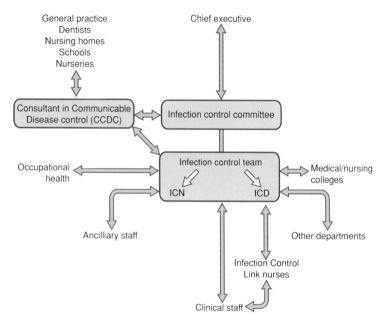

Figure 11.2 The management of infection control in hospitals.

• **Preparation of policy documents.** Written guidance on the prevention and control of infection needs to be developed and regularly updated. This includes clinical activities (e.g. isolation), procedures for specialist departments, (e.g. theatre) and policies giving guidance on antibiotic use and the purchase of equipment.

• **Formulation and implementation of an annual infection control programme.** This defines the focus of infection control activity for the year and identifies policies that require development or revision, plans for audit and surveillance and education targets. The infection control team are responsible for co-ordinating the actitiviy and ensuring that the targets are met.

• **Monitoring clinical practice to ensure that infection prevention and control procedures are in place**, e.g. management of invasive devices, decontamination of medical equipment, cleaning of the environment and waste disposal.

• **Developing standards and an audit programme.** This can be used to systematically evaluate procedures of importance to infection control, e.g. food handling

- **Education.** In addition to the advisory service there should be a planned education programme for staff.
- **Surveillance of infections.** This should be carried out routinely to detect outbreaks of infection, identify trends (e.g. of antibiotic resistance) and monitor for infectious disease. In addition there should be a planned programme of surveillance targeted at specific HAI.
- **Detecting and controlling outbreaks of infection.** Systems should be in place to facilitate the early detection of outbreaks of infection and plans for controlling outbreaks should be prepared. The team is then responsible for the implementation of the outbreak plan and co-ordination of the control activities.

As well as co-ordinating the main components of the infection control programme the infection control team provides advice in its area of responsibility by visiting wards and departments, by phone and by attendance at various committees, e.g. Health and Safety, Waste Management, Supplies and Laundry Users

The infection control nurse (ICN)

The ICN usually works full-time in infection control and carries the main responsibility for ensuring that the infection control programme is carried out, liaising with a wide range of departments and different categories of staff within the Trust. The ICN is a Clinical Nurse Specialist, the characteristics of which have been defined by Hamric (1989; List 11.5). A key component of the role is the ability to act as an expert practitioner, interpreting laboratory and other relevant data and providing expert advice to clinical staff, patients and their families (Prieto, 1994). The ICN is usually a registered nurse who has further specialist training and experience; a number of courses are available for training nurses in the role (List 11.6). It is recommended that every hospital should appoint at least one ICN and, in practice, many employ more (NHS Executive 1995). The SENIC project indicated that the most effective infection control programmes in the USA employed one ICN for every 250 hospital beds (Haley et al 1985).

More ICNs are now being appointed to positions in community healthcare trusts or public health, where they provide an advisory service and infection control programme for community

List 11.5   Defining characteristics of the Clinical Nurse Specialist role (Source: Hamric, 1989)

Primary criteria
- Graduate study in speciality
- Certification
- Focus of practice on patient/client/family

Skills and competencies
- Change agent
- Collaborator
- Clinical leader
- Role model
- Patient advocate

Subroles
- Expert practice
- Education
- Consultation
- Research

List 11.6   Training for Infection Control Nurses

Professional certificates
- ENB 329 Foundation course in infection control nursing
- ENB 910 Principles of infection control
- N26 Developments in infection control nursing

Academic courses
- Diploma in Infection Control
- BSc (Hons) Infection Control
- Postgraduate Diploma in Infection Control
- MSc Infection Control

healthcare staff, nursing homes, general practitioners and practice nurses.

Infection control doctor (ICD)

This is usually a consultant microbiologist based in an acute hospital and with access to microbiology laboratory facilities, but usually does not work full-time in the role as ICD. S/he should have specialist training in infection control and often provides leadership for the team. The ICD can influence the prescribing of antimicrobial agents and treatment of hospital-acquired infection and is usually involved in the training of medical students and newly qualified doctors.

Consultant in Communicable Disease Control (CCDC)

This is a doctor appointed in the Department of Public Health Medicine of each health authority to co-ordinate the surveillance, prevention and control of all communicable diseases in the area. S/he is usually designated as the 'proper officer' defined in the 1984 Public Health Act to whom infectious diseases must be notified, and acts as the link between the health service and the local authority. The CCDC works closely with community-based ICNs and liaises with hospital ICTs to co-ordinate infection prevention and control activities within and outside the hospital. S/he has an important role in ensuring that outbreaks of infection are managed effectively and advising the health authority on contractual arrangements for infection control. In Scotland a similar role is performed by the Consultant in Public Health Medicine (Communicable Disease and Environmental Health).

Infection control link nurses

In many hospitals, link nurses who have a special interest in infection control are being used to provide a link between the ICT and clinical areas. They undertake the role alongside their normal duties but receive some basic training in the principles of infection control. ICLNs can help to provide information to other staff, undertake surveillance and audit, and report on infection control problems (Teare & Peacock 1996).

Infection control committee (ICC)

Every hospital should have an Infection Control Committee NHS Executive 1995). In addition to the infection control team, the committee will draw its membership from the chief executive (or a senior member of the management team), director of nursing, consultant in Communicable Disease Control, occupational health physician or nurse, senior clinical medical staff, pharmacy and sterile services supplies. The role of the committee is to support the ICT and to act as a forum through which the ICT can consult with key groups within the hospital. The ICC will discuss, advise on and approve the infection control programme and infection control policies.

Advisory services

There are a number of organisations that can be consulted for expert advice on infection control, the diagnosis and treatment of unusual infection and the investigation of infections.

Public Health Laboratory Service (England and Wales)

Central Public Health Laboratory (CPHL), Colindale, London. This is a specialist centre providing a wide range of microbial reference services that assist in the identification of pathogenic strains and the investigation of outbreaks of infection. It is staffed by scientists who are experts in clinical and public health microbiology, and doctors and nurses with experience in hospital infection control, surveillance of hospital-acquired infections and outbreak management.

Regional Public Health Laboratories. A network of 53 laboratories located thoughout England and Wales is linked to CPHL. They monitor infectious disease occurring within their area, report on them centrally and disseminate information from the centre to their local area. Most regional laboratories provide a full microbiological service to the hospital in which they are based and specialist testing for neighbouring health authorities, local authorities, environmental health departments, water and food suppliers. They will undertake public health microbiology such as testing food, milk and water and environmental and outbreak specimens.

Communicable Diseases Surveillance Centre (CDSC), Colindale, London. This centre is responsible for co-ordinating the management of national outbreaks of infection, and will help in the investigation and control of localised outbreaks. It offers expert advice on epidemiology, immunisations and infections acquired abroad. It is also responsible for the surveillance of infections in England and Wales, publishing data weekly in the Communicable Disease Report and via computer networks.

Regional epidemiologists. These doctors are based in Regional offices of the NHS Executive. They are involved in the monitoring and control of communicable diseases within the population and are available to provide expert advice to the CCDC and ICT.

Scottish Centre for Infection and Environmental Health (SCIEH)

This centre is based in Glasgow and is responsible for the surveillance of infection, publication of reports and expert advice on the investigation and control of outbreaks of infection in Scotland. Data on infections are published in the SCIEH weekly report.

Notifiable diseases

The importance of monitoring the occurrence of infectious diseases has been recognised since the early 1900s when the statutory requirement of doctors to notify cases of infectious disease was introduced. In England and Wales these are reported to the proper officer (usually the CCDC), collated and analysed by the Office for National Statistics (ONS) and published by the CDSC in the weekly Communicable Disease Report. In Scotland, notifications are reported to the Consultant in Public Health Medicine, and the data collated and analysed by the Common Services Agency (CSA) and published by SCIEH in the weekly report. The infectious diseases for which notification is required are listed in List 11.7.

SURVEILLANCE OF HOSPITAL-ACQUIRED INFECTION

Surveillance is a term applied to the systematic monitoring of the occurrence of disease in a population; to be of value the data collected must be analysed and the results disseminated. The importance of surveillance in the control of infectious diseases prevalent in the community was recognised at the beginning of the 20th century and there is now a statutory requirement for doctors to notify cases of infectious disease, enabling data to be collected on their incidence, upward trends to be detected and preventative action taken. Surveillance in a hospital setting has, until recently, been focused on detecting cases of infectious disease that have the potential to cause outbreaks of infection

---

List 11.7 Notifiable diseases (England and Wales)

Public Health (Control of Diseases) Act 1984
- Cholera
- Food poisoning
- Plague
- Relapsing fever
- Smallpox
- Typhus

Public Health (Infectious Diseases) Regulations 1988
- Acute encephalitis
- Acute poliomyelitis
- Anthrax
- Diphtheria
- Dysentery
- Leprosy
- Leptospirosis
- Malaria
- Measles
- Meninigitis
- Meningococcal septicaemia
- Mumps
- Ophthalmia neonatorum
- Paratyphoid fever
- Rabies
- Rubella
- Scarlet fever
- Tetanus
- Tuberculosis
- Typhoid fever
- Viral haemorrhagic fever
- Viral hepatitis
- Whooping cough
- Yellow fever

Local authorities have the power to add to, or subtract from this list, in order to prevent the spread of infectious diseases. AIDS is not a notifiable disease but doctors are asked to report cases to a voluntary, confidential scheme at CDSC. Sexually transmitted diseases are reported anonymously by genitourinary clinics to the Department of Health.

(see List 11.2). Now, many more hospitals are using surveillance to assess the quality of care provided as part of the clinical audit process and the introduction of clinical governance into the management of health care recognises the importance of the process (Figure 11.3). If the data is disseminated to clinical staff whose practice is key in preventing infection, it can help to reinforce good practice and identify areas where improvements could be made (Glynn et al 1997).

Purchasers of health care are increasingly interested in measures of quality of care, and rates of infection have been used for this purpose. However, although surveillance can be helpful in focusing infection control activity on to specific problems, the data needs to be interpreted with care. Differences in methods of data collection, criteria for defining infections and the mix of patients can all affect the results and need to be considered when comparing data from different hospitals (Wilson, 1995).

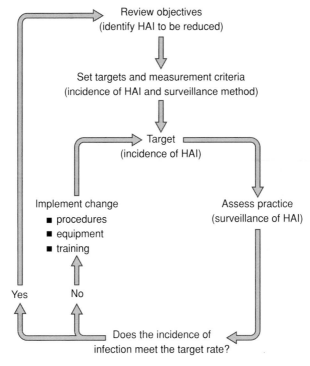

Figure 11.3 The role of surveillance in the audit process.

The Nosocomial Infection Surveillance Unit (NISU), based at the Central Public Health Laboratory in London, co-ordinates a programme to help hospitals in England to collect data on specific HAI using standard methodology and definitions, and to make national data on their incidence available for comparison.

DETECTION, INVESTIGATION AND CONTROL OF OUTBREAKS OF INFECTION

Outbreaks or epidemics of infection can occur in any community but are a particular problem in institutions where many people live in close proximity, e.g. schools, universities, residential homes and military barracks. The risks are even greater in hospital settings, where many patients have underlying illnesses that make them more susceptible to infection. The deaths of several patients during an outbreak of salmonella at the Stanley Royd Hospital in

---

Box 11.2   Outbreak of *Salmonella* at the Stanley Royd Hospital

---

In 1984, a large number of patients and staff at the Stanley Royd Hospital for mentally ill patients in Wakefield acquired salmonella poisoning after eating beef served by the hospital kitchens. Out of a total of 788 residents, 355 had been ill with suspected salmonella and a further 81 were symptom-free but had positive specimens. Of the 980 staff, 109 had been ill with suspected salmonella and a further 29 had positive specimens but no symptoms. Many of the affected patients were elderly and there were 19 deaths due to, or in part contributed to by, the infection. The inquiry that followed identified many deficiencies in the way that food was handled, stored and prepared, and in the way that the outbreak of infection was managed.

At the time of this incident hospitals were protected from prosecution by Crown immunity so that, while environmental health officers could inspect hospital kitchens, they had no means of enforcing their recommendations or preventing the continuation of unsafe practices. Following the Stanley Royd enquiry Crown immunity was removed from health-service catering facilities in 1987 and formal requirements for infection control advice and the management of outbreak of infection were established (Department of Health and Social Security 1988).

Wakefield in 1985 (Box 11.2) highlighted deficiencies in the management of outbreaks of infection and led to advice to introduce more careful controls and clearer lines of responsibility in the future (NHS Executive 1995). In England and Wales, health authorities (HA), and in Scotland health boards, have responsibility for controlling communicable diseases. The Director of Public Health appointed by each HA leads the Public Health department and will work with the Consultant in Communicable Disease Control (CCDC) (Consultant in Public Health Medicine, Communicable Disease and Environmental Health in Scotland), who has responsibility for monitoring, preventing and controlling outbreaks of infection. The CCDC will liaise between the environmental health officers of the LA, who have responsibility for food hygiene and pollution control within the local area, and the HA (NHS Management Executive 1993). When an outbreak of infection occurs within a hospital, the ICT will usually take the lead in the management of the outbreak, but will work closely with the CCDC. If the outbreak has significant implications for the community the CCDC should take the lead. The team will investigate the source of infection, identify people who have been in contact with the infection, advise on the control measures that are required and monitor their implementation. The ICT may establish an Outbreak Control

Group, involving clinicians and senior nurses from affected departments, the CCDC, occupational health physician and other staff whose help may be required to ensure that the outbreak is controlled effectively (NHS Executive, 1995). Clinical staff can be crucial in the early detection of outbreaks of infection. They should be aware of symptoms indicative of infection amongst patients or staff and report to the ICT where two or more cases with similar symptoms occur. Relevant clinical specimens can also help to determine the cause of infection and whether cases are related to the outbreak (Box 11.3).

Box 11.3 Key steps in the control of suspected outbreaks of gastrointestinal infection

Where more than one patient or member of staff is affected by unexplained diarrhoea or vomiting, the following actions should be taken:

1. In a hospital:
   - Inform the doctor in charge of the patients
   - Inform the infection control doctor/nurse
   - Ensure sufficient supplies of gloves/aprons
   - Collect stool specimens from affected patients for viral and bacterial culture
   - Wash hands after contact with affected patients
   - Use protective clothing for handling body fluids
   - Change gloves and wash hands between patients
   - Transfer affected patients to single rooms and follow isolation precautions
   - Ensure affected staff attend Occupational Health

2. In a nursing home
   - Inform the GP responsible for affected patients
   - Inform the CCDC
   - Ensure sufficient supplies of gloves/aprons
   - Collect stool specimens from affected patients for viral and bacterial culture
   - Wash hands after contact with affected patients
   - Use protective clothing for handling body fluids
   - Change gloves and wash hands between patients
   - Ensure affected staff consult their GP

Role of occupational health department (OHD)

The OHD has an important role to play in ensuring that staff are protected from infections by immunisation and are managed appropriately when they may present a risk of infection to patients (e.g. gastrointestinal infection, hepatitis B carriage, severe skin conditions). The OHD is also there to provide advice and support to staff who have been exposed to infection, such as those concerned about acquiring a blood-borne virus following a needlestick injury, and those who may be particularly susceptible to infection themselves, e.g. with HIV infection.

POLICIES AND PROCEDURES TO PREVENT AND CONTROL INFECTION

Although the infection control team is available much of the time to provide advice and information about infections and their control and prevention, the subject is complex and staff need to have access to written information to reinforce the guidance. Written material helps to clarify the routine practices and the standards of care expected by the organisation. This is important, for the protection of patients and staff, for example the safe management of sharp instruments and prompt and appropriate management of sharps injuries.

Many of the procedures carried out on patients are associated with a risk of infection, particularly when invasive devices are used. Infection control advice therefore needs to be incorporated into many of the procedures used in clinical areas. Policies also provide guidance on how to manage patients with infectious diseases, where particular care may be required because of the risk of transmitting infection to other vulnerable patients being cared for in the same area. The safe and effective management of equipment, the environment and waste materials will also need to be addressed in specific policies.

The infection control team, in conjunction with other staff, is responsible for developing many of these policies. The infection control committee will decide on the priorities for policy development and revision, and approve them when completed. Other staff may develop their own policies e.g. for the management of urine catheters or IV cannulae, but seek the advice of the infection control team on recommended practice. There are often conflicting views about what constitutes best practice in terms of infection control, as was clearly demonstrated in a recent analysis of policies from 19 hospitals across England and Wales (Glynn et al 1997). The publication of some simple clinical guidelines for preventing infection associated with a range of commonly used invasive devices may help to focus on those practices which have been most clearly demonstrated to reduce the risk of infection (Ward et al 1997).

The written policy alone may not be sufficient to ensure effective practice. Policies and guidelines must be carefully developed, taking into account local practices and attitudes. There must also be a system for implementation and dissemination, to ensure that the relevant staff know about the policy and understand its contents (Cheater & Closs 1997, Seto et al 1991).

Education and training

Clearly, the availability of a range of written policies on infection control is of little value if the staff are not aware of them or do not understand their content. Infection control procedures are much easier to adopt if staff understand the risks of infection and the rationale for recommended practice.

ICNs spend a considerable proportion of their time in the education of a wide range of the staff who work in clinical settings (Griffith Jones 1991). This can take place informally, e.g. discussing the management of a particular patient, as a ward-based seminar, or more formally as lectures and study days. Infection control should also form part of the basic training of all groups of healthcare professionals, and infection control nurses are usually involved in the training of domestic, portering and other ancillary staff.

There is a close relationship between health and safety and many aspects of infection control. The Health and Safety legislation acknowledges the importance of training in ensuring that staff understand the procedures and know what is expected of them. Staff who join a healthcare organisation should be made aware of local infection control policies, and the infection control team should be involved in their orientation programmes.

A basic knowledge of microbiology underpins the practice of infection control and several workers have pointed to the lack of this knowledge amongst qualified nurses. The fears and misunderstandings that built up around the management of the first patients with AIDS demonstrate how important education is if such problems are to be avoided. (Välimäki et al 1998). Staff who have received education are in a better position to educate others, both patients and other staff. Ching & Seto (1990) used infection control link nurses (ICLNs) to support the teaching activity of the ICN and were able to demonstrate significant improvements in adherence to an infection control policy when ICLNs were providing tutorials on the ward.

Monitoring clinical practice

The ICN will monitor infection control practice in routine visits to clinical areas. However, a systematic approach to the observation of infection control practice has been used to measure the quality of care and identify where improvements could be made (Millward et al 1993). Such audits take the form of checklists of key standards related to a particular area of practice (Figure 11.4). The ICN visits a clinical area and marks where the criteria on the checklist are met. Such a process can identify where information about infection control policies, additional equipment or in-service education may be required. The score generated from this process is fed back to the clinical staff in the department concerned, problems identified are discussed and solutions are agreed (Friedman et al 1984).

They are also involved in educating staff in personal hygiene and safety. The review of records of sharps injuries or other accidents helps to identify trends and contributory factors that may be addressed.

Standard: sharps will be handled safely to negate the risk of sharps injury

- A container as specified by the Infection Control Committee is in use ☐

- The container is less than 2/3rds full ☐

- The box is free from protruding sharps ☐

- Sharps box is available on the arrest trolley ☐

- Sharps box available on the medicine trolley ☐

- Sharps box is correctly assembled ☐

- Sharps box is labelled according to hospital policy ☐

- Sharps are disposed of directly into a sharps box ☐

- What action would you take following a needlestick injury? (question to a member of staff at random) ☐

Comments:

Figure 11.4 An infection control audit tool (Source: Millward et al 1993).

The infection control team have a close working relationship with the occupational health department. Routine visits to clinical areas may alert the ICN to staff who could present a risk of infection (e.g. with diarrhoea). The OHD will be closely involved in outbreaks of infection, monitoring staff and ensuring that they remain off work while suffering from an illness that may affect patients.

REFERENCES

Barness, S., O'Mahoney, M., Socket, P.N. *et al.* (1989) The tangible cost implications of multiply-resistant salmonella. *Epidemiol. Infect.*, **103**, 227–234.
Bowell, B. (1992). Protecting the patient at risk. *Nurs. Times*, **88**(3), 32–35.
Cheater, F. M. and Closs, S. J. (1997) The effectiveness of methods of dissemination and implementation of clinical guidelines for nursing practice: a selective review. *Clin. Effect. Nurs*, **1**, 4–15.
Ching, T. Y. and Seto, W. H. (1990) Evaluating the efficacy of the infection control liaison nurse in the hospital. *J. Adv. Nurs.*, **15**, 1128–1131.
Coello, R., Glenister, H., Fereres, J. *et al.* (1993) The cost of infection in surgical patients: a case control study. *J. Hosp. Infect.*, **25**, 239–250.
Communicable Disease Report (1997). Epidemic methicillin resistant *Staphylococcus aureus. Commun. Dis Rep.*, **7**(22), 191.
Cox, R. A., Conquest C., Mallghan, C. *et al.* (1995) A major outbreak of methicillin-resistant *Staphylococcus aureus* caused by a new phage type (EMRSA 16). *J. Hosp. Infect.*, **29**, 87–106.
Currie, E. and Maynard, A. (1989) *Economic Aspects of Hospital Acquired Infection. Discussion Paper 56.* Centre for Health Economics, University of York, York.
Daschner, F. D. (1991) Unnecessary and ecological costs of hospital infection. *J. Hosp. Infect.*, **18**(Suppl. A), 73–78.
Department of Health (1998) *A First Class Service in the New NHS.* Stationery Office, London.
Department of Health and Social Security (1988) Hospital infection control. *HC(88)33*, HMSO, London.
Dickson, G. (1995) Principles of risk management. *Qual. Health Care*, **4**, 75–79.
Elliston, P. R. A., Slack, R. C. B., Humphreys, H. *et al.* (1994) The cost of postoperative wound infections. *J. Hosp. Infect.*, **28**(3), 241–242.
Emmerson, A. M., Enstone, J. E., Griffin, M. *et al.* (1996) The second national prevalence survey of infection in hospitals – overview of the results. *J. Hosp. Infect.*, **32**, 175–190.
Friedman, C., Richter, D., Skylist, T., Brown, D. (1984) Process surveillance: Auditing infection control policies and procedures. *Am. J. Infect. Control*, **12**, 228–232.
Glenister, H. M., Taylor, L. J., Cooke, E. M. *et al.* (1992) *A Study of Surveillance Methods for Detecting Hospital Infection.* PHLS, London.
Glynn A., Ward V., Wilson, J. *et al.* (1997) *Hospital Acquired Infection: Surveillance Policies and Practice.* Public Health Laboratory, Service, London.
Griffith Jones, A. (1991) Are we giving value for money? *Nurs. Times*, **87**(11), 64–68.
Haley, R. W. (1992) A cost benefit analysis of infection control activities. In: *Hospital Infections* (eds Brachman, P.S. and Bennett, J.V.). Little, Brown & Co., Boston, MA.

Haley, R. W., Culver, D. H., White, J. W. *et al.* (1985) The efficacy of infection surveillance and control programs in preventing nosocomial infections in US hospitals (SENIC Study). *Am. J. Epidemiol.*, **121**, 182–205.

Hamric, A. B. (1989) History and overview of the CNS role. In: *The Clinical Nurse Specialist in Theory and Practice*, 2nd edn (eds Hamric, A. B. and Spross, J. A.). W. B. Saunders, Philadelphia, PA.

Kingsley, A. (1992) First step towards a desired outcome. Preventing infection by risk recognition. *Prof. Nurse*, **7**(11), 725–729.

Millward, S., Barnett, J. and Thomlinson, D. (1993) A clinical infection control audit programme: evaluation of an audit tool used by infection control nurses to monitor standards and assess effective staff training. *J. Hosp. Infect.*, **24**, 219–232.

Moss, F. (1995) Risk management and the quality of care. *Qual. Health Care*, **4**, 102–107.

NHS Executive (1995) *Hospital infection control. Guidance on the control of infection in hospitals.* Infection Control Working Group. *HSG(95)10*. Health Publications Unit, Heywood, Lancs.

NHS Management Executive (1993) Public health: responsibilities of the NHS and roles of others. *HSG (93)56*. Health Publications Unit, Heywood, Lancs.

Nightingale, F. (1863) *Notes on Nursing*. Longman, London.

Plowman, R. M. Graves, N. and Roberts, J. A. (1997) *Hospital-acquired Infection.* Office of Health Economics, London.

Prieto, J. (1994) The specialist role of the ICN. *Nurs. Times*, **90**(38), 63–66.

Selwyn, S. (1991) Hospital infection: the first 2500 years *J. Hosp. Infect.*, **18**(Suppl. A), 5–65.

Seto, W. H., Ching, R. N., Yuen, K. Y. *et al.* (1991) The enhancement of infection control in-service education by ward opinion leaders. *Am. J. Infect. Control*, **19**, 86–91.

Simpson, J. Y. (1869). Some propositions on hospitalism. *Lancet*, **16 Oct**, 535–538.

Teare, E. L. and Peacock, A. (1996) The development of an infection control link-nurse programme in a district general hospital. *J. Hosp. Infect.*, **34**, 267–278.

Wade, J. J., Desai, N., Casewell, M. W. (1991) Hygienic hand disinfection for the removal of epidemic vancomycin-resistant *Enterococcus faecium* and gentamicin-resistant *Enterobacter cloacae*. *J. Hosp. Infect.*, **18**, 211–218.

Ward, V., Wilson, J., Taylor, L. *et al.* (1997) *Preventing Hospital-acquired Infection. Clinical Guidelines*. Public Health Laboratory Service, London.

Wilson, J. (1995) Infection control: surveying the risks. *Nurs. Stand.*, **9**(15 Suppl NU); 3–8.

Wilson, J. (1998) Clinical governance. *Br. J. Nurs.*, **7**(16), 987–988.

World Health Organisation (1993) *Global programme on AIDS. The HIV/AIDS Pandemic: 1993 overview.* WHO, Geneva.

Välimäki, M., Suominen, T. and Peate, I. (1998) Attitudes of professionals, students and the general public to HIV/AIDS and people with HIV/AIDS: a review of the research. *J. Adv. Nurs.*, **27**, 752–759.

FURTHER READING

Infection Control Standards Working Party (1993) *Standards in Infection Control in Hospitals*. Laboratory of Hospital Infection, CPHL, London.

12

The principles of infection prevention and control

INTRODUCTION

Hospital patients are vulnerable to developing infection while in hospital: at least 6% will be affected and the associated morbidity and mortality is considerable (Glenister et al 1992). Preventing infection is important, not only to the patients themselves but also to the health service as a whole since infections increase the costs of care and divert limited resources (Plowman et al 1997). There is evidence that up to a third of hospital-acquired infection could be prevented through the use of effective infection control measures (Haley et al 1985).

Healthcare workers are healthy and therefore not especially vulnerable to infection, but contact with infectious body fluids and exposure to infectious patients can place them at risk of infection. Infections acquired occupationally by healthcare workers include: infections of the skin, e.g. streptococci, herpes simplex virus; respiratory infections such as tuberculosis; enteric infections; and blood-borne viruses (Greaves et al 1980, George et al 1986, Ross et al 1998). The routine application of infection control procedures is therefore also important to protect staff from infection.

The concept of using precautions for the care of all patients, regardless of whether or not they are known or suspected to have an infection, was recommended in response to the AIDS epidemic and became known as universal precautions (Box 12.1). This approach has now been widely adopted and has been seen as a means of minimising the transmission of a wide range of pathogens in all healthcare settings (Wilson & Breedon 1990, Garner 1996). A key component of universal precautions is an assessment of the risk of exposure to pathogens and so implies that the level of precaution can vary according to the particular activity involved. This is important, as 'universal precautions' is often perceived incorrectly to mean the routine use of extensive protective clothing.

Box 12.1 Universal blood and body fluid precautions

Universal precautions were first recommended by the Centers for Disease Control in Atlanta, USA in 1985 in response to growing concerns about the risk to healthcare workers from the Human immunodeficiency virus (HIV) (Centers for Disease Control, 1987). Until then, special precautions had only been taken with body fluids from patients known or suspected to be infected. HIV had highlighted the difficulty of identifying people who were incubating a disease and infectious but had no outward signs of the infection. Universal precautions also recognised that there were a few simple practices that could be employed in the care of all patients to prevent direct contact with potentially infectious body fluids. These included the safe management of sharps, the use of protective clothing in situations where open skin lesions or mucous membrane contact with blood or body fluid was likely, use of waterproof dressings to cover cuts and hand washing after any contact with body fluids.

Since universal precautions were first proposed, other workers have recognised their benefit in protecting staff and patients from other pathogens that have a propensity to spread in clinical settings. Lynch et al (1990) recommended that universal precautions should be incorporated into routine practice and used in combination with other isolation practices in a system called body substance isolation. In the UK the Department of Health advised similar measures to protect staff against infection with blood-borne viruses and endorsed their use with all patients (UK Health Departments, 1998). More recently, the concept has been described as 'standard precautions', and its significance in the general prevention of cross-infection in clinical settings, rather than just blood-borne viruses, has been recognised (Garner 1996).

This chapter reviews key infection control practices that, if used routinely, can help to protect both patients and their carers from infection. Chapter 13 then focuses on preventing infection associated with important invasive devices and procedures.

HAND WASHING

The importance of hands as a route of transmission of infection was first described by Ignaz Semmelweis, an Austrian obstetrician. In the 1850s he noticed that large numbers of women were succumbing to puerperal fever after delivering their babies in the obstetric hospital. He surmised that there might be an association between doctors performing post-mortems on women who had died of puerperal fever and their subsequent contact with women in labour. He therefore issued instructions for doctors to wash their hands in chlorinated lime between contact with the cadavers and labouring women. This new policy brought about a dramatic reduction in mortality from puerperal fever and demonstrated clearly the role of hands in the transmission of infection (Newsom 1993). Since then, hands have been implicated as an important route of transmission in many outbreaks of infection among hospital patients (Reybrouck 1983, Ansari et al 1991, Larson 1988).

There are two categories of microorganism found on the skin. The resident organisms inhabit the hair follicles, sebaceous glands and crevices on the surface of the skin; transient organisms are acquired by contact and do not survive on the surface of skin for long.

Resident skin flora

The microorganisms that form the resident flora of the skin mostly comprise micrococci, streptococci, corynebacteria and staphylococci and are generally of low pathogenicity. They are not easily removed by the mechanical action of washing but their numbers can be reduced by antiseptics such as chlorhexidine and povidone-iodine (Lowbury & Lilly 1973). As these organisms are not readily transferred by touch and are an unusual cause of infection, their removal is unnecessary for routine clinical care. However, some could cause infection if introduced into sterile tissues, e.g. during surgery or other invasive procedures, and for this reason detergents containing antiseptics are recommended for hand washing prior to invasive procedures, or for handling vulnerable sites on patients who are at increased risk of infection, e.g. critically ill adults or neonates (Hoffman & Wilson 1995).

Transient skin flora

Microorganisms are acquired on the hands through contact with contaminated surfaces, excretions or secretions and most are readily transferred to the next object or person that is touched (Mackintosh & Hoffman 1984). The type of microorganism making up the transient flora reflects microorganisms that are prevalent in the environment. Thus, antibiotic-resistant strains of bacteria are commonly found on the hands of staff when they are caring for a patient infected with the organisms (Cookson et al 1989). Studies in clinical environments have shown that a wide range of pathogens are acquired during routine procedures such as bed making, nappy changing, lifting or washing patients, or using the sluice (Sanderson & Weissler 1992, Casewell & Phillips 1977, Samadi et al 1983). Tomlinson (1987) showed that, even where forceps are used to dress wounds, microorganisms present in the wound are still transferred to the hands. These transient organisms are unable to survive for long in the arid environment of the skin and are also easily removed by washing with soap and water (Sprunt et al 1973).

Indications for hand washing

Ideally hands should be washed with soap and water between all contacts with patients. However, as a minimum, hands should always be washed before procedures that could place the patient at risk of acquiring infection, e.g. handling an invasive device, or after procedures during which the hands could have been contaminated, e.g. contact with body fluids. List 12.1 summarises some of the main indications for hand washing. Antiseptic soap solutions (e.g. Hibiscrub) are not intended for routine use in clinical areas as they remove the resident as well as the transient flora and their harsh effect on the skin can cause damage which may subsequently increase the number of bacteria present (Ojajärvi et al 1977). They may have a place in the control of outbreaks of antibiotic-resistant bacteria (Wade et al 1991). The hands should be washed systematically to ensure that all parts are covered by the soap and

---

List 12.1   Indications for hand-washing

- Before and after contact with susceptible sites, e.g. wounds
- Before and after manipulation or insertion of invasive devices, e.g. intravenous cannula, urinary catheters
- Before and after preparing or handling food
- Before leaving a work area
- After contact with contaminated items, e.g. linen, equipment
- After contact with body fluids
- After contact with a patient being isolated
- After using the toilet

water. Taylor (1978) observed that some parts of the hands are frequently missed during hand washing (Figure 12.1). Drying is an important part of the procedure, probably removing more microorganisms, while inadequate drying tends to make the skin dry and cracked and more prone to infection and colonisation.

Rings should be removed, as they may harbour microorganisms, especially Gram-negative bacteria (Hoffman et al 1985). Cuts, abrasions or damaged skin act as a focus for bacteria to multiply and enable pathogens to penetrate. Hand creams help to maintain the skin in good condition but communal creams, which can become contaminated, should be avoided (Morse & Schonbek 1968).

Numerous studies have indicated that healthcare staff do not wash their hands frequently enough, even after dirty procedures (Gould 1993, Glynn et al 1997). Even extensive education campaigns do not achieve a prolonged improvement in frequency of hand washing (Williams & Buckles 1988), although repeated audit of the practice may be more effective (Dubbert et al 1990). The provision of adequate hand washing facilities is also an important factor in encouraging more frequent hand washing (Kaplan & McGuckin 1986).

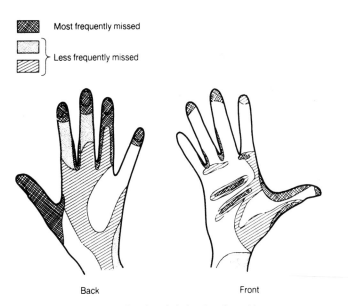

Most frequently missed

Less frequently missed

Back   Front

Figure 12.1   Parts of the hands missed during hand washing.

Alcohol handrubs

Repeated hand washing takes up a considerable amount of time, especially when there is some distance between handwash basins. Alcohol handrubs provide a convenient alternative to washing with soap and water, can be applied quickly without the need for access to water and remove both transient and resident flora (Mackintosh & Hoffman 1984). They are particularly useful before and during procedures requiring an aseptic technique, for isolation procedures and in intensive care units where frequent hand washing is often required. They are also useful when staff attend patients in their own home, where hand washing facilities may be inadequate. However, they should not be used if hands are physically soiled as soap and water is required for mechanical removal of dirt.

PROTECTIVE CLOTHING

Some body excretions are heavily contaminated with pathogenic bacteria and present an important risk of infection. In addition, exposure to blood, tissues and body fluids may result in the transmission of blood-borne viruses (UK Health Departments 1998). List 12.2 illustrates the hazards presented by different body sub-

---

List 12.2 Infectious body fluids

Body fluids that may contain blood borne viruses
- Blood
- Cerebrospinal fluid
- Peritoneal fluid
- Pleural fluid
- Pericardial fluid
- Synovial fluid
- Amniotic fluid
- Semen
- Vaginal secretions
- Breast milk
- Any other body fluid containing visible blood (eg saliva associated with dentistry)
- Tissues and organs

Body fluids that may contain other pathogens
- Faeces
- Urine
- Vomit
- Sputum
- Saliva

stances. Protective clothing is recommended to prevent skin becoming contaminated with pathogens and reduce the risk of their transmission to staff or via staff to patients. Microorganisms cannot penetrate intact skin, but can readily pass through mucous membranes such as the mouth or conjunctiva and protection of these sites may be required if exposure to body fluids is anticipated. The choice of protective clothing should be dictated by the anticipated risk of exposure to body fluids during particular activities (Figure 12.2).

These principles are in line with the Health and Safety legislation, in particular the Control of Substances Hazardous to Health Regulations (COSHH), which dictate that measures should be taken to protect staff against exposure to substances, including body fluids, that may be hazardous to health. An important principle of these regulations is that procedures should be assessed to establish the likely exposure and to define the measures required to prevent and control exposure (p. 110).

Gloves

Clean disposable gloves should be readily available in all clinical areas and worn for any activity likely to involve direct contact with body fluids or moist body sites, such as mucous membranes (e.g. mouth, vagina). They prevent contamination of the skin and protect cuts and abrasions from infection, but to successfully

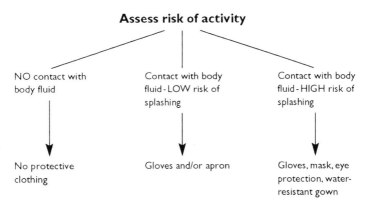

Figure 12.2 Risk assessment in the selection of protective clothing. The risk of exposure to blood or body fluid should be assessed before commencing a procedure. Source: Wilson 1995.

interrupt the transmission of infection to others they must be changed after each procedure. Hands should always be washed after gloves have been removed as the gloves may have been punctured during the procedure and the hands may be contaminated when the gloves are removed (Olsen et al 1993). Washing or disinfecting gloved hands between procedures has been advocated (Grinnell 1998), but is not to be encouraged as microorganisms that survive will be transmitted to others. In addition, gloves that are punctured unknowingly may have allowed body fluids to reach and remain in contact with the skin for prolonged periods, exposing the wearer to the risk of infection (Adams et al 1992).

Disposable gloves are made of either latex or vinyl. Latex gloves conform well to the hands and enable dexterity to be maintained; however, latex sensitisation can make their use inappropriate for some staff (Medical Devices Agency 1996). Vinyl gloves have a much looser fit but are not associated with sensitisation reactions.

Gloves cannot prevent percutaneous injuries but reduce the risk of infection by blood-borne viruses by reducing the volume of blood reaching the punctured skin (Rhodes & Bell 1995). Wearing two pairs of gloves can prevent some percutaneous injuries (Gerberding et al 1990) and has been advised for certain procedures where the risk of injury is high, e.g. orthopaedic and gynaecological surgery (UK Health Departments, 1998).

Masks and eye protection

Masks were introduced in the early 1900s and were advocated for surgical procedures and for caring for patients with infectious diseases such as diphtheria. Although improvements have been made to the filtering efficacy of these early models, modern masks are effective only if they fit closely around the mouth and nose, otherwise air is inhaled and exhaled around the edge of the mask and so is not filtered. Masks worn for prolonged periods become damp with exhaled air, preventing air passing easily through the mask and increasing the amount that flows around the edges (Belkin 1997). In addition, it is now recognised that health staff do not expel pathogens from the upper respiratory tract (Ayliffe 1991).

Masks are now rarely used in ward areas, but widely used in operating theatres, despite studies questioning their value for those not directly involved in the operation, and no evidence that they reduce the incidence of surgical wound infection (Hubble et al 1996). Masks and eye protection should be worn by personnel likely to be splashed by blood or body fluids, as there is a small risk of acquiring blood-borne viruses after splashes into the eye or mouth (Communicable Disease Report 1998). This includes some surgical and obstetric procedures, endoscopy and cleaning of surgical instruments. A wide range of protective eye wear and face shields is available for use in clinical areas.

Aprons and gowns

Plastic disposable aprons provide an effective and convenient method of protecting the clothing from contamination by microorganisms. The front of the body is most prone to contamination and most likely to transmit infection to others; aprons therefore provide adequate protection in most circumstances (Babb et al 1983). However, if cross-infection is to be avoided, they must be changed between procedures and especially between caring for different patients.

Cotton gowns are not water-repellent and provide minimal protection against contamination. Their main use is as sterile outer clothing for use in operative procedures, where, provided they are made from closely woven material they can reduce the dispersal of bacteria from the operator's skin (Whyte et al 1990). Wet cotton allows bacteria to pass through readily (Holborn 1990). In operating theatres, some surgical procedures involve considerable contamination with blood or body fluids and the use of disposable or reusable water-repellent gowns should be considered.

DECONTAMINATION OF EQUIPMENT

Inadequately decontaminated equipment is frequently responsible for the transmission of infection between patients. The risk of transmission depends on the degree of contamination with body fluids, the number of microbes present and the type of contact between the equipment and susceptible sites on the patient. Items that have contact with intact skin, e.g. sphygmomanometer cuffs, are unlikely to be heavily contaminated or to have contact with susceptible sites and therefore have a low risk of transmitting infection. On the other hand, surgical instruments will be heavily contaminated with blood or body fluids after use and if used without prior decontamination inside a subsequent patient's body present a major risk of introducing infection.

Equipment that is used to contain fluids is particularly vulnerable to contamination and can act as an effective source of infection if not decontaminated properly. Cefai et al (1990) reported an outbreak of respiratory tract infections caused by acinetobacter due to inadequate disinfection of ventilation equipment and Botman & de Krieger (1987) described how contaminated nebulisers caused pathogens to colonise the oropharynx. Even disinfectant or soap solutions can support the growth of microorganisms and act as a source of infection (Oie & Kamiya 1996). Equipment should not be stored in solutions of disinfectant but should be thoroughly cleaned and dried and then stored dry.

The level of decontamination required for a piece of equipment therefore needs to be assessed, taking into account its potential as a source or vehicle of infection. The principles of this risk assessment and methods of decontamination are discussed in Chapter 6.

It is important to have a written policy clearly defining the level, method and frequency of decontamination of each item after use. This is often described as a disinfection policy and is drawn up by the infection control team. The recommended methods should be applied in all situations and not only after equipment has been used on an infectious patient. Advice on decontamination should be sought from the infection control team when there is doubt and before introducing new pieces of equipment. Consideration must also be given to staff who service or repair clinical equipment. The equipment should be thoroughly decontaminated beforehand and a certificate should be completed when this has been carried out (NHS Management Executive 1993).

MAINTAINING A CLEAN ENVIRONMENT

While the environment may contain many microorganisms, the majority are not harmful and they are not readily transferred into susceptible sites where they could cause infection. This was demonstrated in a study by Maki et al in 1982, who sampled the environment of an old hospital building for several months before the hospital moved into a new building. Subsequent sampling from the new building showed that initially there were far fewer pathogens but after 12 months the numbers had risen and were similar to those found in the old building. The incidence of hospital-acquired infection did not change either before or after the move and was the same 12 months later and the authors concluded that organisms in the hospital environment did not make a major contribution to endemic infection in hospital patients. Collins (1988) pointed out that a microbe-free environment is neither practicable nor desirable. The aim of good environmental control should be to 'minimise the number of organisms present' and make the surroundings unfavourable to those organisms most likely to cause problems. Most bacteria will not survive for long in a clean and dry environment; surfaces should therefore be kept in good condition, intact, smooth and dry so that they cannot harbour dirt and bacteria. Moist surfaces can present a microbiological hazard because bacteria are able to survive on them more easily; however to cause infection there must be a suitable vehicle to carry them to a susceptible site on the patient.

The environment may play a part in the transmission of pathogens that are highly resistant to desiccation. *Clostridium difficile* survives for long periods in dry environments because it forms spores. Extensive contamination of the environment may occur where a patient has a colitis due to *Clostridium difficile* and this has been implicated as the source of infection in outbreaks of infection (Hoffman 1993). There is still considerable debate about the role of the environment in the transmission of some antibiotic-resistant pathogens such as methicillin-resistant *Staphylococcus aureus* (MRSA). These bacteria survive for long periods in dust on surfaces and may then be transferred to other patients. However, transient carriage on the hands of staff is responsible for most cases of cross-infection with this organism and neither the environment nor airborne particles are an important route of transmission (Mylotte 1994, Barrett et al 1993).

Floors

These may be contaminated with a wide variety of microorganisms, mostly introduced with dust as it settles on the surface. Dust is largely composed of skin scales and fabric fibres; some particles carry microorganisms, but not many of these are able to survive for long without moisture. Regular removal of dust, either by vacuum cleaner or dust-control mop, ensures that the number of microorganisms is kept to a minimum and that they are not re-dispersed into the air. Wiping with a damp mop tends to redistribute rather than remove dust; however it is required for the removal of heavy soiling or spillages. Disinfectants remove a significant proportion of bacteria from floors but are of no value for routine use as bacterial numbers return to the same level within a short time (Ayliffe et al 1967). They do have a place in the treatment of body fluid spills: in particular, spills of blood should be covered with sodium dichloroisocyanurate granules (e.g. Presept) or 1% hypochlorite solution to ensure that any blood-borne virus present is destroyed before the spillage is removed (UK Health Departments 1998, Coates & Wilson 1989). These chemicals should not be put on urine spills as irritant chlorine vapour may be released (Department of Health, 1990). They should also not be used on fabrics or carpets as they will damage the material.

Mops become heavily contaminated with bacteria if not cleaned regularly. They should be laundered and dried at least daily. Water used for mopping should be changed regularly and discarded after use, mops should always be stored dry, as microorganisms will multiply rapidly on mops left in buckets of dirty water (Maurer 1985).

There is no evidence that carpets present a risk of infection, but they should be washable and have short, water-repellent fibres to enable spills to be dealt with easily. They can be cleaned routinely with a vacuum cleaner but will be damaged by many chemical disinfectants. Detergent and water and a cleaning machine should be used to remove spillages, and carpeting in clinical areas where frequent spills occur is therefore impractical.

Furniture

Furniture and fittings simply require regular dusting of horizontal surfaces and spot cleaning of spills or splashes with detergent. Dust accumulates on bed frames and as they are particularly vulnerable to the collection of dust they must be included in cleaning schedules. Mattresses with smooth impermeable covers do not support the growth of microorganisms. If contaminated with body fluid they should be cleaned with detergent and water. Some chemicals, e.g. phenol, should not be used as they damage the cover. Mattresses can become a hazard if the cover is damaged and bacteria gain access (Loomes 1988). Outbreaks of infection related to damaged mattresses have been reported and it is therefore important to check the condition of the covers and turn the mattresses over regularly to prolong their life (Department of Health 1991a, Sherertz & Sullivan 1985)

Sinks, baths and toilets

Bacteria survive easily in these moist environments but are not readily transferred to susceptible sites on a patient and as a result are an unlikely source of infection. Most species of bacteria colonising taps and washbasins are environmental and not human pathogens (Orsi et al 1994).

Baths will become contaminated if used by patients with large open wounds. Dowsett & Wilson (1981) reported an outbreak of infections in episiotomy wounds, caused by group A streptococci, associated with the use of two baths in the ward. Bath water was found to be moderately contaminated with coliforms and streptococci before patients got into the water and heavily contaminated after bathing. The badly scratched and chipped enamel in these baths probably contributed to microbial contamination, especially as patients were expected to clean the bath themselves after use, as a smooth surface is essential for effective cleaning. Baths should be thoroughly cleaned with detergent between patients and harsh scouring agents or salt, which can damage the enamel surface, should be avoided. Bath hoists have also been associated with cross-infection and should be cleaned with detergent after each use (Murdoch 1990).

Regular cleaning with detergent should be sufficient to minimise the risk of basins and toilets acting as a source of infection; disinfectants have not been shown to have any advantages (Newsom 1972, Nystrom 1981).

Ventilation systems

In most situations airborne microorganisms do not present a significant infection hazard. Some hospitals have isolation rooms with negative pressure ventilation systems. These maintain a lower pressure inside the isolation room so that air flows from other ward areas into the isolation room rather than in the reverse direction. Air is extracted from the room to the outside or through filters. This helps to contain pathogens in the isolation room and ensure that they are ventilated outside the building not into adjacent rooms in the ward. However, most infectious diseases are not spread by an airborne route and special ventilation is therefore not often necessary.

Microbes can also be removed from air by filtration. This is most important in operating theatres, where the risk of introducing microorganisms into susceptible sites is high. Burns are also particularly vulnerable to infection, as pathogens readily gain access to the bloodstream and cause septicaemia. Ayliffe & Lowbury (1982) demonstrated that the number of bacteria in the air increased during the removal of dressings from burns. The use of filtered air and a ventilation system to change the air volume 20 times per hour reduced the number of airborne bacteria and minimised the risk of introducing them into wounds.

Operating theatre ventilation

In the operating theatre tissues that are normally protected by the skin are exposed for a considerable time. It is therefore important for the air to be as free from microorganisms as possible. The greatest source of airborne bacteria is people. Bacteria are constantly shed on tiny flakes of skin (squames), with as many as 10 000 squames being released from one person in a minute (Howarth 1985) 10% of which may carry microorganisms. Friction of the clothing against the skin during movement is particularly likely to increase skin squame release. The number of bacteria in the air is therefore related to the number of people present in the room (Suzuki et al 1984). Microorganisms in the air settle into the exposed tissues or on to instruments and those introduced into the wound can subsequently cause infection of the surgical site (Barrie et al 1992). To reduce the number of microorganisms, air is passed through very fine high-efficiency particulate (HEPA) filters, which trap the majority of microorganisms. Air is extracted, filtered and delivered to the operating room at a measured rate, usually equivalent to changing the volume of the room 20 times an hour. This ensures that the air in the room is continuously passed through the filters.

The direction in which air flows is also important and is controlled by pressure gradients between different zones. The pressure is highest in the cleanest areas, i.e. preparation and operating rooms; and lowest in the changing and sluice rooms so that air flows from clean to dirty areas.

Ultraclean ventilation systems aim to produce very highly filtered air in the operating zone. The demonstration of their value in reducing the incidence of deep infections following orthopaedic joint replacement surgery has resulted in their widespread use for orthopaedic surgery in the UK (Gosden et al 1998). This type of ventilation introduces fast-flowing air through a bank of filters on the wall or ceiling and produces a laminar flow of highly filtered air across the operating site at a rate of 600 air changes per hour. Staff standing in the laminar flow will cause turbulence and the skin squames released can enter the wound. This problem can be overcome by the use of ventilated air-proof suits, although these have the disadvantage of hindering movement and being uncomfortable to wear.

Environmental sampling

Sampling of the environment is of very limited value in hospitals and should only be undertaken on the advice of the infection control team and with a clear purpose in mind. Sometimes it may be necessary when investigating an outbreak of infection (Box 12.2) or testing the quality of food production or efficacy of air filtration. However, specialist knowledge is required to devise the sampling method and to interpret the results. Sampling may also be used as part of an education programme to demonstrate the presence of bacteria and the significance of infection control measures.

SAFE HANDLING OF SHARP INSTRUMENTS

Injuries with contaminated sharp instruments present a major hazard to healthcare workers. They can result in localised skin infections or septicaemia, but more seriously are associated with transmission of the blood-borne viruses. The risk of acquiring human immunodeficiency virus (HIV) after a single injury with a contaminated needle is low, less than 1%, but it depends on the volume of blood transferred and the infectivity of the source patient. Since the epidemic of AIDS was first recognised, four healthcare workers in the UK are known to have acquired HIV following a percutaneous injury with a contaminated sharp; a further eight have probably acquired the virus in this way, although evidence for the source is not complete (Public Health Laboratory Service 1998). The risk of acquiring Hepatitis B after single injury with a contaminated sharp

---

Box 12.2 The use of environmental sampling in an outbreak investigation (Source: Barrie et al 1992)

This case report illustrates how environmental sampling can sometimes be of value in the investigation of an outbreak.

Following neurosurgery two patients developed meningitis caused by an organism not usually associated with meningitis, *Bacillus cereus*. The infections occurred a few days after surgery, before dressings were changed or drains were handled, and they were caused by unrelated strains of the organism. It seemed likely that the *B. cereus* was acquired from a common source in the operating theatre, and sampling of the air, environment and equipment was therefore carried out.

Swabs were taken from surfaces, equipment and air filters in the theatre, nine yielded a few colonies of *B. cereus* and small numbers were also found in sampled air. However, the impression plates taken from linen, including theatre scrub suits, strongly indicated the probable source of the organism. A heavy growth of *B. cereus* was found on 25 plates and a moderate growth on a further 16 impression plates. This was a highly unusual finding as freshly laundered linen would be expected to contain very few bacteria; indeed impression plates taken from linen laundered at other hospitals grew fewer than five colonies of *B. cereus*. More than half of the impression plates taken from the hands of staff in theatre also grew *B. cereus*, one plate taken from a surgeon who had just put on a scrub suit grew 24 colonies. The organisms on staff hands were probably acquired as a result of contact with contaminated linen.

The two cases of meningitis probably occurred as a result of *B. cereus* from contaminated scrub suits becoming airborne on small particles of lint and settling directly in the wound or on surgical instruments that were subsequently inserted into the wound. In both cases, the surgery lasted more than 6 hours, so that there was considerable opportunity for the organism to enter the wound in this way.

---

instrument is much higher. In the case of blood from an e-antigen-positive hepatitis B carrier the risk is one in four (Royal College of Pathologists, 1992). Several healthcare workers have been reported to have acquired hepatitis B infection occupationally each year (Ross et al 1998). Many other cases probably go unrecognised. Hepatitis C screening tests only became available in 1990 and currently little is known about the risk of transmission to healthcare workers, although cases have been reported (Neal et al 1997, Cariani et al 1991).

Causes of sharps injuries

In clinical areas, injuries commonly occur while sharp instruments are being used, for example when inserting needles or giving injections, and are often due to the patient moving unexpectedly (Eisenstein & Smith 1992). However, as many as a third of injuries occur during re-capping of a needle (Jagger 1988), which still appears to be a commonplace practice (Becker et al 1990). 25% of injuries occur as a result of sharps being left on beds, trolleys or locker tops, or discarded into waste or laundry bags, and highlights the importance of the person using the sharp being responsible for its safe disposal (Eisenstein & Smith, 1992). Even where appropriate sharps containers are used, careless assembly or overfilling results in sharps protruding from the bin and injury to people who use or dispose of them (Saghafi et al 1992).

The risk of sharps injury is particularly high in operating theatres, although it varies according to the type of surgical procedure being performed, with the highest rates being reported in gynaecological procedures. Percutaneous injuries have been reported in as many as 21% of vaginal hysterectomies (Tokars et al 1992). They are commonly associated with suturing, particularly if fingers are used to hold tissue, or when used needles or scalpel blades are replaced (Jagger et al 1990). Assistants are vulnerable to injury when instruments are passed from the surgeon.

Prevention of sharps injuries

Many percutaneous injuries could be prevented by proper preparation for procedures involving the use of sharps. Appropriate containers must be readily available and should either be taken to the point of use or the used sharps returned to the container in a receiver or tray, not carried by hand. Sharps must never be left on trolleys or locker tops or in makeshift containers, a particular problem with lancets used for blood glucose monitoring. The most important principles of safe sharps management are summarised in List 12.3.

Sharps containers must conform to the British Standard specification (List 12.4) and must be of sufficient size to contain the largest disposable sharp instrument used in the department. Procedures need to be in place to ensure that sharps containers are securely closed and replaced when three-quarters full. Most containers require assembly and this must be done thoroughly to ensure that they do not come apart during use or disposal (Medical Devices Agency 1993).

Needles are often re-capped in order to carry them to a container. This dangerous procedure is unnecessary if the sharps container is taken to the point of use. If re-capping is essential, it is safer to place the cap on a flat surface and insert the needle into it without holding the cap in a hand. Unnecessary handling of sharps, e.g. disconnecting needles and syringes, should be avoided.

List 12.3   Important principles of safe sharps management

- Discard sharps immediately after use into an appropriate container
- Use sharps bins that comply with BS7320
- Ensure a sharps bin is available at the point where the sharp is used
- Do not re-cap needles
- Do not disassemble needles, syringes or intravenous cannulas
- Always report sharps injuries to the Occupational Health Department
- Assemble sharps bins properly and seal when three-quarters full

In the operating theatre:
- Do not pass sharps from hand to hand: use a tray
- Use blunt suture needles where possible
- Use a thimble or needle-guard for suturing
- Remove scalpels carefully on a flat surface
- Wear two pairs of gloves for procedures with a high risk of needlestick injury
- Keep needles and blades safe prior to disposal
- Ensure that plenty of sharps bins of sufficient size are available

---

List 12.4   British standard for sharps containers (Source: British Standard 7320 – British Standards Institute 1990)

Suitable containers intended to hold used sharps should:
- be resistant to penetration
- not leak or break open when dropped
- have a closure device that does not open when carried or dropped
- be yellow
- be marked with the words: *Danger. Contaminated sharps only. Destroy by incineration.*
- have an indication of when 70–80% full
- have a handle

A number of measures can be used to prevent sharps injuries in operating departments:

- Blunt tipped needles can be used for suturing and stapling devices used for skin and bowel closure (UK Health Departments 1998)

- Needle holders with integral guards and thimbles have been recommended for the protection of fingers during suturing (Smith & Grant 1990)

- Sharps containers must be readily available and of appropriate size

- Sharp instruments should not be passed from hand to hand but picked up from a surface such as a tray or magnetic mat

- Blades should be removed by using a disarming device or pressing downwards on to a firm surface so that they do not fly off; they should then be stored safely
  - Disposable sharps can be added to instrument counting procedures to help ensure that all in use are safely discarded
  - Clear responsibility for sharps disposal should be established.

Double gloving can significantly reduce the risk of the inner glove becoming punctured and is particularly recommended for procedures associated with a high risk of injury, e.g. gynaecology (UK Health Departments 1998, Gerberding et al 1990). Telford & Quebberman (1993) recommend combining an outer glove of the usual size with an inner glove one size larger, for greatest comfort.

Management of sharps injuries

Although most hospitals have systems in place for reporting sharps injuries to their Occupational Health Department, as many as 70% are not reported (Mangione et al 1991). Reporting such injuries is important, firstly, to ensure that the appropriate treatment and follow-up is provided, e.g. Hepatitis B vaccination or immunoglobulin and secondly, to collate data on the incidence of sharps injuries and identify factors that contribute to injuries so that further injuries can be prevented. All healthcare workers, including those working in the community, should be aware of the procedures for reporting and receiving treatment for sharps injuries incurred at work (Department of Health, 1993; Figure 12.3).

Hepatitis B vaccination

All staff who have contact with blood and body fluids should be vaccinated against hepatitis B (Department of Health 1996). Vaccination comprises a course of three injections and confers protection in the majority of people, although a booster dose is recommended after 5 years. Vaccination is important, not only to protect the healthcare worker from a potential serious disease but also to protect patients from staff who may otherwise become carriers of the virus and transmit it to patients during invasive procedures. Numerous incidents of patients who have acquired hepatitis B following an invasive procedure performed by an infected member of staff have been reported (Heptonstall 1991).

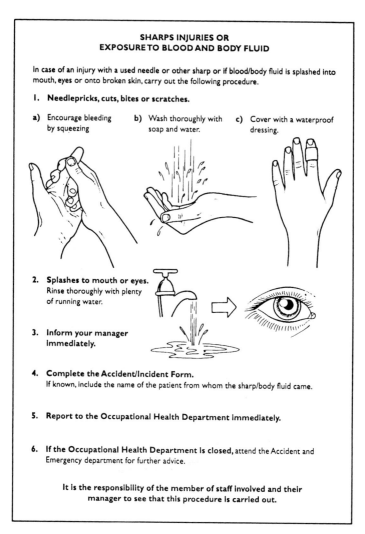

Figure 12.3 Management of sharps injuries or exposure to blood or body fluids. Source: Wilson 1995.

Sharps injuries involving blood infected or strongly suspected to be infected with HIV

Postexposure prophylaxis with an antiviral drug may reduce the risk of developing infection if given very soon after the exposure. Advice on how to assess the risk of acquiring HIV and when to administer postexposure prophylaxis has been issued by the Department of Health, and local policies based on this advice should be in place for health care workers (Department of Health 1997).

MANAGEMENT OF WASTE

Waste from hospitals, clinics, pharmacies or other healthcare facilities may be infectious or toxic and therefore requires careful disposal. Although microorganisms are unlikely to be transmitted from such clinical waste it is important to manage it in such a way that the risk is eliminated (Griffiths 1989).

The Environmental Protection Act 1990 defines the responsibilities of those who produce waste and the Health and Safety Executive has recommended how clinical waste should be handled and discarded safely (Health and Safety Executive 1992). There is a national colour-coding system for waste to ensure that any hazardous material reaches the correct disposal destination (Table 12.1). Any waste contaminated with blood or body fluids or used on an infectious patient should be placed in yellow bags for destruction. Human tissue is also incinerated but should be segregated from other waste. Sharp instruments must be discarded into rigid, puncture-proof containers and disposed of by incineration.

Since the introduction of higher standards for the design of incinerators and control of their emissions, many hospitals, which previously incinerated a large volume of their waste on site, are unable to comply with the regulations (Department of Health

Table 12.1 Colour coding for the disposal of clinical waste (Source: Health and Safety Executive, 1992)

Colour of bag	Type of waste	Method of disposal
Black	Household waste; uncontaminated paper, plastic, food, etc.	Landfill
Yellow	Material contaminated with blood or body fluid, human or animal tissue	Incineration
Yellow sharps containers	Needles, syringes, broken glass and any other contaminated sharp item	Incineration
Blue or transparent with blue inscription	Material from microbiology laboratories	Autoclave, then incineration

1991b). It is now common for hospitals to employ external contractors to collect and dispose of their waste. However, a considerable proportion of waste generated in clinical areas is not contaminated and as such can be considered as household waste suitable for disposal in landfill sites. Household waste is much cheaper to dispose of and efficient segregation of this waste can have considerable advantages in terms of both costs and harm to the environment (Audit Commission 1997). Supplies department should take disposal into account when selecting products as purchasing those with minimal packaging can significantly reduce the volume of waste produced (Daschner & Dettenkofer 1997). List 12.5 details items that should be considered clinical waste and require incineration.

List 12.5 Definition of clinical waste (Source: London Waste Regulation Authority)

- Soiled surgical dressings, swabs and instruments
- Material (other than linen) from patients with infectious disease
- Human and animal tissue, blood and excretions
- Discarded syringes, needles, cartridges, broken glass and other sharp surgical instruments in contact with the above
- Pharmaceutical and chemical products used for treatment purposes
- Used disposable bedpan liners, urine containers, incontinence pads, sanitary towels and other items contaminated with body fluid

---

Microbiological laboratory waste, including specimens, culture plates and media, requires sterilisation by autoclaving before it is incinerated. Such waste is marked by placing in blue bags or transparent bags with blue writing.

Management of waste collection

Simple written policies for operating and controlling waste collection are essential. All staff should understand how and where different types of waste should be discarded and the importance of not overfilling bags so that they can be securely closed. Portering and domestic staff who may be involved in removal of waste from clinical areas should be trained in how to handle bags safely. Sharp instruments should never be placed into plastic or paper bags as they can protrude and cause injury to people subsequently handling the bag. Sharps containers must be clearly marked so that they can be handled with care and staff must be trained on what action to take in the event of spillage or injury. Some hospitals label bags and sharps containers with the point of origin so that if problems subsequently occur the source of the bag can be identified (Gibbs 1990).

Areas where waste is stored need to be secure from animals and inquisitive children and must be easy to clean. Different-coloured bags should be stored in designated areas.

Disposal of clinical waste in the community

Waste produced at home and handled only by patients or their families (e.g. incontinence pads) is considered household waste and is therefore exempt from the duty of care prescribed by the Environmental Protection Act (Department of the Environment, 1990). The volume of such waste is minimal and when mixed with large quantities of ordinary household waste it does not present an infection hazard. Contaminated needles, such as those used by insulin-dependant diabetics, could be more dangerous and these should be discarded into sharps containers where possible. Some pharmacies and clinics provide facilities for collection of sharps containers, but where this is not available some other form of rigid container, e.g. a can, should be used.

However, healthcare workers who produce clinical waste in the patient's own home are obliged to arrange for its proper disposal. Portable sharps containers can be used to contain used sharps and small dressings for incineration. Local authorities have a legal obligation to collect infectious waste if requested, but this usually only applies to waste from dialysis patients or those infected with HIV.

Disposal of excreta

With very few exceptions (e.g. excreta from patients with viral haemorrhagic fever) urine, faeces and waste water from hospitals can be released into the sewage system without any special treatment. Excreta should never be covered with disinfectant prior to disposal as it is both ineffective and increases the possibility of spillage occurring while the bedpan and its contents remain in the sluice. Excreta should be discarded directly into the drainage system, either in a toilet, bedpan washer or macerator. To prevent the transmission of microorganisms between patients, bedpans must either be disposable or heat-disinfected in a bedpan washer.

Faults in either type of machine must be reported promptly. Bedpan washers that do not reach 80°C for at least 1 minute will not decontaminate the bedpan (Central Sterilising Club 1986). Macerators should have an effective seal around the lid to prevent the escape of contaminated aerosols and the plastic bedpan holders must be thoroughly washed in detergent and water to prevent any risk of residual contamination resulting in cross-infection.

MANAGEMENT OF LINEN

In the past many hospitals had their own laundry. Now it is more common for the laundering service to be contracted to commercial laundries. Linen is sent to the laundry in bags and sorted into batches of sheets, blankets, pillow cases, etc. Each batch is usually washed in large, continuous tunnel washers that can process as many as ten batches of linen at one time (Barrie 1994). Laundry staff are exposed to microorganisms on linen during the sorting process and microbiologically hazardous linen, e.g. from patients with particular infections, must be disinfected by washing without prior sorting. It should be put into water-soluble or alginate stitched bags at the bedside, then into an outer red bag, transported to the laundry and placed directly into a designated washing machine without opening. The recommended categorisation of linen is described in Table 12.2.

Table 12.2   Categories of hospital linen (Source: NHS Executive 1995)

Category	Bag colour	Description	Recommended process
Used	White linen or clear plastic	Soiled and foul linen	Thermal disinfection by washing at 65°C for 10 minutes or 71°C for 3 minutes
Infected	Water-soluble bag, with red outer bag	Linen used by patients with certain infectious diseases or as advised by ICT	Not sorted prior to washing; thermal disinfection as 'used linen'
Heat-labile	Orange stripe	Fabrics damaged by thermal disinfection, e.g.wool	Washing at 40°C and addition of hypochlorite to penultimate rinse

Microorganisms contaminating the linen are removed by the action of detergent and water and the linen is disinfected by the temperature in the wash, which must reach a minimum of 65°C for 10 minutes or 71°C for 3 minutes. There must be sufficient time for mixing to ensure that all parts of the load reach the correct temperature. A prewash at a temperature below 40°C is used to remove blood and faeces. Fabrics that are damaged by high temperatures should be disinfected by adding hypochlorite to the rinse cycle (NHS Executive 1995).

Risks to laundry workers

Protective clothing, including gloves, overalls and boots, should be used by laundry workers to avoid contamination with the normal faecal flora, which may be present on used linen (NHS Executive 1995). Combined with good personal hygiene, especially hand washing, this should be an adequate safeguard against infection. The danger from contaminated objects inadvertently discarded into linen bags is a much greater hazard and occurs surprisingly frequently (Figure 12.4). Sharp instruments present particular problems because of the risk of transmitting blood-borne viruses. Healthcare staff have a responsibility to ensure that such equipment is not put into laundry bags. Labelling bags with the ward name can help to identify the source of incorrectly bagged linen.

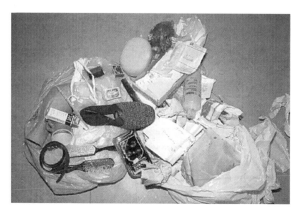

Figure 12.4   Examples of objects discarded into laundry bags.

Handling linen on the ward

On the ward used linen should be handled carefully to minimise the release of microorganisms; the important principles are summarised in List 12.6 (Overton 1988).

List 12.6   Safe handling of linen

- Linen should not be shaken but should be placed carefully into a linen bag
- Soiled linen should be bagged according to local guidelines and these should comply with health service guidance (HSG(95)18)
- Bags should be securely fastened
- Linen heavily soaked in body fluid should be contained in a plastic bag to prevent leakage
- Plastic aprons should be worn when handling soiled linen
- Hands should be washed after contact with soiled linen

Bedding used in clinical areas must be made of fabrics able to withstand heat disinfection and this should be considered when new linen is purchased. Wards sometimes use their own domestic washing machines to wash patients' clothing. Such machines must not be used to launder bedlinen as the wash temperatures are insufficient to ensure heat disinfection and proper drying and ironing facilities are not available.

Duvets are becoming more popular, with two types in common use: PVC-coated and fabric (Croton 1990, Ayton, 1983). PVC-coated duvets should be cleaned with detergent and water between patients. Fabric duvets should be able to withstand heat disinfection and must comply with fire retardancy standards (Barrie 1994). They should be laundered at least every 3 months and when soiled (Webster et al 1986). Fabric duvet covers should be laundered between patients.

FOOD HYGIENE

Several hundred outbreaks of food-borne gastrointestinal infections, in addition to sporadic cases, are reported in England and Wales every year (Cowden et al 1995). The microorganisms most commonly associated with food-borne infection are listed in Table 12.3.

Table 12.3 Common food-borne infections (Source: PHLS Salmonella Committee 1995)

Micro-organism	Common source	Symptoms
Bacillus spp.	Cereals, dried foods, dairy products	Vomiting, 1–5 h after ingestion; diarrhoea few hours after ingestion
Campylobacter spp.	Raw or undercooked meat, poultry, untreated water, unpasteurised milk	Profuse diarrhoea, severe abdominal pain; incubation 2–5 d; prodromal phase of headache and photophobia
Clostridium perfringens	Cooked meats, gravy, fish, dried foods, vegetables	Diarrhoea, abdominal pain 8–22 h after ingestion
Escherichia coli (toxogenic strains)	Raw or undercooked beef, milk, vegetables, infected animals	Diarrhoea (can progress to haemolytic uraemic syndrome). Incubation period 1–6 d
Salmonella typhi/paratyphi	Food in contact with an infected human carrier or contaminated by sewage	Fever, malaise, constipation followed by diarrhoea. Incubation 1–3 weeks
Other salmonellas	Meat, especially poultry, eggs, milk, dairy products	Diarrhoea, vomiting, fever, 12–72 h after ingestion
Shigella spp.	Faecally contaminated water and food eg salads	Diarrhoea, fever, abdominal pain, 1–7 d after ingestion
Staphylococcus aureus	Cold food handled during preparation, dairy products	Vomiting, abdominal pain 1–7 h after ingestion
Gastrointestinal viruses, e.g.SRSV, Norwalk agent, rotavirus	Contaminated water, shellfish, cold foods handled during preparation	Vomiting, diarrhoea, fever, abdominal pain 24–48 h after ingestion

Gastrointestinal infection is commonly acquired through the ingestion of contaminated food or water; however transmission from person to person can also occur, particularly in hospital settings where patients are in close proximity to each other and have regular contact with staff. The effects of the infection may be more severe in people who are debilitated or frail and either the disease itself or associated dehydration can cause or accelerate the patient's death.

There are many ways in which poor practice in the handling or preparation of food can result in contamination by pathogens and subsequent cases of food poisoning. The most common causes of food poisoning are given in List 12.7. The essential aspects of safe food production from animal slaughter to the point of sale are defined in the Food Safety Act 1990. The Food Safety (General Food Hygiene) Regulations 1995 apply to food premises and specify the mandatory training of people who handle food. Specific guidance on the management of food in healthcare establishments is contained in the guidance document *Management of Food Services and Food Hygiene in the National Health Service* (NHS Management Executive 1992). The important principles of food hygiene are described below and summarised in List 12.8.

List 12.7   Common causes of food poisoning Source: Roberts 1982

- Food prepared too far in advance
- Food stored at room temperature
- Food cooled too slowly prior to refrigeration
- Food not reheated to a high enough temperature to destroy food poisoning bacteria
- Cooked food contaminated with food-poisoning bacteria
- Meat and meat products undercooked
- Frozen meat and poultry not thawed completely
- Cross-contamination from raw to cooked foods
- Hot food stored below 63°C
- Food handlers with gastrointestinal infection

Food preparation

Raw food is frequently contaminated with bacteria, some of which are pathogenic for humans. In particular, meat and poultry products may be contaminated with bacteria from the intestine of the animal, such as salmonella, campylobacter, toxigenic strains of *Escherichia coli* and *Clostridium perfringens*. Although these pathogens are found only in approximately 1% of red meat, salmonella has been detected in nearly 50% of raw poultry carcasses and some eggs (Mackey 1989, De Louvois 1993). Vegetables may be contaminated by organisms present in soil e.g. *Clostridium perfringens*, and rice often contains *Bacillus cereus*. Milk and dairy products support the growth of a variety of pathogens and can be contaminated during collection or processing.

List 12.8   Key principles of food hygiene

- Thaw frozen meat before cooking
- Cook food thoroughly
- Do not allow raw food to come into contact with cooked food
- Store cold food below 5°C
- Keep hot food above 63°C
- Reheat food to a temperature of 70°C
- Wash hands before and after handling food and between handling raw and cooked foods
- Wash utensils and chopping boards after each use
- Ensure all kitchen surfaces are intact and are kept clean and dry

---

To establish infection, most gastrointestinal pathogens need to be ingested in reasonably large numbers to overcome the acidic environment of the stomach. Provided food is thoroughly cooked, most microorganisms will be destroyed. However, many cases of food poisoning occur when previously cooked food, such as ham, comes into contact with raw contaminated food. Pathogenic bacteria may then multiply freely and will not be destroyed by further cooking prior to ingestion. Separating cooked and raw foods is therefore an essential principle of good food hygiene. Separation includes the use of separate knives, bowls, chopping boards and washing hands between handling different types of food. Vegetables, fruit and salads that are eaten raw should be washed in running water to remove microorganisms.

Gastrointestinal viruses, such as small round structured viruses (SRSV), are commonly transmitted by affected people who, while still excreting the virus, handle these types of food during the preparation of sandwiches, salads and desserts (Luthi et al 1996). Outbreaks of SRSV are commonly associated with oysters that are contaminated by sewage in the water prior to harvesting and, since they are eaten raw, viruses are not destroyed before ingestion.

Chopping boards, knives and pots become contaminated by raw foods. Chopping boards should be colour-coded, each colour indicating a specific use (e.g. meat, vegetables etc.), designed for easy cleaning and washed with detergent and water after use. Cleaning cloths will harbour many bacteria and should be disposable.

Cooking

Most microorganisms are destroyed at cooking temperatures of 70°C, but the food needs to be held at this temperature for long enough to ensure that the heat penetrates it completely. Frozen food should be completely defrosted prior to cooking so that all parts are subjected to the cooking time and temperature to ensure that undercooking does not occur. This is particularly important for poultry, as such a large proportion are contaminated with salmonella in the raw state.

Cooked hot food should be served immediately or kept at 70°C and eaten within 2 hours. Reheating of cooked food should be avoided as far as possible. If it is essential the food should be re-cooked thoroughly in all parts. This is required to kill bacteria and some toxins, although some toxins are not easily destroyed by heat (e.g. *B. cereus*). A thermometer should be used to check this as some parts of the food, such as gravy, may heat up more quickly than others. Microwave ovens have a tendency to heat food unevenly. If a microwave oven is used to reheat food it should be allowed to stand for several minutes after heating to enable heat to distribute completely through the food (Lund et al 1989).

Food storage

Microorganisms will multiply in food if moisture is present and the temperature is between 20°C and 40°C. Food should therefore always be kept at temperatures either greater than 63°C or less than 5°C. The temperature in refrigerators should not rise above 5°C as most microorganisms will only be able to multiply slowly below this temperature. The exception is *Listeria monocytogenes*, which is frequently present in salads, cold meats and soft cheeses and continues to multiply in the refrigerator. Outbreaks of infection associated with chilled foods, salads and milk have occurred (Jones 1990). The standards for temperature control during storage, processing and distributing food are contained in the Food Safety (Temperature Controls) Regulations 1995.

Another problem is presented by bacteria such as *Bacillus cereus* and *Staphylococcus aureus*, which produce heat-stable toxins. If these bacteria are present in food stored at room temperature, they can multiply and produce large quantities of toxin, which will not be destroyed when the food is cooked or reheated. Cooked food should be cooled as quickly as possible, placed in the refrigerator and not stored for prolonged periods.

Supply and delivery of meals in hospitals

Meal delivery systems should be able to keep hot food above 63°C and cold food in a refrigerated compartment. Many hospitals use a cook–chill catering system. This means that food is prepared and cooked in the usual way but then is rapidly cooled to a temperature between 0 and 3°C. It can then be kept at this temperature for up to 5 days before re-heating immediately prior to consumption. In cook–freeze systems, meals are frozen within 30 minutes of preparation; they can then be stored at –18°C for up to 8 weeks and thawed before re-heating. Cook–chill or cook–freeze meals are delivered to the ward in chilled cabinets and re-heated for a set time and temperature in the cabinet. Provided the appropriate quality checks are in place, these food delivery systems can provide good quality and microbiologically safe meals (Department of Health 1989).

Staff training is a key component of ensuring safe food production, together with a systematic approach to monitoring standards of food safety and hygiene. A common approach is to use HACCP – hazard analysis critical control points. This identifies potential hazards in the production process, decides what controls are necessary and which are critical to consumer safety (the critical control points). Criteria to ensure safety are then defined for each control point (e.g. a particular temperature or checking process) and the system for monitoring the controls is agreed. Microbiological testing of food is sometimes used during the commissioning of a cook–chill or cook–freeze catering system to ensure that the process is safe, and may be used in the investigation of an outbreak of infection where a food-borne source is suspected. Routine microbiological sampling of food is not usually necessary.

Environmental health officers (EHO) are responsible for inspecting food premises to ensure that they comply with the food safety and food hygiene regulations. In general, they inspect all the food handling areas in a hospital twice a year.

Ward kitchens

The principles of food hygiene also apply at ward level and staff involved in handling food or serving meals should receive training. There should be clear policies for the use of microwave ovens, ice-making machines and refrigerators. Refrigerators in ward kitchens should only be used for patients' food and items should be clearly labelled with the patient's name and the date. There should be a local policy about when food should be discarded and who is responsible for this. The temperature inside the refrigerator should be checked regularly (Goldthorpe et al 1991).

Ice-making machines have been associated with outbreaks of infection, particularly among immunosuppressed patients (Ravn et al 1991). They need to be regularly cleaned and maintained and ice should not be removed by hand as this may transfer pathogens on to ice remaining in the machine (Barrie 1994).

Re-heating food in ward kitchens can also present hazards. Food for patients away from the ward at mealtimes should not be saved for more than an hour as bacteria may multiply in the food during this time. Where food has been saved, it must be thoroughly re-heated. Catering departments should be able to offer a flexible service for patients who have missed meals. There should be clear rules about the use and cleaning of microwave ovens and the storage of food at ward level.

Ward kitchens are subject to the food hygiene regulations and can be inspected by the environmental health officer. Many infection control teams also take a keen interest in auditing ward kitchens to ensure that food is being stored and handled correctly. Surfaces should be smooth, clean and dry and soap and paper hand towels should be provided.

Personal hygiene

Microorganisms are readily transferred from the hands during food preparation; thus hand hygiene is an essential part of safe food production. Hands should always be washed before and after handling food and between handling raw and cooked foods. Someone suffering from a gastrointestinal illness can excrete large quantities of the infecting bacteria or viruses in faeces and vomit. In a recent review of food-borne gastrointestinal illness, 20% of outbreaks were associated with an infected food handler (Cowden et al 1995). Food handlers with gastrointestinal illness should therefore not work and must seek advice from the Occupational Health Department before returning. Some bacteria, e.g. salmonella, are excreted in faeces for many weeks after symptoms have resolved; therefore hand washing is of particular importance.

In ward areas, staff should wear clean plastic aprons and wash their hands prior to distributing meals to ensure that pathogens acquired on hands or clothing during the care of patients are not transferred to food.

Enteral feeding

Nasogastric tubes are commonly used to supply seriously ill patients unable to feed themselves. Infection control is an important part of the management of these enteral feeds as they can present considerable microbiological hazards (Crocker et al 1986). The feed solutions will readily support the growth of a wide range of bacteria. If introduced to the gut, some may cause gastroenteritis; others may be able to colonise the gut and are associated with pneumonia, which develops when the organisms are aspirated from the upper gastrointestinal tract (Craven et al 1991).

Most feed solutions are commercially produced and are supplied in prepacked sterile containers. A careful non-touch technique must then be used to transfer feeds to the administration set and reservoir and the solutions used must not be allowed to stand by the bedside for more than 24 hours (Ward et al 1997). Where special feeds are made up in the hospital kitchens, strict asepsis must be used to ensure that they are not contaminated during preparation and they should not be allowed to run over longer than 4 hours (Anderton et al 1986). Opened feed solutions should be refrigerated and discarded after 24 hours.

REFERENCES

Adams, D., Bagg, J., Limaye, M. *et al.* (1992) A clinical evaluation of glove washing and re-use in dental practice. *J. Hosp. Infect.*, **20**, 153–162.
Anderton, A., Howard, J.P. and Scott, D.W. (1986) *Microbiological Control in Enteral Feeding*. British Dietetic Association, London.
Ansari, S.A., Springthorpe, V.S., Sattar, S.A. *et al.* (1991) Potential role of hands in the spread of respiratory viral infections: studies with human parainfluenza virus 3 and rhinovirus 14. *J. Clin Microbiol.*, **29**, 2115–2119
Audit Commission (1997) *Getting Sorted – the Safe and Economic Management of Hospital Waste*. Audit Commission Bookpoint Ltd, Abingdon, Oxon.
Ayliffe, G.A.J. (1991) Masks in surgery? *J. Hosp. Infect.*, **18**, 165–166.
Ayliffe, G.A.J. and Lowbury, E.J.L. (1982) Airborne infection in hospital. *J. Hosp. Infect.*, **3**, 217–240.
Ayliffe, G.A.J., Collins, B.J. and Lowbury, E.J.L. (1967) Ward floors and other surfaces as reservoirs of hospital infection. *J. Hyg.(Lond.)*, **2**, 181.
Ayton, M. (1983) Continental quilts – their use in hospitals. *Nurs. Times*, **79**(30), 64–65.

Babb, J.R., Davies, J.G. and Ayliffe, G.A.J. (1983) Contamination of protective clothing and nurses' uniforms in an isolation ward. *J. Hosp. Infect.*, **4**, 49–57.

Barrett, S.P., Teare, E.L. and Sage, R. (1993) Methicillin-resistant *Staphylococcus aureus* in three adjacent Health Districts of South East England 1986–91. *J. Hosp. Infect.*, **24**, 313–325.

Barrie, D., Wilson, J.A., Hoffman, P.N. and Kramer, J.M. (1992) *Bacillus cereus* meningitis in two neurosurgical patients: an investigation into the source of the organism. *J. Infect.*, **25**, 291–297.

Barrie, D. (1994) How hospital linen and laundry services are provided. *J. Hosp. Infect.*, **27**, 219–235.

Barrie, D. (1996) The provision of food and catering services in hospital. *J. Hosp. Infect.*, **33**, 13–33.

Becker, M.H., Janz, N.K., Band, J. *et al.* (1990) Non-compliance with universal precautions policy: why do physicians and nurses recap needles? *Am. J. Infect. Control*, **18**, 232–239.

Belkin, N.L. (1997) The evolution of the surgical mask: filtering efficiency versus effectiveness. *Infect. Control Hosp. Epidemiol.*, **18**(1), 49–56.

Botman, M.J. and de Krieger, R.A. (1987) Contamination of small volume medication nebulisers and its association with orophayngeal colonisation *J. Hosp. Infect.*, **10**, 204–208.

British Standards Institute (1990) Specification for Sharps Containers. *BS 7320.* British Standards Institute, London.

Cariani, E., Zonaro, A., Primi, D. *et al.* (1991) Detection of hepatitis C virus RNA and antibodies after needlestick injuries. *Lancet*, **337**, 850.

Casewell, M. and Phillips, I. (1977) Hands as a route of transmission for *Klebsiella* species. *Br. Med. J.*, **ii** 1315–1317.

Cefai, C., Richards, J., Gould, F.K. *et al.* (1990) An outbreak of acinetobacter respiratory tract infection resulting from incomplete disinfection of ventilatory equipment. *J. Hosp. Infect.*, **15**, 177–182.

Centers for Disease Control (1987) Recommendations for the prevention of HIV transmission in health care settings. *MMWR*, **21 Aug**, 36 (2S).

Central Sterilising Club (1986) *Washer/Disinfectors. Report No. 1.* Central Sterilising Club, London.

Coates, D. and Wilson, M. (1989) Use of dichloroisocyanurate granules for spills of body fluids. *J. Hosp. Infect.*, **13**, 241–252.

Collins, B.J. (1988) The hospital environment: how clean should a hospital be? *J. Hosp. Infect.*, **11**, (Suppl. A): 53–56.

Communicable Disease Report (1998) Occupational transmission of HIV infection. *Commun. Dis. Rep.*, **8**(22),

Control of Substances Hazardous to Health Regulations (COSHH) 1988. Statutory instrument No. 1657. HMSO, London.

Cookson, B., Peters, B., Webster, M. *et al.* (1989) Staff carriage of epidemic methicillin-resistant *Staphylococcus aureus*. *J. Clin. Microbiol.*, **27**, 471–476.

Cowden, J.M., Wall, P.G., Adak, G. *et al.* (1995) Outbreaks of foodborne infectious intestinal disease in England and Wales: 1992 and 1993. *Commun. Dis. Rep. Rev.*, **5**(8), R109–R117.

Craven, D.E., Steger, K.A., Barber, T.W. (1991) Preventing nosocomial pneumonia: state of the art and perspectives for the 1990s. *Am. J. Med.*, **91** (Suppl. 3B), 3S–44S.

Crocker, K.S., Krey, S.H., Markovic, M. *et al.* (1986) Microbial growth in clinically used enteral delivery systems. *Am. J. Infect. Control*, **14**, 250–256.

Croton CM (1990) Duvets on trial. *Nurs. Times*, **86**(26), 63–67.

Daschner, F.D. and Dettenkofer, M. (1997) Protecting the patient and the environment – new aspects and challenges in hospital infection control. *J. Hosp. Infect.*, **36**(1), 7–16.

De Louvois, J. (1993) Salmonella contamination of eggs. *Lancet*, **342**, 366–367.

Department of the Environment (1990) Environmental Protection Act 1990. Waste Management: The Duty of Care. A Code of Practice. HMSO, London.

Department of Health (1989) *Chilled and Frozen Guidelines on Cook–chill and Cook–freeze Catering Systems*. HMSO, London.

Department of Health (1990) Spills of urine: a potential; misuse of chlorine-releasing disinfecting agents. *SAB 59(90): 41*. HMSO, London.

Department of Health (1991b) Strategic guide to waste management. *Circular EL(90)M/I*. HMSO, London.

Department of Health (1991a) Hospital mattress assemblies: care and cleaning. *Safety Action Bulletin, SAB(91)65*. HMSO, London.

Department of Health (1993) Protecting health care workers and patients from hepatitis B: recommendations of the Advisory Group on Hepatitis. *HSG(93)40 and Addendum (1996) EL(96)77*. HMSO, London.

Department of Health (1996) *Immunisation Against Infectious Disease*. HMSO. London.

Department of Health (1997) Guidance on post-exposure prophylaxis for health care workers occupationally exposed to HIV. *PL/CO(97)1*. HMSO, London.

Dowsett, E.G. and Wilson, P.A. (1981) An outbreak of *Streptococcus pyogenes* infection in a maternity unit. *Commun. Dis. Rep.*, **81**(17), 3.

Dubbert, P.M., Dolce, J., Richter, W. *et al.* (1990) Increasing ICU staff handwashing: effects of education and group feedback. *Infect. Control Hosp. Epidemiol.*, **11**, 191–193.

Eisenstein, H.C. and Smith, D.A. (1992) Epidemiology of reported sharps injuries in a tertiary care hospital. *J. Hosp. Infect.*, **20**(4), 271–280.

Garner, J.S. (1996) Hospital Infection Control Practices Advisory Committee. Guideline for isolation precautions in hospitals. *Infect. Control Hosp. Epidemiol.*, **17**(1), 54–80.

George, R.H., Gully, P.R., Gill, O.N. *et al.* (1986) An outbreak of tuberculosis in a children's hospital. *J. Hosp. Infect.*, **8**, 129–142

Gerberding, J.L., Littell, G., Tarkington, A. *et al.* (1990) Risk exposure of surgical personnel to patients' blood during surgery at San Francisco General Hospital. *New Engl. J. Med.*, **322**, 1788–1793.

Gibbs, J. (1990) Waste line. *Nurs. Times*, **86**(13), 71–73.

Glenister, H.M., Taylor, L.J., Bartlett, C.L.R. *et al.* (1992) An 11 month incidence study of infections in ward of a district general hospital. *J. Hosp. Infect.*, **21**(4), 261–273.

Glynn, A., Ward, V. and Wilson, J. (1997) *Hospital Acquired Infection: Surveillance, Policies and Practice*. Public Health Laboratory Service, London.

Goldthorpe, G., Kerry, P. and Drabu, Y.J. (1991) Refrigerated food storage in hospital ward areas. *J. Hosp. Infect.* **18**, 63–66.

Gosden, P.E, MacGowan, A.P. and Bannister, G.C. (1998) Importance of air quality and related factors in the prevention of infection in orthopaedic implant surgery. *J. Hosp. Infect.*, **39**(3), 173–180.

Gould, D. (1993) Assessing nurses' hand decontamination performance. *Nurs. Times*, **89**(25), 47–50.

Greaves, W.L., Kraiser, A.B., Alford, R.H. *et al.* (1980) The problem of herpetic whitlow among hospital personnel. *Infect. Control*, **1**, 181–185.

Griffiths, G. (1989) Safety in disposal. Nurs Standard 4(8): 52–6.

Grinnell, F. (1998) Disinfection of latex gloves with ethyl alcohol. *Prof. Nurse*, **13**(8), 504–507.

Haley, R.W., Culver, D.H., White, O.W. *et al* (1985) The efficacy of surveillance and control programs in preventing nosocomal infections in US hospitals. *Am. J. Epid.*, **121**, 182–205.

Health and Safety Executive, Health Services Advisory Committee (1982) *The Safe Disposal of Clinical Waste*. HMSO, London.

Heptonstall, J. (1991) Outbreaks of hepatitis B virus infection associated with infected surgical staff. *Commun. Dis. Rep.*, **1**, R81–R85.

Heptonstall, J., Gill, O.N., Porter, K. *et al.* (1993) Health care workers and HIV: surveillance of occupationally acquired infection in the United Kingdom. *Commun. Dis Rep. Rev.*, **3**(11), R147–R153.

Hoffman, P.N. (1993) *Clostridium difficile* and the hospital environment. *PHLS Microbiol. Digest*, **10**(3), 91–92.

Hoffman, P. and Wilson, J. (1995) Hands, hygiene and hospitals. *PHLS Microbiol. Digest*, **11**(4), 211–216.

Hoffman, P.N., Cooke, E.M., McCarville, M. *et al.* (1985) Micro-organisms isolated from the skin under wedding rings worn by hospital staff. *Br. Med. J.*, **290**, 206–207.

Holborn, J. (1990) Wet strike through and the transfer of bacteria through operating barrier fabrics. *Hyg. Med.*, **15**, 15–20.

Howarth, F.H. (1985) Prevention of airborne infection during surgery. *Lancet*, **i**, 386–388.

Hubble, M.J., Weale, A.E., Perez, J.V. *et al.* (1996) Clothing in laminar flow operating theatres. *J. Hosp. Infect.*, **32**, 1–7.

Jagger, J. (1988) Rates of needlestick injury caused by various devices in a University hospital. *New Engl J. Med.*, **318**, 284–288.

Jagger, J., Hunt, E.H. and Pearson, R.D. (1990) Sharp object injuries in the hospital: causes and strategies for prevention. *Am. J. Infect. Control*, **18**, 227–231.

Jones, D. (1990) Foodborne listeriosis. *Lancet*, **336**, 1171–1174.

Kaplan, L.M. and McGuckin, M. (1986) Increasing handwashing compliance with more accessible sinks. *Infect. Control*, **7**, 408–409.

Larson, E. (1988) A causal link between handwashing and risk of infection? Examination of the evidence. *Infect. Control Hosp. Epidemiol.*, **9**(1), 28–36.

Loomes, S. (1988) Is it safe to lie down in hospital? *Nurs. Times*, **84**(49), 63–65.

Lowbury, E.L. and Lilly, H.A. (1973) Use of a 4% chlorhexidine solution (Hibiscrub) and other methods of skin disinfection. *Br. Med. J.*, **1**, 510–515.

Lund, B.M., Knox, M.R. and Cole, M.B. (1989) Destruction of *Listeria monocytogenes* during microwave cooking. *Lancet*, **i**, 218.

Luthi, T.M., Wall, P.G., Evans, H.S. *et al.* (1996) Outbreaks of foodborne viral gastroenteritis in England and Wales: 1992 to 1994. *Commun. Dis. Rep. Rev.*, **6**(10), R131–R135.

Lynch, P., Cummings, M.J., Roberts, P.L. *et al.* (1990) Implementing and evaluating a system of generic infection control precuations: body substance isolation. *Am. J. Infect. Control*, **18**, 1–13.

Mackey, B.M. (1989) The incidence of food poisoning bacteria in red meat and poultry in the United Kingdom. *Food Sci. Technol. Today*, **3**, 246–249.

Mackintosh, C.A. and Hoffman, P.N. (1984) An extended model for the transfer of micro-organisms and the effect of alcohol disinfection. *J. Hyg.*, **92**, 345–355.

Maki, D.G., Alvarado, C.J., Hassemer, C.A. *et al.* (1982) relation of the inanimate environment to endemic nosocomial infection. *New Engl. J. Med.*, **307**, 1562–1566.

Mangione, C.M., Gerberding, J.L. and Cummings, S.R. (1991) Occupational exposure to HIV: frequency and rates of underreporting of percutaneous and mucopercutaneous exposures by medical housestaff. *Am. J. Med.*, **90**, 85–90.

Maurer, I.M. (1985) *Hospital Hygiene*, 3rd edn. Edward Arnold, London.

Medical Devices Agency (1993) Use and management of sharps containers. *Action Bulletin No. 102*. HMSO, London.

Medical Devices Agency (1996) Latex sensitisation in the healthcare setting (Use of latex gloves) *DB9601*. HMSO, London.

Morse, L.J. and Schonbek, L.E. (1968) Hand lotions and potential nosocomial hazard. *New Engl. J. Med.*, **278**, 376–378.

Murdoch, S. (1990) Hazards in hoists. *Nurs. Times*, **86**(49), 68–70.

Mylotte, J.M. (1994) Control of methicillin-resistant *Staphylococcus aureus*: the ambivalence persists. *Infect. Control Hosp. Epidemiol.*, **15**, 73–77.

Neal, K.R., Dornan, J., Irving, W.L. (1997) Prevalence of hepatitis C antibodies among healthcare workers of two teaching hospitals. Who is at risk? *Br. Med. J.*, **314**, 179–180.

Newsom, S.W.B. (1972) Microbiology of hospital toilets. *Lancet*, **ii**, 700–703.

Newsom, S.W.B. (1993) Ignaz Philip Semmelweis. *J. Hosp. Infect.*, **23**, 175–188.

NHS Executive (1995) Hospital laundry arrangements for used and infected linen. *HSG(95)18*. HMSO, London.

NHS Management Executive (1992) Management of food services and food hygiene in the National Health Service. *HSG(92)34*. HMSO, London.

NHS Management Executive (1993) Decontamination of equipment prior to inspection, service or repair. *HSG(93)26*. HMSO, London.

Nystrom, B. (1981) The disinfection of baths and shower trolleys in hospitals. *J. Hosp. Infect.*, **2**, 93–95.

Oie, S. and Kamiya, A. (1996) Microbial contamination of antiseptics and disinfectants. *Am. J. Infect. Control*, **24**, 389–395.

Ojajärvi, J., Mäkelä, P. and Rantasalo, I. (1977) Failure of hand disinfection with frequent hand washing: a need for prolonged field studies. *J. Hyg. (Camb.)*, **79**, 107–119.

Olsen, R.J., Lynch, P., Coyle, M.B. *et al.* (1993) Examination gloves as barriers to hand contamination in clinical practice. *J. A. M. A.*, **270**, 350–353.

Orsi, G.B., Mansi, A., Tomao, P. *et al.* (1994) Lack of association between clinical and environmental isolates of *Pseudomonas aeruginosa* in hospital wards. *J. Hosp. Infect.*, **27**(1), 49–60.

Overton, E. (1988) Bed-making and bacteria. *Nurs. Times*, **85**(9), 69–71.

Plowman, R.M., Graves, N. and Roberts, J.A. (1997) *Hospital-acquired Infection*. Office of Health Economics, London.

Public Health Laboratory Service (1998) Occupational transmission of HIV infection. *Commun. Dis. Rep. Wkly*, **8**(22), 193

Public Health Laboratory Service Salmonella Committee (1995) The prevention of human transmission of gastrointestinal infections, infestations, and bacterial intoxications. *Commun. Dis. Rep. Rev.*, **5**(11), R158–R172.

Ravn, P., Lundgren, J.D., Kjaeldgaard, P. *et al.* (1991) Nosocomial outbreak of cryptosporidiosis in AIDS patients. *Br. Med. J.*, **302**, 277–280.

Reybrouck, G. (1983) Role of the hands in the spread of nosocomial infections: 1. *J. Hosp. Infect.*, **4**, 103–110.

Rhodes, R.S. and Bell, D.M. (eds) (1995) *Surg. Clin. North Am.*, **75**, 1047–1217.

Roberts, D. (1982) Factors contributing to outbreaks of food poisoning in England and Wales. 1970–1979. *J. Hyg.*, **89**, 491–498.

Ross, D.J., Cherry, N.M. and McDonald, J.C. (1998) Occupationally acquired infectious disease in the United Kingdom: 1996 to 1997. *Commun. Dis. Public Health*, **1**(2), 98–102.

Royal College of Pathologists (1992) *HIV Infection: Hazards of Transmission to Patients and Health Care Workers During Invasive Procedures*. Royal College of Pathologists, London.

Saghafi, L., Raselli, P., Francillon, C. *et al.* (1992) Exposure to blood during various procedures: results of two surveys before and after the implementation of universal precautions. *Am. J. Infect. Control*, **20**, 53–57.

Samadi, A.R., Huq, M.I. and Ahmed, Q.S. (1983) Detection of rotavirus in handwashings of attendants of children with diarrhoea. *Br. Med. J.*, **286**, 188.

Sanderson, P.J. and Weissler, S. (1992) Recovery of coliforms from the hands of nurses and patients: activities leading to contamination. *J. Hosp. Infect.*, **21**, 85–93.

Scanlon, J.W. and Leikkanen, M. (1973) The use of fluorescein powder for evaluating contamination in a newborn nursery. *J. Pediatr.*, **82**, 966–971.

Sherertz, R. and Sullivan, M. (1985) An outbreak of infections with *Acinetobacter calcoaceticus* in burn patients: contamination of patients' mattresses. *J. Infect. Dis.*, **151**, 252–258.

Smith, J.R. and Grant, J.M. (1990) The incidence of glove puncture during caesarian section. *J. Obstet. Gynaecol.*, **10**, 317–318.

Sprunt, K., Redman, W. and Leidy, G. (1973) Antibacterial effectiveness of routine handwashing. *Pediatrics*, **52**, 264–271.

Suzuki, A., Namba, Y., Matsuura, M. and Horisawa, A. (1984) Airborne contamination in an operating suite: a 5 year survey. *J. Hyg.*, **93**(3), 567–573.

Taylor, L. (1978) An evaluation of handwashing techniques. *Nurs. Times*, **74**, 108–110.

Telford, G.I. and Quebberman, E.J. (1993) Assessing the risk of blood exposure in the operating room. *Am. J. Infect. Control*, **21**, 351–356.

Tokars, J.I., Bell, D.M., Culver, D.H. *et al.* (1992) Percutaneous injuries during surgical procedures. *J.A.M.A.*, **267**, 2899–2904.

Tomlinson, D. (1987) To clean or not to clean? *Nurs. Times*, **83**, 71–75.

UK Health Departments (1991) *AIDS–HIV Infected Health Care Workers. Occupational Guidance for Health Care Workers, their Physicians and Employers. Recommendations of the Expert Advisory Group on AIDS.* HMSO, London.

UK Health Departments (1998) *Guidance for Clinical Health Care Workers: Protection Against Infection with Blood-borne Viruses. Recommendations of the Expert Advisory Group on AIDS and Advisory Group on Hepatitis.* HMSO, London.

Wade, J.J., Desai, N. and Casewell, M.W. (1991) Hygienic hand disinfection for the removal of epidemic vancomycin-resistant *Enterococcus faecium* and gentamicin-resistant *Enterobacter cloacae*. *J. Hosp. Infect.*, **18**(3), 211–218.

Ward, V., Wilson, J., Taylor, L. *et al.* (1997) *Preventing Hospital-acquired Infection. Clinical Guidelines*. Public Health Laboratory Service, London.

Webster, O., Cowan, M. and Allen, J. (1986) Dirty linen. *Nurs. Times*, **82**, 36–37.

Whyte, W., Hamblen, D.L., Kelly, I.G. *et al.* (1990) An investigation of occlusive polyester surgical clothing. *J. Hosp. Infect.*, **15**, 363–374.

Williams, E. and Buckles, A. (1988) A lack of motivation. *Nurs. Times*, **84**, 60–64.

Wilson, J. (1995) *Infection Control in Clinical Practice*. Baillière Tindall, London.

Wilson, J. and Breedon, B. (1990) Universal precautions. *Nurs. Times*, **86**, 67–70.

FURTHER READING

British Medical Association (1990) *A Code of Practice for the Safe Use and Disposal of Sharps*. British Medical Association, London.

Legge, A. (1996) Sharps disposal systems. *Prof. Nurse*, **12**(1), 57–62.

Jackson, M.M. and Lynch, P. (1986) Education of the adult learner: a practical approach for the infection control practitioner. *Am. J. Infect. Control*, **14**, 257–271.

West, D.J. (1984) The risk of hepatitis B infection among health professionals in the United States: a review. *Am. J. Med. Sci.*, **287**, 26–33.

13

Important nosocomial infections: pathogenesis and prevention

INTRODUCTION

The previous chapter described the infection control practices that should be used in the routine care of all patients. This chapter focuses on the main nosocomial infections: wound, bloodstream, urinary tract and lower respiratory tract infections. It reviews the factors that contribute to their acquisition and the specific practices that are important for their prevention.

The aseptic technique

When the normal defences of the body have been breached the tissues are vulnerable to invasion by microorganisms. Preventing the introduction of microorganisms depends on applying the principle of asepsis. This means ensuring that microorganisms are not introduced during treatment or manipulation of sites, such as wounds and devices. The aseptic technique emerged in the 1940s and became incorporated into nursing ritual. Many aspects of the practice have therefore been based on tradition rather than evidence for their effectiveness (Walsh & Ford 1989). A good example of this is the cleaning of trolleys with alcohol: Thompson & Bullock (1992) have recently illustrated that there are very few bacteria present on the surface of the trolley and that routine trolley cleaning is not necessary.

Technological developments mean that low-cost, good-quality disposable gloves can be produced and many staff now favour the use of sterile gloves, rather than cumbersome forceps, to prevent direct contact between hands and a vulnerable site (Box 13.1). In addition, improved understanding of the mechanisms of wound healing have seen the introduction of a wide range of dressings that are not as easy to use with the conventional aseptic technique. For example, hydrocolloid and alginate dressings are often removed most easily by soaking the wound in bath water. It is also recognised that chronic wounds are heavily colonised by microorganisms and that, while steps should be taken to avoid introducing more microorganisms, preventing their transfer to others is of greatest importance and the use of a rigorous aseptic technique is unnecessary (Ayliffe et al 1990).

Hollinworth & Kingston (1998), in a small study on clean, non-sterile gloves, were unable to detect microbial contamination of the gloves prior to use and recommend using clean, non-sterile gloves in place of forceps for dressing wounds.

Box 13.1 Aseptic technique (Source: adapted from Riverside Health Authority nursing procedures and reprinted with permission)

Aim
To minimise the risk of introducing pathogenic organisms into a wound or other susceptible site and to prevent the transfer of pathogens from the wound to other patients or staff

Indications
• Wounds healing by primary intention (before surface skin has sealed)
• Intravenous cannulation
• Urinary catheterisation
• Suturing
• Vaginal examination during labour
• Medical invasive procedures

Principles
1. Ensure that all required equipment is readily available and there is a clear field in which to carry out the procedure
2. Explain the procedure to the patient, obtain verbal consent and position the patient so that the procedure can be performed easily
3. Wash hands or disinfect clean hands with an alcohol handrub
4. Open the sterile pack carefully to prevent contamination of the contents
5. Wear sterile gloves for the procedure to prevent introducing pathogenic bacteria to the site, direct contact with body fluids and cross-infection
6. When the procedure has been completed discard waste contaminated with body fluid into a yellow waste bag and sharps into a sharps container. Discard protective clothing and wash hands.

INFECTION ASSOCIATED WITH WOUNDS

The skin provides a complete barrier to microorganisms. A wound allows microorganisms to gain entry to the tissues underneath. Wounds occur as the result of trauma (e.g. accidents, burns, surgery) or an underlying disease process (e.g. venous ulceration). Healing occurs in two ways: where there is no loss of tissue and the two edges of skin are together, the two surfaces are quickly repaired by a fibrin mesh, which is gradually filled in by collagen and capillaries. This is called *healing by primary intention*. Where there is loss of tissue, new cells are laid down at the base of the wound and the gap is gradually closed by contraction from the sides. This is called *healing by secondary intention* and takes place over many weeks or months. The risks of infection associated with these two types of wound are quite different and will therefore be considered separately.

Detection of wound infection

Clinical signs and symptoms are important indicators of wound infection and are listed in List 13.1. In wounds healing by secondary intention slough is often difficult to distinguish from pus, and other signs such as inflammation or pain are therefore important in the diagnosis of infection (Hutchinson & Lawrence 1991). The isolation of microorganisms from a wound swab does not necessarily indicate that infection is present as it may simply reflect bacteria colonising the surrounding skin or the wound itself. While the laboratory cannot usually diagnose the infection, culture can be used to identify the organism causing infection and most appropriate antimicrobial therapy. The most accurate information can be obtained by aspirating pus or exudate from the wound. If this is not possible the exudate should be cleaned away and a wound swab should be rubbed over the base of the wound (Burdette-Taylor & Taylor 1993). If the wound is large swabs should be taken from those parts that have signs or symptoms of infection.

List 13.1 Symptoms and signs of wound infection

- Pain in or around the wound
- Inflammation or discoloration spreading from the wound margins
- Oedema
- Pyrexia
- Purulent exudate

Surgical wounds

The balance between the patient's immune defences and the number of bacteria present in the wound at the end of the operation determines whether an infection subsequently develops. Pathogens can be acquired from the patient's own flora, the theatre environment and instruments or personnel taking part in the surgery.

The following factors have an important effect on the risk of wound infection (Figure 13.1).

Bacteria present at the operative site. Operations on sites of the body colonised by large numbers of bacteria will inevitably be associated with bacterial contamination and a higher risk of infection than sites without a normal bacterial flora (Table 13.1). Prophylactic antibiotic therapy is usually prescribed for these operations. Prior to bowel surgery, elemental diets and purgatives are used to minimise the amount of faeces in the bowel.

Table 13.1 Classification of wound contamination

Category	Description	Type of surgery	Approx. no. wound infections per 100 operations
Clean	GI, GU or respiratory tract not entered; no evidence of inflammation/infection; no break in technique	Orthopaedic, neurosurgery cardiac surgery	2–5
Clean–contaminated	GI, GU or respiratory tract entered but no spillage of contents	Abdominal hysterectomy, resection of prostate	8
Contaminated	Open traumatic wounds; major break in technique; spillage from GI tract; inflamed tissue encountered	Reduction of open fracture, some large bowel surgery	15
Dirty	Delayed treatment of traumatic wounds; pre-existing clinical infection, perforated viscera at site of operation	Drainage of abscess	40

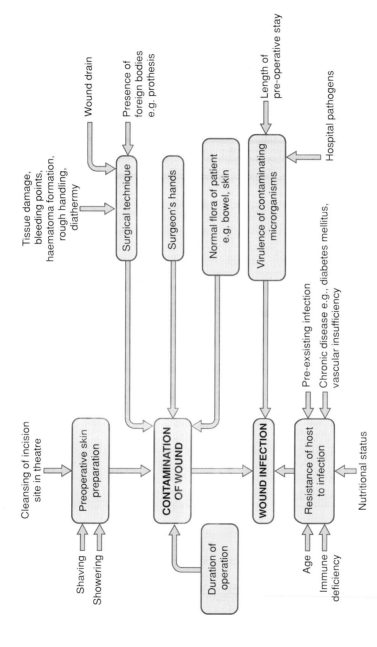

Figure 13.1   Factors influencing the development of wound infection.

Presence of foreign material. Bacteria present in a wound are able to multiply much more effectively in the presence of a foreign body. This was clearly demonstrated by Elek & Conen (1957), who found that in the presence of a suture only 100 bacteria were required for to establish infection, compared to over 6 million when no suture was present. Small areas of inflammation are commonly seen around the sutures in surgical wounds, although these normally resolve soon after the sutures are removed. Implanted material such as joint or valve replacements enables bacteria to adhere and multiply, especially coagulase-negative staphylococci, which produce an extracellular slime. Infection may therefore emerge many weeks after the procedure (Sanderson 1991).

Duration of the operation. The longer the tissues are exposed in the operating theatre, the greater the risk that microorganisms carried on airborne particles will settle into the wound (Whyte et al 1982). Duration of surgery is therefore a major factor in determining the risk of subsequent wound infection (Haley et al 1985a).

Surgical technique. The skill of the surgeon can have a major effect on the risk of subsequent wound infection. A poor technique may result in more damage to tissue, bleeding and haematoma formation, all of which can all encourage the multiplication of bacteria in the wound. The procedure may take longer, providing more opportunity for bacteria to enter the wound, and accidental breaks in technique, such as perforation of the bowel, can increase contamination (Holzheimer 1997).

Susceptibility of the patient. Underlying disease may impair the immune response or increase susceptibility to infection, e.g. diabetes, increasing age (Cruse 1986). Poor nutrition or obesity may delay wound healing (Bucknall 1985).

Preoperative stay. Patients who have been in hospital for a few days prior to surgery gradually replace their normal flora with hospital pathogens. Cruse & Foord (1980) found a greater risk of surgical wound infection associated with prolonged preoperative stay.

Measures to prevent surgical wound infection

Preparation of the patient

If the procedure is elective then the patient should be as healthy as possible at the time of surgery. Infections at other sites should be treated and patients who are malnourished should be given supplementary feeding. Many hospitals now use preadmission clinics to prepare the patient for surgery, take blood for cross-matching, etc., enabling the preoperative stay to be reduced to less than a day.

Preoperative bathing has been part of the routine but evidence for its effectiveness is conflicting (Lynch et al 1992). Ayliffe et al (1990) suggest that two antiseptic baths taken the night before surgery and the morning of surgery may be of more value than one. More important is the application of disinfectants to the surgical site immediately prior to incision. Chlorhexidine and iodine-based antiseptics in alcoholic formulations are applied to reduce the number of bacteria on the skin and thus minimise the number of bacteria entering the wound.

Preoperative shaving of the incision site causes local skin damage, providing sites for bacterial growth, and increasing the risk of infection. When hair removal is essential for proper access to the surgical site it should be removed as close to the time of surgery as possible to minimise the number of bacteria present at the site (Cruse & Foord 1980). Hair clippers cause less damage than razors (Pettersson 1986).

Antibiotic prophylaxis is recommended for surgery involving a significant risk of infection. It should be given 30 minutes before the initial incision and therapeutic levels of the drug should be maintained throughout the procedure. Prophylaxis should not usually be continued for more than 48 hours as this may encourage antibiotic resistant pathogens to develop (Mangram et al 1999).

Hand washing prior to surgery

The resident flora of the skin, although of low pathogenicity, may cause infection if introduced deep into the tissues during surgery. Microbiocidal detergents, known as surgical scrubs, are therefore used to eliminate resident flora from the hands and arms of the surgeon immediately prior to performing the operation. Chlorhexidine and povidone-iodine persist on the skin and continue to destroy microorganisms for several hours after application (Ojajärvi et al 1976). Outbreaks of infection caused by infected staff have been reported, particularly by strains of *Staphylococcus aureus* carried on the skin and group A streptococcus colonising the throat (Garner et al 1981).

Procedures in the operating theatre

Microorganisms carried on airborne particles can settle into open wounds or on instruments during the operative procedure. The number of airborne particles is related to the number of staff present, since most are derived from squames released from the skin. Special ventilation systems are used to filter out airborne microorganisms (p. 284). The number of airborne particles can be minimised by reducing the number of people present in the room and avoiding opening the doors during the procedure, which disrupts the air filtration (Howarth 1985).

Ultraclean air systems are recommended for orthopaedic joint replacements because even small numbers of organisms, including those of low pathogenicity, cause infections in these procedures, with considerable morbidity.

Protective clothing can reduce the dispersal of squames into the air, but they will escape through the openings at the neck, ankles and wrists and can also pass through pores in normal cotton fabric, especially if the material becomes wet (Whyte et al 1990). Disposable non-woven fabrics, close-woven polyester, cotton-polyester and laminated fabrics are more efficient at preventing the passage of squames (Hoborn 1990). Masks probably have little effect since very few bacteria are expelled from the respiratory tract and these can escape around the side of the mask (Belkin 1997). However, they are necessary for those closely involved in the surgery to protect them from splashes of blood. Similarly, studies on punctured sterile gloves suggest that bacteria from surgeons' hands do not readily contaminate the wound; however gloves are an essential protection against contact with blood and may provide some protection against needlestick injury (UK Health Departments 1998; p. 278).

Although the risk of acquiring organisms from the environment is low, horizontal surfaces should be cleaned regularly to remove dust, and blood should be cleaned from surfaces after each patient.

Post-operative care

The majority of wound infections result from contamination of the operative site during surgery. Postoperative care does not usually result in infection but wounds should be covered with a sterile dressing for at least 24 hours until the edges have sealed. After this time, microorganisms are unlikely to gain access and Chrintz et al (1989) suggest that there is no reason why patients should not be allowed to bathe or shower. If the wound has to be inspected or the dressing changed, hands should be washed beforehand and afterwards. Wound dressings should be removed if the patient develops a fever or complains of pain, or if excessive fluid is draining from the site. A study by Tomlinson (1987) illustrated how little effect routine cleaning of surgical wounds had on the number of bacteria present, which tended to be redistributed rather than removed. In addition, bacteria already contaminating the wound were readily acquired on the hands, even when forceps were used, highlighting the risk of cross-infection if hands are not washed after touching wounds.

Wound drains are used to enable blood, pus or necrotic material to drain out, preventing them from collecting in the wound bed, where they may encourage bacterial multiplication. However, the drain itself provides a route of access into the wound, enabling bacteria to be introduced postoperatively (van der Linden et al 1981). Therefore they are usually only inserted when significant amounts of fluid are expected to collect in the wound. They should be inserted via a separate stab wound, so that pus in the drain does not reach the incision and the incision site does not need to be exposed when the drain is shortened or removed. Closed drainage systems attached to a sealed bag or bottle reduce the risk of introducing infection, but these must be handled aseptically.

Surveillance of surgical wound infection

Training of surgeons in the optimum technique is essential to minimise the risk of postoperative complications, including infection. This includes careful handling of tissues, tying off bleeding, reasonable speed and aseptic technique. Reductions in surgical wound infection rates have been demonstrated when surveillance programmes are in place. This involves monitoring the occurrence of surgical wound infection and reporting the rates of infection to individual surgeons, who may then modify their practice if their rates of infection are high (Olsen et al 1984, Haley et al 1985b). Recently, a national surveillance scheme has been established in the UK, based at the Central Public Health Laboratory in Colindale. This enables hospitals to compare surgical wound infection rates in different categories of surgery with national average data (Cooke et al 1999).

Preventing infection in wounds healing by secondary intention

Where there has been loss of tissue in the wound, healing takes considerably longer and the exposed tissue provides an ideal medium in which bacteria can grow and multiply. However, these chronic wounds appear to heal despite becoming rapidly colonised by bacteria, provided that the bacteria remain at the surface of the wound and do not invade the tissue (Hutchinson & Lawrence 1991). A considerable amount of exudate may be produced from the wound and plays an important role in enabling epithelialisation and microcapillary formation. The exudate also contains white blood cells, which help to reduce the number of bacteria present and prevent them from invading tissues (Buchan et al 1980). Many dressings are available that absorb excess exudate while providing a warm and moist environment that will promote healing (List 13.2). These occlusive dressings do not appear to increase the risk of infection or encourage the growth of anaerobic bacteria (Gilchrist & Reed 1989).

List 13.2   Properties of an ideal wound dressing

- Maintains a high humidity: epithelial cells require moist conditions to migrate across wound
- Provides thermal insulation: tissue repair occurs best at a constant temperature of 37°C
- Is impermeable to bacteria: helps to prevent cross-infection
- Removes excess exudate: there is a balance between removal of exudate to prevent tissue maceration while maintaining a moist environment; exudate contains white blood cells, which protect the wound from invasion by bacteria
- Is non-adherent: prevents the removal of newly formed tissue and capillaries when dressing is changed
- Is non-toxic and non-allergenic: avoids interference with healing
- Is comfortable and acceptable to the patient

Use of antiseptics

Traditionally antiseptics have been applied to wounds to remove dead tissue, to kill bacteria and to treat infection. Hypochlorite and hydrogen peroxide have been used as debriding agents, but there is little evidence to suggest that they are effective and other evidence that indicates that they delay wound healing (Brennan et al 1986, Gruber et al 1975). Slough or necrotic tissue in a wound may encourage infection and delay healing but can be removed more effectively by using a scalpel, if necessary under anaesthetic.

Bacteria colonising a wound are not readily removed by the application of antiseptics. Most of these solutions do not have a prolonged antibacterial effect, especially in the presence of wound exudate, and there is some evidence to suggest that even chlorhexidine and povidone-iodine affect the activity of fibroblasts (Niedner & Schopf 1986). It is not necessary to remove bacteria colonising the wound but if infection develops, systemic treatment with an appropriate antimicrobial agent is required. Infection should be diagnosed according to clinical signs and symptoms and not on the identification of bacteria in a wound culture.

Preventing cross-infection

The dressings covering chronic wounds can become heavily contaminated with the bacteria colonising the wound. It is important to ensure that these bacteria are not transferred to another patient and it should be recognised that any contact with the dressings will transfer bacteria on to the hands or clothing. Clean disposable gloves and plastic aprons can be used to prevent contamination but these must be changed immediately after use and the hands washed.

Particular care must be taken in dressing clinics, where the rapid throughput of patients may enable cross-infection to occur if scrupulous infection control is not practised. Creams, dressing materials and instruments must be used for one patient only and equipment such as buckets, used for soaking off old dressings, should be thoroughly cleaned with detergent and water between patients.

Burns

Burns present particular problems as they are readily colonised by a variety of microorganisms, some of which may invade the tissue, and infection is the leading cause of death in patients with burns. Those with burns affecting more than 60% of the surface area of the body are most susceptible, with 70% of these burns becoming infected and most patients developing secondary bloodstream infection (Weber et al 1997). Gram-negative bacteria are a common cause of infection in burns; some, such as *Pseudomonas aeruginosa*, are of low pathogenicity in most wounds but can interfere with skin grafting and cause serious infections, including septicaemia, in severely burned patients. Antimicrobial creams and solutions specifically for topical use (e.g. silver nitrate, silver sulphadiazine) are applied to control colonisation and can help to reduce mortality (Lowbury & Cason 1985).

Cross-infection can occur easily in burns units. Large numbers of bacteria may be released during dressing changes, although special filtered dressing rooms can help to reduce the risk of transmission. Equipment may also be implicated in transmission, as demonstrated by Kolmos et al (1993), who reported an outbreak of pseudomonas infections associated with tubing used for irrigating wounds.

INFECTION OF THE BLOODSTREAM

In the UK bloodstream infections account for at least 6% of all hospital-acquired infections and the national surveillance system in the USA has found that over 40% of all bloodstream infections occur in patients in intensive care units (Beck-Sague & Jarvis 1991). *Septicaemia* is the term used to describe the presence of microorganisms in the blood associated with symptoms such as high fever, chills, rigors or hypotension. *Bacteraemia* is the presence of microorganisms in the blood in the absence of symptoms.

The main source of bloodstream infections are intravascular (IV) devices, although microorganisms can also enter the blood from another site in the body, e.g. from a wound or respiratory or urinary tract infection. The latter are termed *secondary infections* and occur most commonly in low-birthweight infants, the elderly and those who are immunosuppressed or have severe underlying illness, although sometimes it is not possible to determine the exact source (Beck-Sague & Jarvis 1991).

As most bloodstream infections are related to IV therapy this section will focus on preventing infections associated with IV devices.

Microorganisms associated with bloodstream infection

20 years ago most hospital-acquired bloodstream infections were caused by Gram-negative bacteria; now the majority are caused by Gram-positive bacteria, in particular *Staphylococcus epidermidis* (Beck-Sague & Jarvis 1991). This change has been caused by the increase in use of IV devices and the improved survival of critically ill patients, particularly neonates (Freeman et al 1990). *S. epidermidis* is part of the normal flora of the skin and, while not usually a pathogen, causes infection of IV devices because it has a particular ability to adhere to plastic materials such as cannulas. In addition, some strains produce a polysaccharide, called slime, which protects them from host defences and the action of antimicrobial agents (Centers for Disease Control 1996).

Other pathogens emerging as important causes of IV-device-associated infections are enterococci, especially strains resistant to several antibiotics, and fungi, which account for 10% of all bloodstream infections (Beck-Sague & Jarvis 1993). Table 13.2 summarises the main sources of microorganisms associated with bloodstream infections.

Table 13.2 Sources of microorganisms causing IV-device-associated infections

Microorganism	Usual source
Gram-positive bacteria	
Staphylococcus epidermidis	Common skin commensal; adheres to IV devices
Staphylococcus aureus	Common skin commensal; adheres to host proteins present on IV devices
Enterococcus spp.	Commensal of bowel flora; transmitted by hands or equipment
Gram-negative bacteria	
Klebsiella spp.	Common bowel flora; may also contaminate
Pseudomonas spp.	pressure monitoring equipment or IV fluids
Serratia spp.	
Enterobacter spp.	
Fungi	
Candida	Contaminated parenteral nutrition fluids

Routes of IV device infection

The main routes of infection are from the skin, along the outside of the cannula, in contaminated fluids or from colonisation in the cannula hub or administration set (Figure 13.2). The risk of infection varies considerably with the location and type of device being used. Peripheral vascular catheters are usually only in place for short periods and are rarely associated with infection during the initial 72 hours; if phlebitis does occur it is usually of mechanical rather than infectious origin (Centers for Disease Control 1996).

Vascular catheters inserted into central vessels are associated with a much higher rate of infection. The factors that influence the risk of infection are as follows.

Number of lumens. Multilumen lines are more likely to become infected than single-lumen lines, probably because they are manipulated more often (Clark-Christoff et al 1992).

Insertion site. Catheters inserted into the subclavian vein are less prone to infection than those inserted into the internal jugular. The femoral vein is associated with a particularly high risk of infection and should not be used (Ward et al 1997).

Duration of cannulation. The longer the catheter is in place the greater the chance of infection developing, with contamination of the hub an important source of infections (Raad et al 1993). The risk of infection in pulmonary artery catheters (i.e. Swan–Ganz) increases 3 days after insertion (Mermel et al 1991).

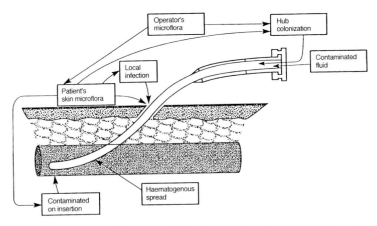

Figure 13.2 Routes of infection in IV devices: a schematic cross-section of the skin and underlying tissue at the site of cannulation. Source: Elliot 1988.

Pressure monitoring. This has been associated with a high risk of infection when the pressure monitoring device is contaminated and transducers are not effectively decontaminated. Disposable transducers have significantly reduced the risk of infection and can be used safely for at least 4 days (Centers for Disease Control 1996).

Cannula material. Microorganisms can adhere more easily to materials with irregular surfaces. Newer materials such as Teflon, silicone elastomer and polyurethane have very smooth surfaces that discourage bacterial adherence and reduce colonisation of the device (Sheth et al 1983). Intravenous catheters impregnated with antiseptic or antibiotic agents such as silver sulphadiazine, chlorhexidine, novobiocin and polymixin have been developed recently. They are probably effective in reducing bacterial colonisation of the device, but their effect on preventing infection has not been fully evaluated (Raad 1997).

Tunnelled or implantable devices. These are commonly used where long-term IV therapy, such as chemotherapy, is required. Tunnelled catheters, e.g. Hickman or Broviac, are inserted into a central vein but are tunnelled under the skin and exit on the chest wall. Tissue grows through a Dacron cuff, situated just beneath the exit site, stabilising the catheter and preventing the migration of microorganisms from the skin. Totally implantable devices, e.g. Port-A-Cath, are also tunnelled but, instead of exiting on the chest wall, have a self-sealing septum just beneath the surface, which can be accessed through the skin by a needle. If the duration of cannulation is taken into account, both types of device are associated with significantly lower rates of infection than conventional central vascular devices (Wurzel et al 1988).

Preventing IV-device-associated infection

Catheter insertion

Asepsis during the insertion of IV devices is important to prevent microorganisms from being inserted into the vein or artery with the cannula. Thorough hand washing prior to the insertion of peripheral catheters and use of a careful aseptic technique is essential. More extensive precautions are recommended for the insertion of central vascular catheters. A recent study has demonstrated the importance of maximal precautions – gloves, gown, mask and sterile drapes – in reducing the risk of colonisation and infection of central vascular catheters. The use of these precautions has a greater effect on preventing device-associated infection than using an operating room rather than ward area for insertion (Raad et al 1994).

Preparation of the skin prior to insertion with antiseptics is widely recommended. Maki et al (1991a) found that a 2% chlorhexidine solution was associated with fewer IV device infections than either 10% povidone iodine or 70% alcohol. However, it is not known whether the solutions with lower concentrations of chlorhexidine currently available have the same effect. Antimicrobial ointments applied to the catheter site at the time of insertion or dressing change have been advocated, but their efficacy has not been demonstrated and they may favour colonisation by fungi (Centers for Disease Control 1996).

Firm anchoring of non-tunnelled catheters with an adherent dressing or tape can help to reduce the risk of mechanical phlebitis (Maki et al 1973).

Maintenance of the insertion site

Transparent, semipermeable polyurethane dressings are now commonly used to cover IV insertion sites. They have the advantage of securing the catheter, protecting it from moisture and enabling the site to be easily checked for signs of inflammation. Their effect on IV-device-associated infection has been widely studied, with conflicting results. Some studies have found an increase in both colonisation of the skin and catheter-associated infections when transparent films have been used (Conly et al 1989). However, a large study by Maki & Ringer (1987) found no difference in the incidence of infection between gauze or transparent film dressings used on peripheral catheters, even when they were left on for the duration of cannulation. Although transparent films on central vascular catheters may increase colonisation of the catheter tip, this does not appear to translate into an increase in bloodstream infection (Hoffmann et al 1992). The apparent effect on colonisation may be resolved by the newer film dressings, e.g. Opsite 3000, which are more permeable to water vapour and less likely to encourage skin colonisation (Maki et al 1991b).

Tunnelled or implanted devices do not need to be covered by a dressing once the insertion site has healed (Johnstone 1982).

Management of the fluid administration equipment

Several outbreaks of infection associated with infusion fluids contaminated during manufacture occurred in the 1970s and demonstrated the capacity of even simple fluids such as dextrose to support the growth of bacteria. Subsequent improvements in quality control have made this an unlikely source of infection in commercially produced fluids. Parenteral nutrition fluids, particularly lipids, encourage the growth of a wide range of microorganisms, including fungi (Beck-Sague & Jarvis 1993), and particular care needs to be taken to prevent contamination during preparation and administration.

The risk of infusion fluids becoming contaminated during administration depends on how frequently the administration set is handled. In intensive care units, where lines are frequently manipulated, 2.5% of fluids were found to be contaminated compared to less than 1% of peripheral lines on general wards (Maki et al 1987). Stopcocks and entry ports are frequently contaminated and may present a portal of entry for organisms. To prevent administration sets becoming a source of infection they should be changed every 72 hours, ensuring that the connectors are not contaminated, and the number of entry ports should be kept to a minimum (Maki et al 1987, Mermel et al 1991). Administration sets should also be changed after they have been used to infuse blood, blood products or lipid emulsions, which readily support the growth of microorganisms if they become contaminated. Lines that are handled frequently, e.g. in intensive care units, may need to be changed more often. In this setting in-line filters may be a cost-effective means of preventing microorganisms colonising the administration set from reaching the patient (Spencer 1990). Parenteral nutrition should be infused in designated tubing which should not be used for administering drugs or withdrawing blood samples.

Administration sets and infusion fluids should be assembled using a non-touch technique. There is no evidence that wrapping connectors in antiseptic-soaked gauze is effective, and in fact this may damage the cannula (Hazard Notice 1993).

Catheter replacement

A marked increase in phlebitis and colonisation occurs in peripheral catheters left in place for longer than 72 hours; re-siting at

72-hour intervals is therefore recommended. Changing a central intravascular device does not appear to affect the risk of developing a bloodstream infection and routine changing is not recommended (Cobb et al 1992). They can be replaced at the existing site over a guidewire, but this may increase the risk of bloodstream infection and should not be carried out if a catheter-related infection is already present (Centers for Disease Control 1996).

Intravascular devices in the community

Advances in medical technology and decreasing hospital stays have resulted in many patients with long-term vascular access being discharged, and renal dialysis, chemotherapy or other treatments being administered via these devices in the patient's own home. The patient is less likely to encounter the antibiotic-resistant microorganisms common in hospitals and readily transmitted between patients. However, the patient remains at risk of endogenous infection from bacteria colonising the skin, which remain a common cause of infection in intravascular devices. The patient must receive thorough training on how to manage his/her intravascular device while at home (Willis 1996). This may involve regular heparinisation or other manipulation of the device and they must therefore be instructed in the importance of hand washing and asepsis when handling the site. Written instructions are important as the patient may not retain detailed information after discharge. Consistent advice must be provided by all health-care workers involved in the patient's care, and where practices between hospital and community settings differ the reasons for these variations must be explained to the patient.

INFECTION OF THE URINARY TRACT

The normal bladder is protected against invasion from bacteria by dilution with fresh urine and by regular emptying. Urine inhibits the growth of many bacteria because of the concentration of urea, salts and organic acids and the presence of white blood cells. Successful bacterial invasion depends on their virulence and on the numbers of bacteria that reach the bladder, and is more likely to occur where the host defences are impaired by incomplete emptying or immunosuppression.

Organisms that cause infection are usually colonising the peri-urethral area and reach the bladder via the urethra (Warren 1997). The most common cause of urinary tract infection (UTI) is *Escherichia coli*, a faecal organism some strains of which are able to invade the urinary tract and multiply in urine. The faecal flora is the main source of uropathogens, but the vagina is also an important reservoir in women. Changes in the pH of the vagina can eliminate the lactobacilli that form its normal flora, enabling Gram-negative bacteria from the faecal flora to establish and subsequently cause urinary tract infection (Stamey & Timothy 1975). The decline in oestrogen production in postmenopausal women affects the vaginal pH and normal flora, contributing to the increase in incidence of UTI in this group.

Incomplete emptying of the bladder also predisposes to UTI and may be due to an enlarged prostate or prolapsed uterus, other factors that increase the risk of UTI in the elderly. Even when an indwelling urine catheter is present the bladder does not empty completely, as a small residual volume of urine remains below the level of the catheter drainage holes and acts as a reservoir for microbial multiplication (Figure 13.3).

Hospital-acquired urinary tract infection

UTI is the most common hospital-acquired infection (HAI), accounting for over 20% of all HAI and affecting 1.6 per 100 admissions to acute specialities (Emmerson et al 1996, Glynn et al 1997). In hospital the single most important cause of UTI is the urethral catheter. Between 10% and 30% of patients with an

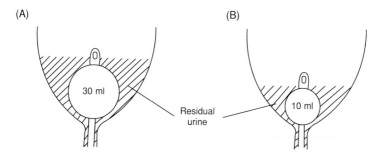

(A)   (B)

30 ml

Residual urine

10 ml

Figure 13.3 The urine catheter retention balloon, illustrating the residual urine in the bladder. A) 30 ml balloon B) 10 ml balloon. Source: Wilson 1995.

indwelling catheter develop bacteriuria, and of these a third develop symptoms of infections such as fever or suprapubic pain. The presence of the catheter increases colonisation of the urethra and as a result the risk of UTI continues for at least 24 hours after the catheter has been removed.

Effects of urinary tract infection

Uncomplicated UTIs in non-catheterised adults can be treated successfully with a short course of antimicrobial agents and are usually not associated with long-term renal problems.

Catheterised patients, especially those with the device in situ for long periods, experience repeated episodes of infection that can damage the urinary tract. Post-mortem studies suggest that 30% of these patients have acute pyelonephritis, urinary stones and perinephritic abscesses (Warren et al 1988). The urinary tract of catheterised patients is also a common source of bacteraemia and septicaemia, which has a high fatality rate, particularly if caused by Gram-negative bacteria. Platt et al (1982) demonstrated a three-times-higher mortality rate among catheterised patients in hospital, even when their age, duration of catheterisation and severity of illness were taken into account.

Symptoms and diagnosis of UTI

Bacterial colonisation of the bladder without symptoms is called *bacteriuria*. Antibiotic therapy is not required for bacteriuria, but may be indicated prior to surgery on the urinary tract or for the immunocompromised. When bacteria invade the tissues and cause inflammation of the bladder or kidneys, clinical symptoms become apparent. Typically these are frequency and urgency of micturition, pain on micturition (dysuria) and sometimes, loin pain, suprapubic pain and fever.

High numbers of bacteria may be found in the urine of patients with either bacteriuria or UTI, the common uropathogens being *Escherichia coli*, *Pseudomonas aeruginosa* and *Proteus mirabilis*. Treatment is usually indicated only when the patient is symptomatic. The typical symptoms may be obscured in elderly or confused patients and catheterised patients do not experience frequency or dysuria. UTI should therefore be considered as a possible cause of unexplained pyrexia. The presence of pus cells in urine can indicate the presence of infection but cannot be relied upon to confirm diagnosis in catheterised patients. In non-catheterised patients there is usually only one organism present in the urine but in catheterised patients there are commonly a mixed group of pathogens, any one of which could be responsible for the infection.

UTI and the urethral catheter

The urethral catheter is no longer widely used as a means of managing incontinence, but is still commonly used in certain surgical specialties. Glynn et al (1997) found that 40% of gynaecology patients, 34% of general surgical patients and 17% of orthopaedic patients were catheterised, compared to only 11% of medical patients. The highest rates of UTI occurred in gynaecological patients, where 16 infections per 1000 days of catheterisation were reported. Since the rates of catheterisation and UTI varied significantly between the 19 hospitals included in the survey, there would appear to be potential for reducing the use of catheters and catheter-associated UTI in some places.

Most infections associated with catheterisation are endogenous. The catheter itself predisposes to infection because it enables bacteria to reach the bladder from the perineum, either through the catheter lumen or via the external surface between catheter and urethral mucosa. The presence of foreign material may interfere with the immune response (Warren 1997). Kass and Schneiderman demonstrated in 1959 that *Serratia marcescens* inoculated on to the perineum at the urethral opening (meatus) of catheterised patients could be isolated in the urine a few days later. This is a particularly important route of infection in women, who are vulnerable to perineal colonisation, particularly the elderly, many of whom are likely to have bacteria in their urine before the catheter is inserted (Nicolle 1997).

Microorganisms are also commonly introduced to the drainage system when the bag is disconnected or emptied. Bacteria introduced to the drainage bag take only a few days to reach the bladder along the tubing (Garibaldi et al 1974). Nickel et al (1985) suggest that the drainage system is the most likely route of infection during the first 7 days of catheterisation (Figure 13.4).

The risk of bacteriuria is related to the period of time that the catheter is in place and increases by between 3% and 10% for

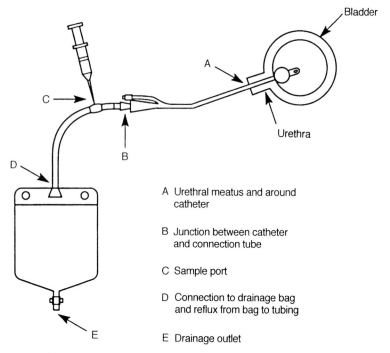

A Urethral meatus and around catheter

B Junction between catheter and connection tube

C Sample port

D Connection to drainage bag and reflux from bag to tubing

E Drainage outlet

Figure 13.4 Potential points of entry of microorganisms into the bladder of a catheterised patient. Source: Wilson 1995.

each day of catheterisation. Thus, by approximately 30 days of catheterisation most patients will have bacteria in their urine. The management of short-term catheters should therefore be focused on preventing bacteria being introduced to the urinary tract, while in the long-term catheterised bacteriuria is inevitable and efforts should be directed at preventing the introduction of new uropathogens that may cause UTI.

Prevention of hospital-acquired urinary tract infection

This section will focus on preventing infection in the management of the urethral catheter, since this device is the most important cause of UTI in hospitalised patients.

Preventing infection at catheter insertion

Between 1% and 30% of catheter insertions introduce bacteria to the bladder, with the severely debilitated patient being most vulnerable (Garibaldi 1993). The application of anaesthetic lubricating gel to the meatus, careful explanation of the procedure and positioning the patient to ensure maximum visibility and accessibility are more likely to result in an aseptic procedure. The catheter should be inserted directly into the urethra, without first touching the periurethral area, which may be colonised with microorganisms. Cleaning the area with soap and water prior to insertion may help to reduce colonisation.

Type of catheter. The catheter selected should be as small as possible to reduce the amount of trauma to the urethral mucosa while maintaining good drainage. Lumens above 16 Charriere are usually only indicated where a significant amount of debris is being passed in the urine, e.g. following prostatic surgery. For routine use a 10 ml retention balloon should be used; the larger 30 ml balloon causes pain and irritation and increases the volume of residual urine in the bladder (Figure 13.3). The balloon must also be inflated with the correct amount of water as under- or overinflation may cause it to become misshapen and irritate the bladder wall. Catheters are made from, or are coated with, a variety of materials designed to reduce the amount of irritation they cause to the urethral mucosa (Table 13.3). Catheters in place for prolonged periods become covered with biofilm, a matrix of sugars and proteins secreted by bacteria and mixed with salts, proteins and cell debris from the urine. This can build up to such an extent that it blocks the internal lumen of the catheter, causing urine to leak around the outside. Certain bacteria, e.g. proteus, are particularly

Table 13.3   Selection of catheters for urine drainage

Catheter material	Indication	Properties
Plastic	Very short-term use only; avoid if possible	Rigid material, irritates mucosa
Latex coated with silicone or Teflon	Up to 3 weeks of catheterisation, e.g. postsurgery	Reasonably non-irritant but prone to encrustation
Latex coated with hydrogel All silicone	More than 3 weeks of catheterisation	Minimal mucosal irritation, resistant to encrustation

associated with biofilm formation. Some catheters, in particular those made of silcone or coated with hydrogel, are more resistant to biofilm formation and are therefore more suitable for long-term catheterisation (Cox et al 1988).

Catheter removal. Indwelling catheters should be removed as soon as possible, yet there is evidence that many are left in far longer than necessary (Garibaldi 1993). Transient bacteraemias may occur when patients with bacteriuria are re-catheterised, and long-term catheters should therefore only be changed when necessary, e.g. when blocked by encrustations (Bryan & Reynolds 1984).

Other methods of urine drainage. Intermittent catheterisation is used for some long-term catheterised patients, particularly those with spinal injuries. Although most patients develop bacteriuria after about 3 weeks, they usually remain asymptomatic and have less long-term renal damage than those with indwelling catheters (Wyndaele & Maes, 1990). Penile sheaths have been associated with high rates of bacteriuria, probably because of an increase in periurethral colonisation (Garibaldi, 1993).

Reducing periurethral infection

Burke et al, in 1981, demonstrated the limited effect that cleansing the urethral meatus had on catheter-associated infection. They found the lowest rate of infection in those patients who received no meatal care, and a lower rate in those where soap had been used rather than povidone-iodine. However, cleansing of the area is important after faecal incontinence, as this markedly increases the number of bacteria present.

Bathing is not likely to introduce infection, provided that steps are taken to prevent reflux of urine from the bag up into the bladder. Antimicrobial creams probably reduce the incidence of infection but their effect is not sufficient to make their use cost-effective (Classen et al 1991).

Management of the drainage system

The importance of maintaining a closed drainage system for the prevention of catheter-associated infection was clearly demonstrated in the 1960s when draining a urethral catheter into a sealed bottle replaced the previous practice of draining into an open bucket. This had a dramatic effect on the infection rate, which prior to closed drainage had resulted in 95% of patients developing bacteriuria within 24 hours.

Even though closed drainage systems have now been in place for several decades, breaks in the system are reported to occur frequently. Crow et al (1988) reported that 42% of patients had their catheter and bag disconnected at least once during the period of catheterisation. Platt et al (1983) used catheters pre-sealed to drainage bags to reduce the rate of disconnection, and found that a third fewer UTIs occurred where pre-sealed catheters were in place. Patients who use a leg drainage bag during the day should connect the leg bag to a larger overnight drainage bag at night to avoid unnecessary disconnection of the catheter and bag.

Once the drainage system has become contaminated, bacteria readily travel from the drainage bag into the bladder. Columns of urine that form above kinks in the tubing cause airlocks and when released, result in bacteria trapped in air bubbles travelling many feet up the tubing (Roberts et al 1965). Preventing kinks forming in the drainage tube by correct positioning is therefore important. The biofilm that forms along the surface of the entire drainage system enables bacteria to pass through devices such as valves or drip chambers designed to prevent reflux of urine. Bacteria introduced to the drainage bag multiply at room temperature and reach the bladder in a few days (Garibaldi et al 1974).

Catheterised patients should be encouraged to drink plenty of fluids to maintain a constant downward flow of urine and dilute the nutrients in urine. Some drinks, e.g. cranberry juice, may help to reduce bacterial growth by changing the acidity of urine (Rogers, 1991). The addition of antiseptic solutions to the drainage bag is probably ineffective, uneconomical and likely to encourage the emergence of resistant bacteria (Stickler 1990).

Patient education. Patients who are managing their own catheters should be advised how to minimise the risk of introducing infection, including the importance of hand washing, positioning the bag and recognising the symptoms of infection (Roe 1990). This is particularly important for those discharged into the community with a urethral catheter.

Preventing cross-infection from urine drainage systems

Most patients with long-term catheters are likely to have a high concentration of bacteria in their urine and great care should be taken to avoid cross-infection after contact with the system. Hands become contaminated with bacteria when the drainage system is emptied, a specimen is taken or the catheter and drainage bag are disconnected. Disposable gloves should therefore always be worn for these procedures. Containers used to collect urine will also become heavily contaminated and should either be disposable or washed in a bedpan washer after each use.

Clusters of infection are frequently associated with catheterised patients in hospital and antibiotic-resistant strains present particular problems, as they are difficult to treat, cause outbreaks and can transfer the DNA coding for antibiotic resistance to other bacteria (Shales et al 1986, Fryklund et al 1997).

Treatment of catheter-associated infection

Bacteria are invariably isolated from the urine when a catheter has been in place for more than a month and such urine is often malodorous and cloudy. Provided the patient is asymptomatic, treatment of this colonisation is not indicated as the effect of antibiotics is likely to be short-lived and encourage the emergence of antibiotic resistant pathogens (Warren 1997). Specimens should therefore only be taken when the patient has symptoms of infection that are suspected to be related to the presence of the catheter. If the catheter can be removed then the urine will become free from pathogens within a day or two and treatment with antibiotics may not be necessary.

Bladder installations. Antiseptic solutions instilled into the bladder may help to prevent infection following urological surgery but are ineffective in the treatment of pre-existing infections (Slade & Gillespie 1985). They are not recommended for routine use in long-term-catheterised patients as they will not prevent bacteriuria and are likely to encourage resistant bacteria to emerge (Stickler 1990). Specimens of urine for culture should be taken from the self-sealing rubber sleeve on the drainage bag tubing. These are more likely to represent the bacteria present in the bladder than if taken from the drainage bag.

INFECTION OF THE LOWER RESPIRATORY TRACT

Infection of the respiratory tract between the larynx and alveoli can be serious and even life-threatening. Such infections account for 23% of all hospital-acquired infection (Emmerson et al 1996).

Whilst *Streptococcus pneumoniae, Haemophilus influenzae* and respiratory viruses account for the majority of community-acquired pneumonias, Gram-negative bacilli predominate as the cause of pneumonia in hospital patients. Nosocomial pneumonia is the main cause of death in a third of affected patients, and the mortality rate approaches 70% if it is caused by Gram-negative bacilli (Wollschlager et al 1988).

Risk factors for hospital-acquired pneumonia

Microorganisms enter the lower respiratory tract by inhalation of minute airborne particles or aspiration from the oropharynx. In healthy people, the ciliated cells covered in sticky mucus that line the tract trap microorganisms and propel them upwards towards the pharynx, where they are coughed out. Aspiration of secretions occurs commonly during sleep, but these natural defences are usually able to remove them (Huxley et al 1973). The risk of pneumonia is increased when the oropharynx and stomach are colonised by Gram-negative bacilli and when factors exist which facilitate their aspiration into the respiratory tract. These are summarised in List 13.3 and Figure 13.5.

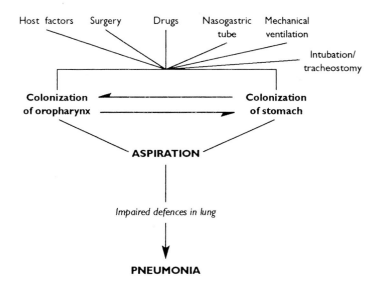

Figure 13.5 Factors that influence the acquisition of hospital-acquired pneumonia. Source: Wilson 1995.

List 13.3 Risk factors for pneumonia

Underlying factors that increase susceptibility of the host
- Extremes of age
- Severe illness
- Immunosuppression

Factors that enhance colonisation of the oropharynx or stomach by Gram-negative bacteria
- Antimicrobial agents
- Critical illness
- Surgery
- H_2 antagonists for stress bleeding prophylaxis
- Nasogastric tube
- Endotracheal tube

Factors that facilitate aspiration
- Supine position
- Depressed consciousness
- Nasogastric tube
- Endotracheal tube

Exposure to contaminated aerosols
- Contaminated respiratory equipment
- Prolonged mechanical ventilatory support

Factors that impede normal microbial clearance from respiratory tract
- Abdominal, thoracic, head and neck surgery
- Immobilisation
- Depressed respiration, e.g. narcotic pain relief
- Underlying respiratory illness

Colonisation of the oropharynx and stomach

Healthy people carry very few Gram-negative bacilli in their oropharynx. Severe illness results in the depletion of fibronectin, a protein that normally prevents bacteria adhering to the epithelial cells; as a result oropharyngeal colonisation with Gram-negative bacilli increases. Surgery also appears to reduce fibronectin production and a third of patients develop Gram-negative oropharyngeal colonisation within 48 hours of major surgery (Johanson et al 1980).

Invasive devices such as nasogastric and endotracheal tubes both enhance colonisation and facilitate aspiration, and the critically ill or unconscious patient is more likely to aspirate because of abnormal swallowing and being in a supine position.

Normally, very few bacteria survive the highly acidic contents of the stomach. However, under certain circumstances the stomach is colonised by increased numbers of bacteria and is then thought to be an important reservoir of organisms that cause hospital-acquired pneumonia. Antacids and H_2 antagonists, used to prevent stress bleeding in the critically ill, allow the pH to increase to levels at which organisms can survive and multiply, and are known to be associated with an increased risk of pneumonia. Increased bacterial colonisation of the stomach is also associated with advanced age, impaired gastrointestinal motility, gastrointestinal disease and enteral feeds, which are also likely to induce gastric reflux because of the increase in fluid volume and pressure in the stomach.

Mechanically assisted ventilation

Patients receiving continuous artificial ventilation have a significantly increased risk of developing pneumonia, with the risk increasing by 1% for each day of ventilation (Fagon et al 1989). A combination of factors contributes to this risk: bacteria may be introduced into the oropharynx during endotracheal intubation; bacteria build up in the biofilm that forms on the surface of the endotracheal tube and can be dislodged into the respiratory tract; and critically ill patients have depressed defences against infection.

Inhalation of contaminated aerosols

Contaminated respiratory or anaesthetic equipment may deliver bacteria in an aerosol to the patient, who subsequently develops pneumonia. Nebulisers are particularly hazardous because they create an aerosol from fluid in the chamber, producing many small droplets that are inhaled deep into the respiratory tract. Their use has frequently been associated with increased oropharyngeal colonisation and hospital-acquired pneumonia (Craven et al 1984a). Humidifiers are less hazardous since they increase the amount of water vapour in the inhaled gas without generating an aerosol of droplets from the fluid. However, fluid tends to collect in the humidified circuits, and bacteria that multiply in the fluid can drain into the patient's trachea (Stucke & Thompson, 1980; Figure 13.6).

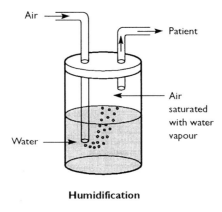

Humidification

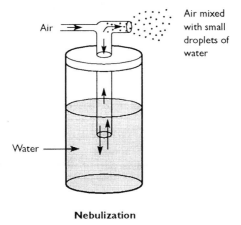

Nebulization

Figure 13.6 Mechanisms of nebulisation and humidification. Source: Wilson 1995.

The prevention of hospital-acquired pneumonia

Measures to prevent hospital-acquired pneumonia should be directed at reducing or preventing colonisation of the oropharynx and stomach, minimising the risk of aspiration and managing respiratory equipment carefully to ensure that contamination and cross-infection do not occur.

Handwashing and the use of protective clothing

Bacteria may be readily transmitted between patients in critical care settings on the hands of staff and via equipment used for respiratory therapy (Craven et al 1984a). This has been illustrated by Cadwallader et al (1990), who found that the hands of staff became contaminated after changing ventilator tubing. Hands should always be washed after contact with these devices, and before and after contact with intubated or ventilated patients. Alcohol handrubs can be used in place of soap to remove transient flora from hands provided they are not visibly soiled.

Clean disposable gloves should be worn for contact with mucous membranes, respiratory secretions and objects contaminated by them. A plastic disposable apron should be worn when contamination of the clothing may occur. Gloves and aprons should be removed after contact and hands washed. The same pair of gloves should never be worn for contact with another vulnerable site on the same patient or for contact with a different patient.

Mechanical ventilator and breathing circuits

Recent studies have shown that breathing circuits can be safely used for at least 48 hours and in one study changing the breathing circuit every 7 days did not appear to increase the risk of pneumonia, although it must be changed between different patients (Kollef et al 1995, Stamm 1998). Heat–moisture exchange filters can be attached to the circuit to protect both the ventilator and patient from contamination, provided a humidifier reservoir is not attached to the circuit. These filters recycle the moisture expired by the patient and obviate the need for a humidifier, although they may increase resistance to breathing. The filter should be changed according to the manufacturer's instructions but the breathing circuit does not need to be changed while in use on a single patient (Tablan et al 1994).

Heated cascade humidifiers cause condensate to collect in the breathing circuit, which can become contaminated and has been associated with outbreaks of infection (Gorman et al 1993). Condensate should therefore be carefully drained out of the tube, not tipped down the patient's trachea or returned to the humidification reservoir. Hands should be washed carefully after handling the tubing and condensate. The humidifier reservoir should be washed with detergent and water, dried and re-filled with sterile water every 48–72 hours (Ayliffe et al 1993).

Resuscitation bags can become contaminated with microorganisms and have been implicated in the transmission of bacteria between patients (Weber et al 1990). They can be protected by a filter, which should be changed between patients; alternatively they should be decontaminated (preferably by autoclave in a sterile supply department) between patients and if the adapter appears soiled. Spirometers, temperature probes and oxygen analysers may also transmit bacteria and should be changed with the ventilator circuits. If re-usable, they should be sterilised between patients (Irwin et al 1980, Weems 1993).

Airway maintenance devices

Tracheal and endotracheal tubes may introduce infection at the time of insertion and while in place accumulate bacteria on their surface in a biofilm that resists antimicrobial agents and the host defences (Sottile et al 1986). Tracheostomies should be performed under aseptic conditions and an aseptic technique should be used to replace the tube.

Secretions should not be allowed to accumulate in the respiratory tract and in ventilated patients these should be removed regularly by suctioning. Secretions that collect above the cuff of the tracheal tube should be removed prior to deflation of the cuff to prevent bacteria draining into the respiratory tract.

Suction should aim to cause the minimum amount of trauma to the respiratory tract. The pressure used should be as low as possible and a Y connector should be attached to enable the catheter to be inserted without suction being applied. The catheter should be withdrawn using a rotating motion and intermittent suction (Ward et al 1997). Outbreaks of infection related to inadequately decontaminated suction equipment or faulty equipment that produces aerosols have been reported and underline the need for effective maintenance and decontamination of suction equipment and an aseptic technique when carrying out the procedure (Creamer & Smyth 1996)

Suction catheters should be sterile and disposable, and each introduced only once using clean disposable gloves. The catheter tubing should be cleaned by sucking through sterile water. Hands may be contaminated by bacteria colonising the oropharynx or respiratory secretions; gloves should therefore be worn for suctioning and should be removed, and the hands washed, as soon as the procedure is finished. Closed-suction catheter systems have been introduced to many intensive care units. They enable a suction catheter to be re-used many times as the catheter is contained inside a sterile sheath and flushed clean with saline. They have the advantage of preventing environmental contamination with condensate and tracheal secretions, which occurs when the breathing circuit is disconnected for open suctioning (Cobbley et al 1991). However, Blackwood & Webb (1998) have reported problems with secretion removal and high levels of hand contamination with condensate where closed-suction systems are in use.

No outbreaks of infection have been associated with suction canisters and these, together with the tubing between catheter and canister can be changed between patients. Canisters do not need to be changed between patients in units where patients only require suction for short periods (Tablan et al 1994).

Nebulisers

Small-volume nebulisers are used for the delivery of medications and can be hand-held or inserted into the breathing circuit of a ventilator. They can become contaminated by the backflow of condensate or inadequate decontamination between use and then will deliver a high concentration of bacteria directly into the lower respiratory tract (Craven et al 1984b). These devices should be changed between patients and washed and dried between uses on the same patient. They should only be filled with sterile solutions, which must be dispensed aseptically into the chamber (Tablan et al 1994).

Large-volume nebulisers are used in intermittent positive pressure breathing (IPPB) and ultrasonic room humidifiers. They can become contaminated by handling, or by inadequate decontamination of the chamber, and are particularly hazardous because, unlike the small-volume nebulisers, they are often in use for prolonged periods. Once introduced, bacteria may multiply to large numbers in a few hours and these types of nebulisers have been associated with the transmission of Gram-negative bacteria and *Legionella* spp. (Mastro et al 1991, Grieble et al 1970). The chamber should only be filled with sterile water which should be dispensed into the chamber aseptically and they should be sterilised daily.

Oxygen delivery equipment

Tubing, nasal prongs and masks should be changed between patients. Wall humidifiers should be maintained by following the manufacturer's instructions and can probably be used safely between patients for several weeks (Golar et al 1993).

Enteral feeding

Patients with an enteral feeding tube in place should have the head of the bed positioned at an angle between 30° and 45° where possible to minimise the risk of reflux and aspiration (Tablan et al 1994). The gastric volume should not be allowed to rise as this will increase the risk of reflux; the intestinal motility will need to be assessed regularly; and the flow of feed must be monitored and adjusted to prevent build-up of fluid in the stomach. The position of the tube should also be checked regularly.

Enteral feeds are a very good medium for the growth of bacteria and are easily contaminated during preparation or administration. They should be prepared and transferred to the feeding reservoir aseptically to avoid contamination of the solution; contamination is less likely if prepacked manufactured feeds are used. The feed should not be allowed to run over a period longer than 24 hours and the reservoir and tubing should then be discarded and new equipment connected. Enteral feed solutions should be stored according to the manufacturer's instructions. Opened containers should be kept in the refrigerator and discarded after 24 hours. Nasogastric tubes should be changed according to the manufacturer's instructions, usually weekly for polyvinyl and 3-monthly for polyurethane (Ward et al 1997).

Anaesthetic equipment

The anaesthetic machine is not considered to be an important source of respiratory infection and routine disinfection is therefore not necessary (Tablan et al 1994). The breathing circuit and accessories may become contaminated with oropharyngeal pathogens, although the risk they present is generally low. Items that have direct contact with the patient's mucous membrane (e.g. laryngoscope, endotracheal tube and face mask) should be cleaned and sterilised between patients. Other parts of the breathing circuit can be protected by a bacterial heat–moisture exchange filter or decontaminated periodically, preferably in an automatic washing machine designed for disinfection of tubing (Das & Fraise 1997).

Prevention of post-operative pneumonia

Patients who are over 70 years of age, are obese or smoke, or have underlying respiratory disease, are at higher risk of developing pneumonia following surgery. The risk is also increased in patients who undergo surgery on the head, neck, thorax or abdomen, which may affect swallowing or normal respiratory tract clearance mechanisms.

The risk of postoperative pneumonia can be reduced by deep breathing exercises and incentive spirometry, which should be taught to patients prior to surgery. Intermittent positive pressure breathing may also be of value and, if oxygen is required, it should always be humidified to avoid drying the respiratory secretions.

Pain control after surgery is also important and has been shown to reduce the incidence of pneumonia after surgery (Wasylak et al 1990). Practical help such as supporting the wound encourages patients to cough up secretions after abdominal surgery.

Management of immobile patients

Patients who are immobile as a result of stroke, critical illness, trauma, coma or mechanically-assisted ventilation are at increased risk of developing pneumonia due to diminished respiratory tract clearing mechanisms and aspiration. Kinetic beds, which continuously rotate the position of the patient, have been recommended to reduce the risk of pneumonia in these patients, but their value has yet to be proved conclusively (de Boisblanc et al 1993)

Therapeutic interventions

Systemic prophylactic antibiotics have been widely used to prevent pneumonia, especially in patients who are critically ill, but are probably ineffective and are associated with the emergence of resistant pathogens (Tablan et al 1994).

Prescribing prophylactic antibiotics to prevent colonisation of the gut and oropharynx with Gram-negative bacilli has been recommended but their efficacy has yet to be clearly demonstrated. Antimicrobial agents in aerosols sprayed on to the oropharynx have been associated with the emergence of other pathogens not affected by the antimicrobial. Selective decontamination of the digestive tract (SDD) aims to remove Gram-negative bacilli but not the normal anaerobic flora. Although it appears to reduce the rate of hospital-acquired pneumonia, it can result in the emergence of antibiotic-resistant organisms and superinfection by fungi (Ward et al 1997). It is therefore probably only of value in small groups of critically ill patients. Routine prophylaxis against pneumonia is not recommended (Tablan et al, 1994).

When stress bleeding prophylaxis is necessary for critically ill patients a cryoprotective agent such as sucralfate should be prescribed, which has minimal effect on the acidity of the stomach. Patients given conventional antacids or H_2 antagonists are more likely to develop bacterial colonisation of the stomach and their risk of pneumonia is therefore increased (Pickworth et al 1993).

Other sources of hospital-acquired pneumonia

More unusual causes of hospital-acquired pneumonia are infections transmitted by an airborne route or contact with respiratory secretions. These include the respiratory viruses, legionnaires' disease and aspergillosis.

Respiratory viruses

These viruses account for a considerable proportion of hospital-acquired pneumonia that, particularly in the severely ill or immunosuppressed, can be severe and sometimes fatal. The most important are Respiratory syncytial virus (RSV) and influenza.

Respiratory syncytial virus. RSV occurs most commonly in children but may also affect adults. Outbreaks in the community usually occur during the winter months and hospital-acquired infections can occur following transmission from children admitted with infection, although visitors and staff may also act as a source. The virus is spread by droplets expelled from the respiratory tract and also by contact with respiratory secretions entering the eyes, nose or mouth from contaminated hands (Hall 1983). Transmission of RSV can be prevented by isolating affected patients who are symptomatic, using gloves and aprons for contact with respiratory secretions and hand washing after any contact with the patient. Additional measures required to protect immunocompromised or cardiac patients, who have a high risk of serious complications following infection, include the early identification, isolation and cohort nursing of infected patients, restricting contact with children under 12, other visitors with respiratory symptoms and symptomatic hospital staff (Garcia et al 1997, Madge et al 1992).

Influenza. Severe infections with influenza may result in viral pneumonia or secondary bacterial infection, and are particularly likely to occur in the very young, the elderly, immunocompromised patients or those with severe underlying heart or lung disease. Outbreaks of infection occur in the community during the winter months and nursing homes are frequently affected (Communicable Disease Report 1998). The virus is spread through close contact with affected people or their respiratory secretions and by small-droplet aerosols (Centers for Disease Control 1994). Affected patients should be isolated or cohorted with others and gloves and aprons should be used to handle respiratory secretions. Annual vaccination of people at high risk of serious infection is recommended before the influenza season begins (Department of Health 1996).

Legionnaires' disease

The causative organism of this infection, *Legionella pneumophila*, can be found in a variety of aquatic environments but only causes infection when aerosols or sprays of heavily contaminated water are inhaled by susceptible individuals. In hospitals and other large buildings with water-cooled air conditioning systems, poor maintenance can result in the build-up of stagnant water in which legionella can multiply and subsequently be released into the air of the building. Hot-water supply systems, humidifiers, nebulisers and other respiratory equipment and ice-making machines have all been implicated in the transmission of legionella (Arnow et al 1982, Medical Services Directorate 1993, Hanrahan et al 1987, Woo et al 1986).

Although it is an uncommon infection, 22 outbreaks of hospital-acquired legionnaires' disease were reported in England and Wales between 1980 and 1992 (Joseph et al 1994). Elderly and immuno-compromised people are normally affected but person-to-person transmission does not occur.

Infection can be prevented by proper maintenance and cleaning of water-cooled air conditioning systems and water tanks, chlorination of the water supply and preventing water stagnating in pipework. Hot water should be maintained at temperatures above 50°C to prevent multiplication of the organism (NHS Estates 1993).

Aspergillosis

This fungus is commonly present in soil, water and decaying vegetation and its spores can be found in the air, particularly when soil is disturbed by building works. Pneumonia following inhalation of the spores usually affects only the immunocompromised, or those with pre-existing lung disease such as cystic fibrosis. The most severely immunosuppressed, for example those receiving bone marrow transplantation, are most at risk and cases are often related to construction near the site of the hospital resulting in increased numbers of airborne spores. A variety of filtered air systems have been used to protect the most vulnerable patients (Rhame 1991, Barnes & Rogers 1989).

REFERENCES

Arnow, P., Chou, T., Weil, D. *et al.* (1982) Nosocomial Legionnaires' disease caused by aerosolised tap water from respiratory devices. *J. Infect. Dis.*, **146**, 460–467.

Ayliffe, G.A.J., Collins, B.J. and Taylor, L.J. (1990) *Hospital Acquired Infection – Principles and Prevention*, 2nd edn. John Wright, London.

Ayliffe, G.A.J., Coates, D. and Hoffman, P.N. (1993) *Chemical Disinfection in Hospitals*. Public Health Laboratory Service, London.

Barnes, R.A. and Rogers, T.R. (1989) Control of an outbreak of nosocomial aspergillosis by laminar air-flow isolation. *J. Hosp. Infect.*, **14**, 89–94.

Beck-Sague, C.M., and Jarvis, W.R. (1991) The epidemiology and prevention of nosocomial infections. In: *Disinfection, Sterilisation and Preservation*, 4th edn (ed. Block, S.S.). Lea & Febiger, Philadelphia, PA.

Beck-Sague, C.M. and Jarvis, W.R. (1993) Secular trends in the epidemiology of nosocomial fungal infections in the United States, 1980–1990. *J. Infect. Dis.*, **167**, 1247–1251.

Belkin, N.L. (1997) The evolution of the surgical mask: filtering efficiency versus effectiveness. *Infect. Control Hosp. Epidemiol.*, **18**(1), 49–57.

Blackwood, B. and Webb, C.H. (1998) Closed tracheal suctioning systems and infection control in the intensive care unit. *J. Hosp. Infect.*, **39**(4), 315–322.

Brennan, S.S., Foster, M.E. and Leaper, D.J. (1986) Antiseptic toxicity in wounds healing by secondary intention. *J. Hosp. Infect.*, **8**, 263–267.

Bryan, C.S. and Reynolds, K.L. (1984) Hospital-acquired bacteremic urinary tract infection. Epidemiology and outcome. *J. Urol.*, **132**, 494–498.

Buchan, I.A., Andrews, J.K., Lang, S.M. *et al.* (1980) Clinical and laboratory investigation of the composition and properties of human skin wound exudate under semi-permeable dressings. *Burns*, **7**, 326–334.

Bucknall, T.E. (1985) Factors affecting the development of surgical wound infections: a surgeon's view. *J. Hosp. Infect*, **6**, 1–8.

Burdette-Taylor, S. and Taylor, T.G. (1993) Wound cultures: what, when and how. *Ostomy Wound Manage.* **39**(8), 26–32.

Burke, J.P., Garibaldi, R.A., Britt, M.R. *et al.* (1981) Prevention of catheter-associated urinary tract infections – efficacy of daily meatal care regimes. *Am. J. Med.*, **70**, 655–658.

Cadwallader, H.L., Bradley, C.R. and Ayliffe, G.A.J. (1990) Bacterial contamination and frequency of changing ventilator circuitry. *J. Hosp. Infect.*, **15**, 65–72.

Centers for Disease Control (1994) Guideline for the prevention of nosocomial pneumonia. *Respir. Care*, **39**(12), 1191–1236.

Centers for Disease Control (1996) Guideline for prevention of intravascular device-related infections. *Am. J. Infect. Control*, **24**, 262–293.

Chrintz, H., Vibits, H., Cordtz, T.O. *et al.* (1989) Need for surgical wound dressing. *Br. J. Surg.*, **76**, 204–205.

Clark-Christoff, N., Watters, V.A., Sparks, W. *et al.* (1992) Use of triple-lumen subclavian catheters for administration of total parenteral nutrition. *J. Parenter. Enteral Nutr.*, **161**, 403–407.

Classen, D.C., Larsen, R.A., Burke, J.P. *et al.* (1991) Daily meatal care for prevention of catheter-associated bacteriuria: results using frequent applications of poly-antibiotic cream. *Infect. Control Hosp. Epidemiol.*, **12**, 157–162.

Cobb, D.K., High, K.P., Sawyer, R.G. *et al.* (1992) A controlled trial of scheduled replacement of central venous and pulmonary artery catheters. *New Engl. J. Med.*, **327**, 1062–1068.

Cobbley, M., Atkins, M. and Jones, P.L. (1991) Environmental contamination during tracheal suctioning. *Anaesthesia*, **44**, 957–961.

Communicable Disease Report (1998) An outbreak of influenza in four nursing homes in Sheffield. *Commun. Dis. Rep. Wkly*, **8**(16), 139.

Conly, J.M., Grieves, K. and Peters, B. (1989) A prospective randomised study comparing transparent and dry gauze dressings for central venous catheters. *J. Infect. Dis.*, **159**, 310–319.

Cooke, E.M., Coello, R. *et al.* (1999). Development of a national surveillance scheme for hospital associated infection: general principles. *J. Hosp. Infect.*

Cox, A., Hukins, D. and Sutton, T. (1988) Comparison of in vitro encrustation on silicone and hydrogel-coated latex catheters. *Br. J. Urol.*, **61**, 156–161.

Craven, D.E., Goularte, T.A. and Make, B.J. (1984a) Contaminated condensate in mechanical ventilator circuits: a risk factor for nosocomial pneumonia? *Am. Rev. Respir. Dis.*, **129**, 625–628.

Craven, D.E., Lichtenberg, D.A. and Goularte, T.A. (1984b) Contaminated medication nebulisers in mechanical ventilatory circuits: a source of bacterial aerosols. *Am. J. Med.*, **77**, 834–838.

Creamer, E. and Smyth, E.G. (1996) Suction apparatus and the suctioning procedure: reducing the infection risks. *J. Hosp. Infect.*, **34**(1), 1–10.

Crow, R.A., Mulhall, A. and Chapman, R.G. (1988) Indwelling catheterisation and related nursing practice. *J. Adv. Nurs.*, **13**, 489–495.

Cruse, P.J.E. (1986) Surgical infection: incisional wounds. In: *Hospital Infections*, 2nd edn (eds Bennett, J.V. and Brachman, P.S.). Little, Brown & Co., Boston, MA.

Cruse, P.J.E. and Foord, R. (1980) The epidemiology of wound infection – a 10 year prospective study of 62,939 wounds. *Surg. Clin. North Am.*, **60**(1), 27–40.

Das, I. and Fraise, A.P. (1997) How useful are microbial filters in respiratory apparatus? *J. Hosp. Infect.*, **37**(4), 263–272.

De Boisblanc, B.P., Castro, M., Everret, B. *et al.* (1993) Effect of air-supported continuous, postural oscillation on the risk of early ICU pneumonia in non traumatic critical illness. *Chest*, **103**, 1543–1547.

Department of Health (1996) *Immunisation Against Infectious Disease*. HMSO, London.

Elek, S.D. and Conen, P.E. (1957) The virulence of *Staphylococcus pyogenes* for men: a study of the problems of wound infection. *Br. J. Exp. Pathol.*, **38**, 573–586.

Elliot,. (1988) Intravascular device infections. *J. Med. Micro.*, **27**, 161–167.

Emmerson, A.M., Enstone, J.E., Griffin, M. *et al.* (1996) The second national prevalence survey of infection in hospitals – overview of the results. *J. Hosp. Infect.*, **32**, 175–190.

Fagon, J.Y., Chastre, J., Domart, Y. *et al.* (1989) Nosocomial pneumonia in patients receiving continuous mechanical ventilation; prospective analysis of 52 episodes with use of a protected specimen brush and quantitative culture techniques. *Am. Rev. Respir. Dis.*, **139**, 877–884.

Freeman, J., Goldmann, D.A., Smith, N.E. *et al.* (1990) Association of intravenous lipid emulsion and coagulase-negative staphylococcal bacteraemia in neonatal intensive care units. *N. Engl. J. Med.*, **323**, 301–308.

Fryklund, B., Haeggman, S. and Burman, L.G. (1997) Transmission of urinary bacterial strains between patients with indwelling catheters – nursing in the same room and in separate rooms compared. *J. Hosp. Infect.*, **36**(2), 147–154.

Garcia, R., Raad, I., Abi-Said, D. *et al.* (1997) Nosocomial respiratory syncytial virus infections: prevention and control in bone marrow transplant patients. *Infect. Control Hosp. Epidemiol.*, **18**, 412–416.

Garibaldi, R.A. (1993) Hospital-acquired urinary infections. In: *Prevention and Control of Nosocomial Infections*, 2nd edn, (ed. Wenzel, R.P.) Williams & Wilkins, Baltimore, MD.

Garibaldi, R.A., Burke, J.P., Dickman, M.L. *et al.* (1974) Factors predisposing to bacteriuria during indwelling urethral catheterisation. *New Engl. J. Med.*, **291**, 215–219.

Garner, J.S., Dixon, R.E. and Aber, R.C. (1981) Epidemic infections in surgical patients. *AORN J.*, **34**, 700–724.

Gilchrist, B. and Reed, C. (1989) The bacteriology of leg ulcers under hydrocolloid dressings. *Br. J. Dermatol*, **121**, 337–344.

Glynn, A., Ward, V., Wilson, J. *et al.* (1997) *Hospital-acquired Infection: Surveillance, Policies and Practice*. Public Health Laboratory Service, London.

Golar, S.D., Sutherland, L.L.A. and Ford, G.T. (1993) Multi-patient use of pre-filled disposable oxygen humidifiers for up to 30 days: patient safety and cost analysis. *Respir. Care*, **38**, 343–347.

Gorman, L.J., Sanai, L., Notman, A.W. *et al.* (1993) Cross infection in an intensive care unit by *Klebsiella pneumoniae* from ventilator condensate. *J. Hosp. Infect.*, **23**, 27–34.

Grieble, H.G., Colton, F.R., Thomas, M.S. *et al.* (1970) Fine particle humidifiers: source of *Pseudomonas aeruginosa* in a respiratory disease unit. *N. Engl. J. Med.*, **282**, 531–533.

Gruber, R.B., Vistnes, L. and Pardoe, R. (1975) The effect of commonly used antiseptics on wound healing. *Plast. Reconstr. Surg.*, **55**, 472–476.

Haley, R.W., Culver, D.H. and Morgan, W.M. (1985a) Identifying patients at high risk of surgical wound infection: a simple multivariate index of patient susceptibility and wound contamination. *Am. J. Epidemiol.*, **121**, 206–215.

Haley, R.W., Culver, D.H., White, J.W. *et al.* (1985b) The efficacy of surveillance and control programs in preventing nosocomial infections in US hospitals. *Am. J. Epidemiol.*, **121**, 182–205.

Hall, C.B. (1983) The nosocomial spread of respiratory syncytial viral infections. *Annu. Rev. Med.*, **34**, 311–319.

Hambreus, A. (1988) Aerobiology in operating rooms. *J. Hosp. Infect.* **11** (Suppl A), 68–76.

Hanrahan, J.P., Morse, D.L., Scharf, V.B. *et al.* (1987) A community hospital outbreak of Legionellosis: transmission by potable hot water. *Am. J. Epidemiol.,* **125**, 639–649.

Hazard Notice (1993) Degradation of silicone tubing by alcohol-based antiseptics. Hazard Notice (93)7 Medical Devices Directorate, London.

Hoborn, J. (1990) Wet strike-through and transfer of bacteria through operating barrier fabrics. *Hyg. Med.,* **15**, 15–20.

Hoffman, K.K., Weber, D.J., Samsa, G.P. *et al.* (1992) Transparent polyurethane film as an intravenous catheter dressing: a meta-analysis of the infection risks. *J.A.M.A.,* **267**, 2072–2076.

Hollinworth, H. and Kingston JE (1998) Using a non-sterile-technique in wound care. *Prof. Nurse,* **13**(4), 226–229.

Holzheimer, R.G., Haupt, W., Thiede, A. *et al.* (1997) The challenge of postoperative infections: does the surgeon make a difference? *Infect. Control, Hosp. Epidemiol.,* **18**, 449–456.

Howarth, F.H. (1985) Prevention of airborne infection during surgery. *Lancet,* **i**, 386–388.

Hutchinson, J.J. and Lawrence, J.C. (1991) Wound infection under occlusive dressings. *J. Hosp. Infect.,* **17**, 83–94.

Huxley, E.J., Viroslave, J., Gray, W.R. *et al.* (1973) Pharyngeal aspiration in normal adults and patients with depressed consciousness. *Am. J. Med.,* **64**, 564–568.

Irwin, R.S., Demers, R.R. and Pratter, M.R. (1980) An outbreak of Acinetobacter infection associated with the use of a ventilator spirometer. *Respir. Care,* **25**, 232–237.

Johanson, W.G., Higuchi, J.G., Chaudhuri, T.R. *et al.* (1980) Bacterial adherence to epithelial cells in bacillary colonisation of the respiratory tract. *Am. Rev. Respir. Dis.,* **121**, 55–63.

Johnstone, J.D. (1982) Infrequent infections associated with Hickman catheters. *Cancer Nurs.,* **5**, 125–129.

Joseph, C.A., Watson, J.M., Harrison, T.G. *et al.* (1994) Nosocomial legionnaires' disease in England and Wales. 1980–1992. *Epidemiol. Infect.,* **112**, 329–345.

Kass, E.H. and Schneiderman, L.J. (1959) Entry of bacteria into the urinary tract of patients with inlying catheters. *New Engl. J. Med.,* **256**, 556–557.

Kollef, M.H., Shapiro, S.D., Fraser, V.J. *et al.* (1995) Mechanical ventilation with or without 7-day circuit changes: a randomised controlled trial. *Ann. Intern. Med.,* **123**, 168–174.

Kolmos, H.J., Thuesen, B., Nielsen, S.V. *et al.* (1993) Outbreak of infection in a burns unit due to *Pseudomonas aeruginosa* originating from contaminated tubing used for irrigation of patients. *J. Hosp. Infect.,* **24**, 11–21.

Lowbury, E.J.L. and Cason, J.S. (1985) Aspects of infection control and skin grafting in burned patients. In: *Wound Care* (ed. Westerby, S.). Heinemann, London.

Lynch, W., Davey, P.G., Malek, M. *et al.* (1992) Cost-effectiveness analysis of the use of chlorhexidine detergent in preoperative whole-body disinfection in wound infection prophylaxis. *J. Hosp. Infect.,* **21**, 179–191.

Madge, P., Patson, J.Y., McColl, J.H. *et al.* (1992) Prospective controlled study of four infection control procedures to prevent nosocomial infection with respiratory syncytial virus. *Lancet,* **340**, 1079–1083.

Maki, D.G. and Ringer, M. (1987) Evaluation of dressing regimens for prevention of infection with peripheral intravenous catheters, gauze, a transparent polyurethane dressing and an iodophor-transparent dressing. *J.A.M.A.,* **258**, 2396–2403.

Maki, D.G., Goldman, D.A. and Rhame, F.S. (1973) Infection control in intravenous therapy. *Ann. Intern. Med.,* **79**, 867–887.

Maki, D.G., Botticelli, J.T., Le Roy, M.I. *et al.* (1987) Prospective study of replacing administration sets for intravenous therapy at 48 hour versus 72 hour intervals. 72 hours is safe and cost-effective. *J.A.M.A.*, **258**, 1777–1781.

Maki, D.G., Ringer, M. and Alvarado, C.J. (1991a) Prospective randomised trial of povidone-iodine, alcohol and chlorhexidine for prevention of infection associated with central venous and arterial catheters. *Lancet*, **338**, 339–343

Maki, D.G., Stolz, S. and Wheeler, S. (1991b) A prospective, randomised, three-way clinical comparison of a novel, highly impermeable, polyurethane dressing with 206 Swan–Ganz pulmonary artery catheters: Opsite IV3000 versus Tegaderm versus gauze and tape. I. Cutaneous colonisation under the dressing, catheter-related infection. In: *Improving Catheter Site Care. Proceedings of a Symposium, Series 179*. Royal Society of Medicine, London, pp. 61–66.

Mangram, A.J., Horan, T.C., Pearson, M.L. *et al* (1999) Guideline for the prevention of surgical wound infection. *Am. J. Infect. Contr.*, **27**, 97–134.

Mastro, T.D., Fields, B.S., Breiman, R.F. *et al.* (1991) Nosocomial legionnaires' disease and the use of medication nebulisers. *J. Infect. Dis.*, **163**, 667–670.

Medical Services Directorate (1993) Ice cubes: infection caused by *Xanthomonas maltophilia. Hazard*, **93**, 42.

Mermel, L., Stolz, S. and Maki, D.G. (1991) Epidemiology and pathogenesis of infection with Swan–Ganz catheters. A prospective study using molecular epidemiology. *Am. J. Med.*, **91**(3b), 197.

NHS Estates (1993) The control of legionellae in healthcare premises – a code of practice. *Health Technical Memorandum 240*. HMSO, London.

Neidner, R. and Schöpf, E. (1986) Inhibition of wound healing by antiseptics. *Br. J. Dermatol.* **115**(S31), 41–44.

Nickel, J.C. Grant, S.K. and Costerton, J.W. (1985) Catheter-associated bacteriuria: an experimental study. *Urology*, **36**, 369–375.

Nicolle, L.E. (1997) Asymptomatic bacteriuria in the elderly. *Infect. Dis. Clin. North Am.*, **11**(3), 647–663.

Ojajärvi, J. (1976) An evaluation of antiseptics used for hand disinfection in wards. *J. Hyg. (Camb.)*, **76**, 75–82.

Olsen, M., O'Connor, M.O. and Schwartz, M.L. (1984) A 5-year prospective study of 20,193 wounds at Minneapolis VA Medical Center. *Ann. Surg.*, **199**, 253–259.

Pettersson, E. (1986) A cut above the rest? *Nurs. Times*, **31**(5), 68–70.

Pickworth, K.K., Falcone, R.E., Hooge-boom, J.E. *et al.* (1993) Occurrence of nosocomial pneumonia in mechanically ventilated trauma patients: a comparison of sulcralfate and ranitidine. *Crit. Care Med.*, **21**, 1856–1862.

Platt, R., Polk, B.F., Murdock, B. *et al.* (1982) Mortality associated with nosocomial urinary tract infection. *New Engl. J. Med.*, **307**, 939–943.

Platt, R., Murdock, B. and Polk, B.F. (1983) Reduction of mortality associated with nosocomial urinary tract infection. *Lancet*, **i**, 1893–1897.

Raad, I. (1997) Vascular catheters impregnated with antimicrobial agents: present knowledge and future direction. *Infect. Control Hosp. Epidemiol.*, **18**, 227–229

Raad, I., Costerton, W., Sabharwal, U. *et al.* (1993) Ultrastructural analysis of indwelling vascular catheters: a quantitative relationship between luminal colonisation and duration of placement. *J. Infect. Dis.*, **168**, 400–407.

Raad, II., Hohn, D.C., Gilbreath, B.J. *et al.* (1994) Prevention of central venous catheter-related infections by using maximal sterile barrier precautions during insertion. *Infect. Control Hosp. Epidemiol.*, **15**, 231–238.

Rhame, F.S. (1991) Prevention of nosocomial aspergillosis. *J. Hosp. Infect.*, **18**, 466–472.

Roberts, J.M.B., Linton, K.B., Pollard, B.R. *et al.* (1965) Long term catheter drainage in the male. *Br. J. Urol.*, **37**, 63–72.

Roe, B.H. (1990) Study of the effects of education on the management of urine drainage systems by patients and carers. *J. Adv. Nurs.*, **15**, 223–231.

Rogers, J. (1991) Pass the cranberry juice. *Nurs. Times*, **87**, 36–37.

Sanderson, P.J. (1991) Infection in orthopaedic implants. *J. Hosp. Infect.*, **18**(Suppl. A), 367–375.

Shales, D.M., Lehman, M.-H., CurrieMcCumber, C.A. *et al.* (1986) Prevalence of colonisation with antibiotic resistant gram-negative bacilli in a nursing home care unit: the importance of cross-colonisation as documented by plasmid analysis. *Infect. Control*, **7**, 538–545.

Sheth, N.K., Rose, H.D., Franson, T.R. *et al.* (1983) Colonisation of bacteria on polyvinyl chloride and Teflon catheters in hospitalised patients. *J. Clin. Microbiol.*, **18**, 1061–1063.

Slade, N. and Gillespie, W.A. (1985) *The Urinary Tract and the Catheter: Infection and Other Problems*. John Wiley & Sons, New York

Sottile, F.D., Marrie, T.J., Prough, D.S. *et al.* (1986) Nosocomial pulmonary infection: possible etiologic significance of bacterial adhesion to endotracheal tubes. *Crit. Care. Med.*, **14**, 265–270.

Spencer, R.C. (1990) Use of in-line filters for intravenous infusions in intensive care units. *J. Hosp. Infect.*, **16**, 281.

Stamey, T.A. and Timothy, M.M. (1975) Studies of introital colonisation in women with recurrent urinary infections I: the role of vaginal pH. *J. Urol.*, **114**, 261.

Stamm, A.M. (1998) Ventilator-associated pneumonia and frequency of circuit changes. *Am. J. Infect. Control*, **26**, 71–73.

Stickler, D.J. (1990) Antiseptics in bladder catheterization. *J. Hosp. Infect.*, **16**, 89–108.

Stucke, V.A. and Thompson, R.E.M. (1980) Infection transfer by respiratory condensate during positive pressure respiration. *Nurs. Times*, **76**(9), 3–4.

Tablan, O.C. (1997) Nosocomial pneumonia. In: *Infection Control and Applied epidemiology. Principles and Practice.* Association for Professionals in Infection Control and Epidemiology (APIC) Inc. Mosby, St Louis, MO.

Tablan, O.C., Anderson, L.J., Arden, N.H. *et al* (1994) Guideline for the prevention of nosocomial pneumonia. Part 1. Issues on prevention of nosocomial pneumonia. *Am. J. Infect. Control*, **22**(4), 247–292.

Thompson, G. and Bullock, D. (1992) To clean or not to clean? *Nurs. Times*, **88**(34), 66–68.

Tomlinson, D. (1987) To clean or not to clean? *Nurs. Times*, **83**(9), 71–75.

UK Health Departments (1998) *Guidance for Clinical Health Care Workers: Protection Against Infection with Blood-borne Viruses. Recommendations of the Expert Advisory Group on AIDS and the Expert Advisory Group on Hepatitis.* HMSO, London

Van der Linden, W., Gedda, S., Edlund, G. *et al.* (1981) Randomized trial of drainage after cholecystectomy: suction versus static drainage through a main wound versus a stab incision. *Am. J. Surg.*, **141**, 289–294.

Walsh, M. and Ford, P. (1989) *Nursing Rituals, Research and Rational Actions.* Butterworth-Heinemann, Oxford.

Ward, V., Wilson, J., Taylor, L. *et al.* (1997) *Preventing Hospital-acquired Infection. Clinical Guidelines.* Public Health Laboratory Service, London.

Warren, J.W. (1997) Catheter-associated urinary tract infections. *Infect. Dis. Clin. North Am.*, **11**(3), 609–617.

Warren, J.W., Muncie, H.L., Hall-Craggs, M. (1988) Acute pyelonephritis associated with bacteriuria during long-term catheterisation: a prospective clinico-pathological study. *J. Infect. Dis.*, **158**, 1341–1346.

Wasylak, T.J.C., Abbott, F.V., English, M.J.M. *et al.* (1990) Reduction of postoperative morbidity following patient-controlled morphine. *Can. J. Anaesth.*, **37**, 726–731.

Weber, J.M., Sheridan, R.L., Pasternack, M.S. *et al.* (1997) Nosocomial infections in pediatric patients with burns. *Am. J. Infect. Control*, **25**, 195–201.

Weber, D.J., Wilson, M.B., Rutala, W.A. *et al.* (1990) Manual ventilation bags as a source for bacterial colonisation of intubated patients. *Am. Rev. Respir. Dis.*, **142**, 892–894.

Weems, J.J. (1993) Nosocomial outbreak of *Pseudomonas cepacia* associated with contamination of reusable electronic ventilator temperature probes. *Infect. Control Hosp. Epidemiol.*, **14**, 583–586.

Willis, J. (1996) Home parenteral nutrition. *Nurs. Times*, **92**(47), 50–51.

Whyte, W., Hodgson, R. and Tinkler, J. (1982) The importance of airborne bacterial contamination of wounds. *J. Hosp. Infect.*, **2**, 349–354.

Whyte, W., Hamblen, D.L., Kelly, I.G. *et al.* (1990) An investigation of occlusive polyester surgical clothing. *J. Hosp. Infect.* **15**, 363–374.

Wilson, J. (1995) *Infection Control in Clinical Practice.* Baillière Tindall, London.

Wollschlager, C.M., Conrad, A.R. and Khan, F.A. (1988) Common complications in critically ill patients. *Disease-a-month*, **34**, 221–293.

Woo, A.H., Yu, V.L., Goetz, A. *et al.* (1986) Potential in-hospital modes of transmission of *Legionella pneumophila*. Demonstration experiments for dissemination by showers, humidifiers and rinsing of ventilation bag apparatus. *Am. J. Med.*, **80**, 567–573.

Wurzel, C.L., Halom, K., Feldman, J.G. *et al.* (1988) Infection rates of Broviac–Hickman catheters and implantable venous devices. *Am. J. Dis. Child*, **142**, 536–540.

Wyndaele, J.-J. and Maes, D. (1990) Clean intermittent self-catheterisation: a 12-year follow up. *J. Urol.*, **143**, 906–908.

FURTHER READING

Henry, L. (1997) Parenteral nutrition. *Prof Nurse*, **13**(1), 39–42.

Orr, J. and Hain, T. (1994) Burn wound management: an overview. *Prof. Nurse*, **10**(3), 153–155.

Sobel, J.D. (1997) Pathogenesis of urinary tract infection: role of host defences. *Infect. Dis. Clin. North Am.*, **11**(3), 531–549.

Taylor, D. and Littlewood, S. (1998) Respiratory system part 1: pneumonia. *Nurs. Times*, **94**(7), 48–51.

Winder, A. (1990) Intermittent self-catheterisation. *Nurs. Times*, **86**(43), 63–64.

14

The management of infectious patients (isolation nursing)

INTRODUCTION

Some microorganisms cause infections which spread readily between people, commonly referred to as infectious or contagious diseases. Special precautions to prevent the spread of such infections date back thousands of years. The principle of segregating people with infectious diseases, such as leprosy and plague, was described in the Bible long before bacteria were recognised as the cause of infections (Selwyn 1991). In hospitals, infectious diseases present particular problems because they can be readily transmitted to other sick and vulnerable patients. Some pathogens take advantage of invasive devices such as urinary catheters and intravenous devices, or cause infection in wounds. Special precautions may be required to control the transmission of strains of antibiotic-resistant bacteria, which have emerged in recent years.

Isolation precautions are intended to prevent the spread of infectious diseases and nosocomial pathogens, among patients in hospital and the staff caring for them. They are required when routine infection control measures cannot contain microorganisms infecting or colonising patients.

HISTORICAL CONTEXT

Several approaches to isolation precautions have been employed since the concept was introduced to hospitals in the UK in the mid-19th century. The early methods involved the use of gloves and gowns and became known as barrier nursing. Florence Nightingale recognised the significance of contact with body substances, rather than the role of air or environment, in the transmission of infection. Her approach to 'fever nursing' emphasised the importance of barrier precautions when caring for patients with infection (Jackson & Lynch 1985). Attitudes altered in the early 20th century when the emphasis shifted towards considering everything in the patient's room as contaminated. In the 1970s the use of categories of isolation became popular. Infections were allocated to a particular category according to their principal route of transmission (Table 14.1). The disadvantage of this approach was that it did not enable individualised patient care or take account of infections requiring elements of more than one category of isolation. For example, antibiotic-resistant bacteria may be present in many body excretions and secretions, depending on the site of infection or colonisation. As a consequence there was a tendency to use too many or too few isolation practices (Garner 1996). In the 1980s, as understanding of the transmission of microorganisms increased and changes in the approach to nursing required patients to be cared for as individuals, many hospitals adopted a disease-specific approach. This tailored precautions towards preventing the transmission of each type of infection and left more of the decision-making about the measures required to the staff responsible for the particular patient's care (Garner & Simmons 1983).

Table 14.1 Example of isolation categories (Source: Control of Infection Group 1974)

Category of isolation	Indication	Diseases
Standard	Most infectious diseases requiring isolation	MRSA, Group A streptococcus, meningitis, tuberculosis
Stool, urine, needle	Infections spread by faeces, urine or blood	Salmonella, shigella, viral hepatitis, acute poliomyelitis
Strict	Serious diseases that spread very easily	Diphtheria, anthrax, generalised chickenpox, staphylococcal pneumonia
Protective	Patients who are highly susceptible to infection	Leukaemia, lymphoma, agranulocytosis, severe burns

In the mid-1980s the introduction of universal precautions to prevent the transmission of blood-borne viruses was recommended for the care of all patients (Centers for Disease Control 1987; p. 270). Widespread adoption of this approach means that additional isolation precautions are not necessary for many infectious diseases and has led some workers to review and simplify the whole concept. This was first suggested by Lynch et al (1987), who used the term 'body substance isolation' to describe a standard level of precautions for the management of all moist body substances, with some additional measures for those patients infected by microorganisms spread by an airborne route. Unlike conventional isolation precautions this system was not diagnosis-driven, so that appropriate precautions could be taken for contact with body substances even before a patient was diagnosed with an infection. For example, the precautions required for a patient with enteric infection would be the use of gloves and apron for contact with excreta, a single room not being essential to prevent transmission. If gloves and aprons were being used routinely for contact with body fluids then no additional precautions would be necessary for such patients. This approach also conferred considerable advantages for some types of infection, such as antibiotic-resistant bacteria, where infection could be transmitted from asymptomatically colonised patients before the need for isolation was recognised. The benefits of a standard level of precautions used in the care of all patients has now been widely recognised (Wilson & Breedon 1990, UK Health Departments 1990, Garner 1996). Its key components are summarised in List 14.1 and discussed in detail in Chapter 12.

A variety of approaches may be taken to provide an enhanced level of precaution for isolating patients with infectious disease, but these are now usually disease-specific or based on only a few simple categories of isolation (Garner 1996).

THE PRINCIPLES OF ISOLATION PROCEDURES

The objective of isolation is to prevent microorganisms from being transmitted from infected or colonised patients to others. While the term implies the separation of the individual from others, it is important to keep in mind that it is the microorganism, rather than the patient, that requires isolation. Thus precautions should be directed towards interrupting the spread

---

List 14.1 Standard precautions (Source: Garner 1996)

- **Handwashing**. After touching body fluids and contaminated items, regardless of whether gloves have been worn. Wash hands between procedures on the same patient to avoid cross-infection
- **Gloves**. Wear clean gloves when touching body fluids and contaminated items and before touching mucous membranes or non-intact skin. Change gloves between patients and between tasks on the same patient
- **Mask and eye protection**. Wear to protect the eyes and mouth during procedures likely to generate splashes of body fluid
- **Plastic apron or gown**. Wear to protect clothing or skin during activities likely to contaminate the clothing or generate splashes of body fluid
- **Equipment**. Wear gloves to handle contaminated equipment and ensure it is cleaned and decontaminated properly after use. Wear eye protection if cleaning is likely to generate splashes.
- **Environment**. Keep surfaces clean and free from dust
- **Linen**. Wear gloves and apron to handle contaminated linen; decontaminate by laundering
- **Sharps**. Handle used sharp instruments carefully to avoid injury and discard into designated containers

---

of the particular microorganism concerned, taking into account its usual route of transmission. The appendix to this chapter provides a guide to the routes of transmission and requirements for isolation of common infectious disease encountered in hospitals in the UK.

Many isolation procedures are based on tradition rather than scientific evidence and their value has not been fully evaluated (Jackson & Lynch 1985). Since isolation can be a disturbing experience for the patient, only appropriate and reasonable precautions should be taken and used for as short a period as possible.

The infection control team should always be consulted when considering placing a patient in isolation. There are a number of factors that need to be taken into account when determining the precautions required. These include:

- the infecting/colonising microorganism
- the site(s) of the body affected
- how it might spread to other patients
- whether other patients or staff are vulnerable to the infection
- measures required to contain the microorganism.

Underlying illness in the patient and his/her physical, psychological and emotional state may all influence how isolation precautions are applied.

In many cases, isolation precautions are only implemented once a diagnosis of an infectious disease is made. However, they should also be used when a patient presents with an undiagnosed rash or pyrexia, diarrhoea or vomiting or suspected tuberculosis, or if a patient is readmitted to hospital having had methicillin-resistant *Staphylococcus aureus* (MRSA) in the past. Precautions should be continued until the diagnosis has been confirmed.

The application of isolation measures may vary according to the risks presented by the particular ward or unit. A patient colonised with MRSA on an intensive care unit or orthopaedic ward requires single-room isolation to protect other vulnerable patients in the unit, while in a rehabilitation ward it may be possible to take adequate precautions without confining the patient.

Routes of transmission

There are several routes by which different microorganisms may be transmitted; the same microorganism may be able to take advantage of more than one route. In healthcare settings, the most important route of transmission is through contact, although a few pathogens may spread by an airborne route.

Contact transmission

This occurs by touching the skin or body fluids of an affected person, or via contaminated equipment. The hands can act as a means of transmission if, following contact with an infectious patient, they are not washed before contact with another person. Infectious diseases spread by contact can be isolated by using protective clothing to handle infectious body substances and contaminated equipment, and washing hands when gloves are removed and after contact with the patient. A single room is not essential to prevent transmission of these infections. Some respiratory infections, e.g. influenza, are transmitted by droplets expelled from the respiratory tract during sneezing or coughing. The droplets may be carried short distances to the oral mucosa of another person but these infections are also commonly transmitted by touching nasal or oral secretions.

Airborne transmission

This occurs when pathogens suspended in droplet nuclei are inhaled by a nearby, susceptible host. Droplet nuclei are small droplets expelled from the respiratory tract and evaporate to particles of less than 5 µm in size. These minute particles remain suspended in the air for prolonged periods and if inhaled can pass deep into the respiratory tract. Only a few pathogens likely to cause serious disease e.g. tuberculosis, are transmitted through inhalation of airborne droplet nuclei. Isolation in a single room, protective clothing for handling infectious respiratory secretions and hand washing when gloves are removed and after contact with the patient are necessary for patients with such infections. In some circumstances a mask may be necessary.

Isolation measures

Single room accommodation

Physical separation of patients is really only necessary where their infection is transmitted by an airborne route and, of the infections commonly encountered in the healthcare setting, only tuberculosis, measles and chickenpox fall into this category. Isolation rooms used to control airborne infections should have negative-pressure ventilation, especially if they are in close proximity to other highly susceptible patients, e.g. on an AIDS unit (Breathnach et al 1998). Negative-pressure ventilation means that air flows from the corridors into the room, not vice versa, minimising the risk of staff or other patients inhaling airborne pathogens. To create this negative pressure, air is extracted from the room to the outside of the building or through filters.

Patients who cannot be expected to follow infection control measures, (e.g. children, psychologically disturbed patients) or those whose illness causes them to contaminate the environment (e.g. profuse diarrhoea and vomiting) should also be placed in a single room. Some bacteria are able to survive for long periods in the environment (e.g. *Clostridium difficile*, MRSA) and for patients with these infections a single room may be required to limit the area affected (Hoffman 1993).

In practice, single-room accommodation is also often preferred for patients with infectious diseases transmitted by contact, as it may help to ensure that control measures are adhered to. A card displayed at the door can be used to indicate to others that special precautions are required (Figure 14.1). However, in many circumstances it should be possible for many patients to leave their room periodically, especially for physiotherapy, exercise and treatment in other departments.

In outbreaks of infection, several patients infected with the same organism can be placed in the same ward or bay. Some hospitals have special wards for caring for patients with infectious diseases, where physicians who specialise in their management are based. Such facilities can be particularly helpful when outbreaks of hospital-acquired infection occur. Regional infectious disease units (IDUs) have high-level isolation facilities with strict controls on air flow and complete bed isolators. These facilities are required for the care of patients suspected to be suffering from highly infectious disease, e.g. viral haemorrhagic fever (Advisory Committee on Dangerous Pathogens 1996). They may also be required to manage cases of multi-drug-resistant tuberculosis.

Handwashing

This is probably the single most important means of preventing transmission of infections, particularly those spread by contact (Garner & Hierholzer 1993). Hands should be washed immediately after contact with the patient, their body fluids and any equipment used by them. In most circumstances, washing with soap and water removes these transient microorganisms. Some hospitals recommend antiseptic detergents for hand washing after contact with isolated patients, especially for antibiotic-resistant microor-

STANDARD ISOLATION

Visitors please check with nurse
before entering

- Remove white coats before entering

- **Wash hands before leaving**

For further information refer to Isolation Policy

Figure 14.1 Example of an isolation notice. Source: Wilson 1995.

ganisms, which may be removed more effectively by these agents (Wade et al 1991). Alcohol handrubs can also be used to disinfect hands, provided that they are physically clean.

Protective clothing

Ayliffe et al (1979) concluded that staff clothing is not an important mode of transfer of microorganisms, after an investigation into its use in a source and protective isolation unit over an 18-month period. Although microorganisms are not readily transmitted on clothing, heavy contamination can occur after some procedures, such as dressing infected wounds (Hambraeus 1973). Plastic aprons are therefore recommended to protect clothing during such procedures.

Many episodes of care are not likely to result in clothing becoming contaminated with infective material and protective clothing is therefore not necessary on these occasions, e.g. serving meals. Where contact with infective material is likely to occur, the level of protection should be selected according to the anticipated exposure (see Figure 12.2). However, it is also important to change protective clothing between different procedures on the same patient to ensure that bacteria are not transferred from an infected to a susceptible site, e.g. between emptying a urine drainage bag and dressing a wound. A supply of clean gloves and aprons should always be readily available both inside and outside rooms used for isolation.

Gloves should be worn to prevent hands becoming contaminated with blood, body fluids or other infectious material. To prevent cross-infection, they must be removed after contact with the patient. Hands should then be washed, as they may be contaminated during removal of the gloves (Olsen et al 1993). Gloves should always be changed after handling excreta or contaminated sites, e.g. wounds.

Aprons and gowns. Plastic aprons are impermeable and disposable, easy to put on and inexpensive. They offer an effective means of protecting staff clothing at bed height, the area most likely to become contaminated. Disposable, water-repellent gowns are available but are relatively expensive and should be reserved for situations where protection against considerable splashing of body fluid is required. Cotton gowns are an inadequate barrier: when they become wet microorganisms pass through easily (Babb et al

1983). However, they can be useful over a plastic apron where additional protection of the arms and shoulders is considered necessary, e.g. in the care of babies to protect the shoulders from dribbling or regurgitation of feeds.

Masks. These are recommended for protecting healthcare workers from acquiring tuberculosis (Vesley 1995). The main risk is from prolonged contact with an infectious patient or during procedures with an increased risk of exposure to infected sputum, e.g. collection of an induced sputum specimen from a patient with pulmonary tuberculosis. However, although improvements have been made to their filtering efficacy, masks are effective only if they fit closely around the mouth and nose, since air inhaled around the edge of the mask will not be filtered (Belkin 1997), but this can make breathing uncomfortable for the wearer. The standard for filtering masks is described in the European Standard EN 149 (1991). Better protection against infection is probably provided by natural or acquired immunity to tuberculosis and by adequate negative-pressure room ventilation (British Thoracic Society 1990). This is particulary important where immunocompromised patients are in the same ward (Interdepartmental Working Group on Tuberculosis 1998).

Chickenpox (varicella) is highly transmissible and masks are unlikely to provide adequate protection against infection. Transmission to healthcare workers can be more reliably prevented by ensuring that only immune staff care for the patient, and these staff will not therefore need the protection of a mask. Most people born in the UK have acquired natural immunity to this infection through exposure in childhood. However, the level of immunity is lower in other countries, e.g. the West Indies, Hong Kong. Vulnerable patients and non-immune staff are at risk of acquiring, and subsequently transmitting, infection. Staff who work in units where patients may be particularly vulnerable to infection (e.g. haematology, renal units, AIDS units) should be assessed for immunity to Varicella-zoster virus so that they can be identified quickly should an outbreak occur (Jones et al 1997).

Cleaning

Domestic staff are unlikely to have direct contact with the patient or their body fluids and their risk of acquiring infection is usually low. This should be explained to them to ensure that the rooms of patients in isolation are cleaned properly. The patient's sense of isolation is likely to be increased if misunderstandings arise and the room is not cleaned regularly. Domestic staff should have their immunity to tuberculosis assessed and they should be instructed on the use of masks where this is recommended.

Contaminated inanimate objects do not play a major part in the transmission of most pathogens, although a few can survive for prolonged periods in dust (e.g. *Clostridium difficile*). Contaminated furniture and equipment, such as fluidized beds, have been implicated in the transmission of vancomycin-resistant enterococci, particularly when the patient has diarrhoea (Weber & Rutala 1997).

Surfaces should be kept clean and dry in the same way as other clinical areas. Disinfectants are not usually necessary but a separate mop, bucket and cleaning cloth may be recommended. When the period of isolation has finished or the patient is discharged, the room should be cleaned with detergent and water before the next patient is admitted. Airing the room is not necessary and laundering of curtains is rarely indicated as they are not a likely vehicle for the transmission of infection.

Waste, linen and excreta

Waste contaminated with infectious material should be discarded into yellow bags for incineration (Health and Safety Executive 1982). It does not require any special labelling and, since the risk of the outside of the bag becoming contaminated is minimal, does not need to be placed inside a second bag (Maki et al 1986). Linen from patients with an infectious disease should not be sorted by laundry staff prior to washing. It should therefore be separated at the bedside by placing it into a water-soluble plastic bag and red outer bag (NHS Executive 1995; p. 292). Once sealed in the appropriate bag, waste and linen can be stored with other waste ready for disposal or transport to the laundry.

Excreta from patients with enteric infections can be discarded into the bedpan washer or macerator in the usual way. It must be placed directly into the machine and not left unattended in the sluice, where it may be inadvertently handled. Pathogens will be destroyed in the bedpan washer provided temperatures of 80°C are achieved for at least 1 minute. This should be checked regularly by looking at the temperature display gauge. Gloves and aprons used to handle or transport excreta should be discarded imme-diately after use and hands washed. Spills of excreta should be wiped up promptly, wearing gloves and aprons, and the area thoroughly cleaned with detergent and water. Chlorine-releasing granules should be used for dealing with spills of blood, but should not be put on to urine as a chemical reaction may release chlorine gas (Department of Health 1990).

Equipment

In most situations normal decontamination procedures are ad-equate for equipment used on a patient with an infectious disease. Advice can be obtained from the local disinfection policy or infection control team. Some items that easily become conta-minated by infectious material, e.g. commodes, must be thoroughly cleaned with detergent before they can be used by another patient.

Items which have not been contaminated, e.g. sealed packs, unused equipment, do not require special cleaning or decontami-nation and do not usually need to be discarded when the patient is discharged. The risk of transmission on crockery and cutlery is negligible and these items should be returned to the catering department in the usual way, where they can be thoroughly washed in an automatic washer (Jackson 1984, Barrie 1996).

Transport of infected patients

The risk of transmission should be minimised by avoiding visits to other departments, but if this is necessary any infected lesions should be covered and personnel involved in the transport should be requested to wash their hands afterwards. Portering staff are unlikely to have contact with infectious material and therefore do not need to wear protective clothing. The receiving department should be informed in advance about the precautions required.

Infrequently, patients who have died may present a risk of infection to mortuary staff or funeral directors. The mortuary will need to be informed when a patient has had tuberculosis, a blood-borne virus or Creutzfeldt–Jakob disease; this will enable them to take the appropriate precautions when handling the body (Healing et al 1995).

Visitors

In most circumstances visitors are unlikely to have contact with infectious material from the patient and do not have contact with other patients on the ward. They should be advised to wash their hands before leaving the room, but do not usually need to wear protective clothing. In the case of infections spread by the airborne route, visitors should be restricted to close relatives while the patient remains infectious. In the case of tuberculosis, close family will already have been exposed to the microorganism and will be followed up by the local authority to establish whether they have already acquired the infection.

Psychological care

Isolation from others is an experience that most people do not enjoy and some find highly stressful. Denton (1986) describes a variety of psychological disorders, including anxiety and hallucinations, that have been reported in isolated patients. More often the patient may become withdrawn, demanding or irritable, behaviours that should be recognised as a response to isolation. Oldman (1998) interviewed patients in isolation and recorded feelings of loneliness, stigmatisation and being forgotten. Different people reacted to isolation in a variety of ways, often depending on their personality. Although some patients enjoyed the privacy, others found it boring and frustrating. Healthcare workers need to be sensitive to the feelings of patients in isolation and adapt their care towards the needs of the individual.

Preparation of the patient for a period of isolation is important. S/he should understand why the precautions are necessary and be given accurate information about the infection and how it is spread. The infection control team will be able to help with this if necessary and educational leaflets may also be available. The psychological care of the patients should therefore be a key part of the care plan of patients in isolation although Knowles (1993) found that this was frequently overlooked.

Isolation is often continued for much longer than necessary and it is important to liaise regularly with the infection control team to ensure that unnecessary or prolonged precautions are not used.

PROTECTION FOR THE IMMUNOCOMPROMISED

Some patients whose immune response has been seriously affected by disease or chemotherapy are particularly at risk of acquiring infection and may need extra protection from normally harmless microorganisms.

Susceptibility to infection depends on the part of the immune system affected. T-cell suppression increases susceptibility to intracellular pathogens such as salmonella, cryptococcus and viruses, while B-cell suppression reduces protection against bacterial pathogens such as staphylococci and pneumococci. The key marker for immunosuppression are the phagocytic cells, in particular neutrophils, since they are essential for the activity of both B and T cells (p. 54). In the past, patients with low neutrophil cell counts were often placed in protective isolation and some hospitals used complex facilities with air filtration systems or plastic isolater tents. Special decontamination procedures and catering facilities were also often provided.

Studies in the 1980s showed that most infections acquired by immunocompromised patients were caused by their own flora, and that the use of simple infection control measures in an open ward were as effective in protecting them from infection as full protective isolation (Nauseef & Maki 1981, Pizzo 1981, Armstrong 1984). The majority of infections acquired by immunocompromised patients are associated with surgical wounds or invasive devices, such as catheters, intravenous cannulas and endotracheal intubation. Efforts at preventing infection should therefore be directed at the care of these devices and the principles of infection control should be rigorously applied (Fishman & Rubin 1998).

Most immunocompromised patients can be managed in a conventional single room. The use of filtered air reduces the risk of aspergillus infection and may be required in hospitals where cases of aspergillosis have occurred (Manuel & Kibbler 1998). Equipment does not usually need special decontamination prior to use, but surfaces should be cleaned regularly to ensure that dust does not accumulate. The principles of routine infection control practice should dictate the use of protective clothing. Staff and visitors with respiratory infections should avoid contact with the patient rather than use masks, which are unlikely to protect patients effectively.

The past practice of autoclaving or irradiating food for these patients has been replaced by carefully selecting the type of food to provide a low-bacteria diet (Barrie 1996). Meat should be thoroughly cooked, fruit and vegetables washed and peeled, and foods likely to be contaminated (e.g. soft cheeses, salads) avoided or, in the case of eggs, well cooked (de Louvois 1993). Food should be eaten fresh and not stored or re-heated. Fresh tap water is safe to drink, but care should be taken with ice in ice-making machines, which can become contaminated and has been associated with outbreaks of infection (Medical Devices Directorate 1993, Ravn et al 1991). Bottled water is frequently contaminated with bacteria and should be stored in the refrigerator and discarded after 3 days (Hunter, 1993).

The key principles of caring for immunocompromised patients are illustrated in List 14.2.

List 14.2 Infection control and the immunocompromised patient

- Advise staff and visitors who have an infection to avoid contact with the patient
- Wash hands before any contact with the patient
- Wear gloves for any contact with invasive devices or susceptible sites
- Remove gloves and wash hands before and after handling invasive devices, body fluids or susceptible sites
- Ensure equipment has been decontaminated properly before use by the patient
- Ensure food is well cooked and served without delay; avoid raw fruit and vegetables, pasteurised milk and delicatessen food

---

APPENDIX: GUIDE TO TRANSMISSION AND MANAGEMENT OF COMMON INFECTIONS/DISEASES

This table provides a guide to the routes of transmission for infections that may be encountered in hospital patients and whether isolation precautions are indicated. Routine infection control precautions should be used in the care of all patients. ICT = infection control team; IDU = infectious diseases unit; NA = not applicable

Infection/disease	Route of transmission	Period of infectivity to others	Isolation precautions	Comments
AIDS: *see* human immunodeficiency virus				
Amoebic dysentery: *Entamoeba histolytica*	Ingestion of faecally contaminated food/water	While cysts being excreted (may be years)	No	
Bronchiolitis (infants)	Respiratory droplets and direct contact with secretions	While symptomatic (5 days or longer)	Yes	Commonly caused by respiratory viruses, e.g. RSV, parainfluenza
Campylobacter	Usually food-borne, also contact with contaminated animals/meat. Person-to-person transmission unlikely	Excreted in faeces for several weeks	No	
Candidiasis	Contact with lesions and secretions	Duration of illness	No	Can be spread by hands or equipment
Cellulitis, e.g. group A streptococci	Direct contact with lesion	Until culture negative or after completion of course of antibiotics	Yes	Organism may be difficult to eradicate from chronic wounds
Chickenpox: Varicella-zoster virus	Inhalation or direct contact with vesicle fluid or respiratory secretions	1–2 days before rash and 5 days after lesions first appear (longer in immunosuppressed)	Yes (single room essential)	Staff attending patient must be immune

Infection/disease	Route of transmission	Period of infectivity to others	Isolation precautions	Comments
Chlamydia trachomatis				
• conjunctivitis	Sexual contact, contact with discharge from eye	May be carried on mucous membranes for months	No	
• genital	Sexual contact		No	
• respiratory	Infected mother to baby during birth		No	
Chlamydia pneumoniae	Not defined but probably airborne, respiratory droplets and direct contact with secretions		No	Spread may occur among families
Cholera	Ingestion of faecally contaminated food or water	During illness (although persistent asymptomatic carriage may occur)	Yes	Case-to-case transmission can occur, so diligence is required
Clostridium perfringens				
• food poisoning	Contaminated food (usually inadequately heated meat)	N/A	No	Heavy bacterial contamination required for transmission to occur
• gas gangrene	Traumatic wounds contaminated by soil; endogenous infection of surgical wounds	N/A	No	Poorly perfused, necrotic wounds required for gangrene to develop
Clostridium difficile – toxigenic strains (pseudomembranous colitis)	Direct/indirect contact with faeces	Duration of diarrhoea	Yes (if symptomatic)	Spores may survive in the environment for prolonged periods. Infection commonly associated with disruption of gut flora due to antibiotic activity

Infection/disease	Route of transmission	Period of infectivity to others	Isolation precautions	Comments
Creutzfeldt–Jakob disease (CJD)	Unknown. Can be transmitted by grafts of human brain tissue, corneas or growth hormone derived from pituitary glands	Duration of illness	No	New-variant CJD probably acquired through ingestion of meat contaminated with bovine spongiform encephalopathy agent
Cryptococcosis: Cryptococcus neoformans	Found in pigeon faeces and soil	Not transmitted from person to person	No	Usually affects immuno-compromised. Causes chronic meningitis but can also infect lungs, kidneys and bone
Cytomegalovirus (CMV)	Intimate contact with mucous membranes. Fetus may be infected in utero, during delivery or by breast milk	Virus excreted in urine and saliva for months. May persist episodically for years	No	Severe disease more likely in immunosuppressed
Diphtheria: Corynebacterium diphtheriae (toxigenic strains)	Direct contact with oral/nasal secretions of infected person	Until throat swabs negative (usually 2 weeks)	Yes	Immunisation in infancy protects against systemic disease; local nasopharyngeal infection may occur
Escherichia coli gastroenteritis				
• enterohaemorrhagic (O157, verotoxin)	Usually food/water-borne, can be transmitted by contact with animals and from person to person	Excreted in faeces for 1 week (longer in children)	Assess risk of trans-mission for individual patients	Associated with haemolytic–uraemic syndrome, usually in under-5s

Infection/disease	Route of transmission	Period of infectivity to others	Isolation precautions	Comments
• enterotoxigenic	Food-borne (developing countries)	Prolonged excretion in faeces	No	Major cause of traveller's diarrhoeas
• enteropathogenic	Food-borne (baby milk and weaning foods). Transmission via hands, especially in nurseries	Prolonged excretion in faeces	No	Causes severe prolonged diarrhoea in infants, especially in developing countries
Ebola virus see Viral haemorrhagic fever				
Erysipelas see Streptococci				
Giardiasis: *Giardia intestinalis*	Ingestion of contaminated drinking water; contact with faeces	Duration of infection (may be months)	Assess risk of transmission for individual patients	Often acquired abroad. Can be transmitted from person to person, especially among children
Glandular fever (infectious mononucleosis): Epstein–Barr virus	Contact with saliva	Oropharyngeal carriage may persist for months or years	No	Infection may be transmitted on hands of staff if contaminated with saliva
Gonorrhoea: *Neisseria gonorrhoeae*				
• genital infection	Sexual contact with infected mucous membranes of genital tract	Until organism eradicated by appropriate therapy	No	
• ophthalmia neonatorum	Infection acquired from infected birth canal during delivery	While discharge persists	Yes	Can be spread by contact with conjunctival discharge

Infection/disease	Route of transmission	Period of infectivity to others	Isolation precautions	Comments
Hepatitis A	Faecal–oral route; food contaminated by infected handler; contaminated water	Maximum infectivity immediately prior to, and for approximately 7 days after onset of jaundice	Assess risk of trans-mission for individual patients	Hepatitis A vaccine or immunoglobulin can be used to protect family contacts from infection
Hepatitis B	Sexually transmitted; blood inoculation through skin or on to mucous membranes; acquired transplacentally or intrapartum from infected mother	May persist indefinitely as carrier state	No (unless uncontrolled bleeding)	Main risk to healthcare workers is from contaminated sharps. All healthcare workers should be protected by vaccination – specific immunoglobulin available
Hepatitis C	As hepatitis B	May persist indefinitely	No	
Hepatitis E	Contaminated water; probably transmitted from person to person by faecal–oral route (not commonly)	Probably similar to hepatitis A	No	
Herpes simplex • cold sores, herpetic whitlow	Direct contact with lesion, exudate or saliva	Virus may be shed into saliva for several weeks after symptoms resolve	No	Staff may develop herpetic whitlow through contact with active cold sores. Staff with active lesions should avoid contact with immunosuppressed patients

Infection/disease	Route of transmission	Period of infectivity to others	Isolation precautions	Comments
• genital herpes	Sexually transmitted	Active lesions infectious for 7–12 days. Transient asymptomatic viral shedding common	No	
• neonatal herpes	Via infected birth canal; can be transmitted congenitally if mother acquires primary infection during pregnancy	Duration of illness	Yes	Separate infant from other neonates. Handle secretions from mother and baby using gloves and aprons
Herpes-zoster virus see Shingles				
Human immunodeficiency virus (HIV)	Sexually transmitted; inoculation of blood/body fluid though skin or on to mucous membranes; transmitted from mother to baby in utero during delivery or shortly after birth	Indefinitely	No	Main risk to healthcare workers is from contaminated sharps
Impetigo: *Staphylococcus aureus*, group A streptococcus	Direct contact with lesion	Duration of lesion (until culture negative or after completion of course of antibiotics)	Yes	Young children often highly susceptible
Lassa fever see Viral haemorrhagic fever				
Legionnaires' disease: *Legionella pneumophila*	Inhalation of contaminated aerosols. Not spread from person to person	NA	No	

Infection/disease	Route of transmission	Period of infectivity to others	Isolation precautions	Comments
Leptospirosis (Weil's disease)	Contact of abraded skin or mucous membranes with water/soil/vegetation contaminated by urine of animals	NA	No	Hazard to farmers, sewer workers etc., water-sports participants, bathers
Listeriosis: *Listeria monocytogenes*	Ingestion of contaminated food; from mother to baby in utero or during delivery	Shed in faeces for several months; shed in vaginal discharge for 7–10 days	Neonates	Outbreaks of infection in nurseries have been reported. Elderly, neonates and immunocompromised particularly susceptible
Lyme disease: *Borrelia burgdorferi*	Transmitted by tick bite	NA	No	Not spread from person to person
Malaria	Transmitted by mosquito bite; transfusion of blood from infected person	NA	No	No person-to-person spread except (rarely) by transfusion of blood
Marburg virus *see* Viral haemorrhagic fever				
Measles	Airborne by respiratory droplets; direct contact with nose/throat secretions	From just before rash appears until 4 days after	Yes	Highly infectious. May cause severe illness in immunosuppressed children. Immunoglobulin available for susceptible patients
Meningitis				
• *Neisseria meningitidis* (meningococcal meningitis)	Direct contact with respiratory droplets, nasal/oral secretions	Until organism no longer present in nasal/oral secretions	Yes (first 24 h of antibiotic therapy)	Most infections subclinical. Rifampicin prophylaxis offered to close *family* contacts

Infection/disease	Route of transmission	Period of infectivity to others	Isolation precautions	Comments
• *Haemophilus influenzae*	Direct contact with respiratory droplets, nasal/oral secretions	Until organism no longer present in nasal/oral secretions (after 48 h of antibiotics)	Not usually	Most common in children between 2 months and 5 years
• viral (e.g. enteroviruses, mumps)	Faecal–oral or respiratory spread (depends on agent)	Before and during acute illness	No	
MRSA *see Staphylococcus aureus*				
Mumps	Transmitted by respiratory droplets and direct contact with saliva	7 days before symptoms appear and up to 9 days after	Yes	Highly infectious. Previous infection confers lifelong immunity
Pneumonia (pneumococcal): *Streptococcus pneumoniae*	Respiratory droplets; direct contact with nasal/oral secretions		No (unless antibiotic-resistant strain)	Susceptibility increased by underlying lung disease, aspiration, immuno-suppression, very young, elderly
Poliomyelitis	Mainly by the faecal–oral route but transmission through direct contact with nasal/oral secretions also occurs	Most infectious for the few days before and after onset of symptoms. Virus persists in faeces for several weeks	Yes (IDU)	Vaccine strain of virus shed in faeces following immunisation: non-immune contacts may be at risk of infection with vaccine virus

Infection/disease	Route of transmission	Period of infectivity to others	Isolation precautions	Comments
Psittacosis: *Chlamydia psittaci*	Inhalation of dust contaminated by bird droppings, secretions or feathers	Birds may shed organisms for weeks	No	Person-to-person transmission by contact with respiratory secretions is unlikely but has been reported. Laboratory staff may acquire infection by handling cultures
Rotavirus	Mainly by faecal–oral route but possibly also through contact with respiratory secretions	Virus shed in faeces for up to 8 days after onset of symptoms (longer in immunocompromised)	Yes	Outbreaks in elderly care and paediatric units reported
Respiratory syncytial virus (RSV)	By direct contact with respiratory secretions or droplets	While symptomatic	Yes	Highly transmissible on paediatric wards
Rubella	Direct contact with respiratory secretions or droplets. Also shed in urine of infants with congenital infection	7 days before and at least 4 days after onset of rash	Yes	Carers should be rubella-immune. In congenital rubella, babies excrete virus for months
Salmonella • enteric fever (*S. typhi* or *S. paratyphi*) • other species	Usually food-borne but can be transmitted from person to person via hands	Excreted in faeces for several weeks (especially infants)	Assess risk of trans-mission for individual patients	Carriers may inadvertently infect food

Infection/disease	Route of transmission	Period of infectivity to others	Isolation precautions	Comments
Scabies	Prolonged skin-to-skin contact	Until mite destroyed by treatment	No (unless Norwegian scabies)	Norwegian scabies only occurs in immuno-compromised, but is highly contagious
Scarlet fever *see* Streptococci				
Shigella	Direct or indirect contact with faeces; can also be water/food borne	Infectious while organism present in faeces	Yes (until symptom-free and normal stool)	Highly infectious. Outbreaks in nurseries caused by transmission on hands
Shingles (herpes zoster)	Contact with lesion exudate	7 days after lesions first appear	Yes	Seronegative contacts develop chickenpox and should be excluded while patient is infectious
Staphylococcus aureus, methicillin-resistant (MRSA)	Direct contact with infected or colonised lesions or skin	While organism present in lesions, in nose or on skin	Yes (seek advice from ICT)	Epidemic strains may cause outbreaks of infection
Streptococci (groups A, C and G)	Direct contact with lesions	Until culture negative (or after course of antibiotics completed)	Yes	
Syphilis: *Treponema pallidum*	Direct contact with lesions during sexual contact; from infected mother to baby	During primary and secondary stages	No	Infectivity rapidly reduced by treatment. Wear gloves for contact with lesions

Infection/disease	Route of transmission	Period of infectivity to others	Isolation precautions	Comments
Tetanus: *Clostridium tetani*	Direct inoculation from contaminated source. Not transmitted from person to person	NA	No	Booster immunisation not required after five doses in childhood or as adult
Toxoplasmosis: *Toxoplasma gondii*	Ingestion of infective oocysts in dirt or tissue cysts in undercooked meat. Primary infection in early pregnancy can result in transplacental infection of fetus	NA	No.	Most infections asymptomatic; immunity develops readily
Tuberculosis (pulmonary) *Mycobacterium tuberculosis*	Inhalation of airborne droplet nuclei	While viable bacilli in sputum	Yes	Prolonged exposure usually required to transmit infection. Infectivity reduced after first 14 days of treatment. Multi-drug-resistant strains should be transferred to IDU
Viral haemorrhagic fever • Lassa • Ebola–Marburg • Crimean–Congo (tick-borne)	Person-to-person transmission by direct contact with blood, pharyngeal secretions or urine, and by sexual intercourse	Variable; depends on virus	Yes – transfer to regional IDU	Crimean–Congo fever is tick-borne; Lassa fever transmitted by direct contact with rat urine. Source of Ebola–Marburg unknown
Whooping cough: *Bordetella pertussis*	Direct contact with respiratory secretions and probably airborne droplets	Highly infectious in early stages; non-infectious 3 weeks after onset of paroxysms	Yes	Children under 5 years most susceptible

REFERENCES

Advisory Committee on Dangerous Pathogens (1996) *Management and Control of Viral Haemorrhagic Fevers*. Stationery Office, London.

Armstrong, D. (1984) Protected environments are expensive and do not offer meaningful protection. *Am. J. Med.*, **76**, 685–689.

Ayliffe, G.A.J., Babb, J.R., Taylor, L. and Wise, R. (1979) A unit for source and protective isolation in a general hospital. *Br. Med. J.*, **ii**, 461–465.

Babb, J.R., Davies, J.G. and Ayliffe, G.A.J. (1983) Contamination of protective clothing and nurses' uniforms in an isolation ward. *J. Hosp. Infect.*, **4**, 49–57.

Barrie, D. (1996) The provision of food and catering services in hospital. *J. Hosp. Infect.*, **33**, 13–33.

Belkin, N.L. (1997) The evolution of the surgical mask: filtering efficiency versus effectiveness. *Infect. Control Hosp. Epidemiol.*, **18**, 48–57.

Breathnach, A.S., de Ruiter, A., Holdsworth, G.M.C. *et al.* (1998) An outbreak of multi-drug resistant tuberculosis in a London teaching hospital. *J. Hosp. Infect*, **39**(2), 111–118.

British Thoracic Society, Joint Tuberculosis Committee (1990) An updated code of practice. *Br. Med. J.*, **30**, 995–1000.

Centers for Disease Control (1987) Recommendations for the prevention of HIV transmission in health care settings. *MMWR*, **21 Aug**, 36(2S).

Control of Infection Group, Northwick Park Hospital and Clinical Research Centre (1974) Isolation system for general hospitals. *Br. Med. J.*, **2**, 41–46.

Denton, P. (1986) Psychological and physiological affects of isolation. *Nursing*, **3**(3), 88–91.

De Louvois, J. (1993) Salmonella contamination of eggs. *Lancet*, **342**, 366–367.

Department of Health (1990) Spills of urine: potential risk of misuse of chlorine-releasing disinfecting agents. *SAB*, **59**(90), 41.

European Standard (1991) Specification for filtering half masks to protect against particles. *BS EN149*. British Standards Institute, London.

Fishman, J.A. and Rubin, R.H. (1998) Infection in organ-transplant recipients. *New Engl. J. Med.*, **338**(24), 1741–1751.

Garner, J.S. (1996) Guideline for isolation precautions in hospital. *Infect. Control Hosp. Epidemiol.*, **17**, 53–80.

Garner, J.S. and Hierholzer, W.J. (1993) Controversies in isolation policies and practice. In: *Prevention and Control of Nosocomial Infections*, 2nd edn (ed. Wenzel, R.P.) Williams & Wilkins, Baltimore, MD.

Garner, J.S. and Simmons, B.P. (1983) Guideline for isolation precautions in hospitals. *Infect. Control*, **4**, 245–325.

Hambraeus, A. (1973) Transfer of *Staphylococcus aureus* via nurses' uniforms. *J. Hyg. (Lond.)*, **71**, 799–714.

Healing, T.D., Hoffman, P.N. and Young, S.E.J. (1995) The infection hazards of human cadavers. *Commun. Dis. Rep. Rev.*, **5**(5), R61–R68.

Health and Safety Executive (1982) The safe disposal of clinical waste. *HN (82)22*. HMSO, London.

Hoffman, P.N. (1993) *Clostridium difficile* and the hospital environment. *PHLS Microbiol. Digest*, **10**(2), 91–92.

Hunter, P. (1993) The microbiology of bottled natural mineral waters. *J. Appl. Bacteriol.*, **74**, 345–352.

Interdepartmental Working Group on Tuberculosis (1998) *The prevention and control of tuberculosis in the United Kingdom. UK guidance on the prevention and control of transmission of I. HIV–related tuberculosis. 2. Drug–resistant, including multiple drug–resistant tuberculosis*. Department of Health Stores, Wetherby.

Jackson, M.M. (1984) From ritual to reason – with a rational approach for the future: an epidemiological perspective. *Am. J. Infect. Control.*, **12**(4), 213–220.

Jackson, M.M. and Lynch, P. (1985) Isolation practices: a historical perspective. *Am. J. Infect. Control*, **13**(1), 21–31.

Jones, E.M. Barnett, J., Perry, C. *et al.* (1997) Control of varicella-zoster infection on renal and other specialist units. *J. Hosp. Infect.*, **36**(2), 133–140.

Knowles, H.E. (1993) The experience of infectious patients in isolation. *Nurs. Times*, **89**(30), 53–56.

Lynch, P., Jackson, M.M., Cummings, M.J. *et al.* (1987) Re-thinking the role of isolation practices in the prevention of nosocomial infections. *Ann. Intern. Med.*, **107**, 243–246.

Maki, D.G., Alvarado, C. and Hassemer, C. (1986) Double bagging of items from isolation rooms is unnecessary as an infection control measure: a comparative study of surface contamination with single and double bagging. *Infect. Control*, 7, 535–537.

Manuel, R.J. and Kibbler, C.C. (1998) The epidemiology and prevention of invasive aspergillosis. *J. Hosp. Infect.*, **39**(2), 95–110.

Medical Devices Directorate (1993) Ice cubes: Infection caused by *Xanthomonas maltophilia. Hazard (93)42.* Medical Devices Directorate, London.

Nauseef, W.M. and Maki, D.G. (1981) A study of the value of simple protective isolation in patients with granulocytopenia. *New Engl. J. Med.*, **304**(8), 448–453.

NHS Executive (1995) Hospital laundry arrangements for used and infected linen. *HSG(95)18.* HMSO, London.

Oldman, T. (1998) Isolated cases. *Nurs. Times*, **94**(11), 67–69.

Olsen, R.J., Lynch, P., Coyle, M.B. *et al.* (1993) Examination gloves as barriers to hand contamination in clinical practice. *J. A. M. A.*, **270**(3); 350–353.

Pizzo, P.A. (1981) The value of protective isolation in preventing nosocomial infections in high risk patients. *Am. J. Med.*, **70**, 631–637.

Ravn, P., Lundgren, J.D., Kjaeldgaard, P. *et al.* (1991) Nosocomial outbreak of cryptosporidiosis in AIDS patients. *Br. Med. J.*, **302**; 277–279.

Selwyn, S. (1991) Hospital infection – the first 2500 years. *J. Hosp. Infect.*, **18**(Suppl. A), 5–65.

UK Health Departments (1990) *Guidance for Clinical Health Care Workers: Protection Against Infection with HIV and Hepatitis Viruses. Recommendations of the Expert Advisory Group on AIDS.* HMSO, London.

Vesley, D. (1995) Respiratory protective devices. *Am. J. Infect. Control*, **23**, 165–168.

Wade, J.J., Desai, N. and Casewell, M.W. (1991) Hygienic hand disinfection for the removal of epidemic vancomycin-resistant *Enterococcus faecium* and gentamicin-resistant *Enterobacter cloacae. J. Hosp. Infect.*, **18**; 211–218.

Weber, D.J. and Rutala, W.A. (1997) Role of environmental contamination in the transmission of vancomycin-resistant enterococci. *Infect. Control. Hosp. Epidemiol.*, **18**; 306–309.

Wilson J. (1995) *Infection Control in Clinical Practice.* Baillière Tindall, London.

Wilson, J. and Breedon, P. (1990) Universal precautions. *Nurs. Times*, **86**(37), 67–70.

FURTHER READING

Bowell, E. (1986) Nursing the isolated patient: Lassa fever. *Nurs. Times*, **33**, 72–81.

Bowell, B. (1992) A risk to others. *Nurs. Times*, **88**(4), 38–40.

Curran, E.T. (1993) Taking down the barriers; a new approach to barrier nursing. *Prof. Nurse*, **9**(7), 472–478.

Edmund, M. (1997) Isolation. *Infect. Control Hosp. Epidemiol.*, **18**, 5–64.

Worsley, M. (1993) A major outbreak of antibiotic-associated diarrhoea. *PHLS Microbiol. Digest*, **10**(2), 97–99.

Glossary

Abscess: a localised collection of pus.

Active immunity: immunity which develops in response to a stimulus, e.g. infection or vaccine, and is dependant on the production of B and T lymphocytes memory cells depending on the production.

Acute infection: an infection which runs its course in a relatively short period.

Aerobe: a microbe that grows in the presence of oxygen. A *strict aerobe* requires oxygen. See anaerobe.

Agar: a polysaccharide made from seaweed and used to solidify bacteriological media.

Agglutinate: to stick to one another, clump (of particles, red cells, etc.); the result is agglutination.

Algae: photosynthetic microbes; the blue-green algae are procaryotes and the others eucaryotes.

Allergy: an undesirable immune response due to hypersensitivity. (See hypersensitivity).

Amoeba: a eukaryotic organism that lacks a rigid cell wall and moves using pseudopods.

Anaerobe: a microbe that grows in the absence of oxygen. A *strict anaerobe* will not grow in the presence of oxygen, a *facultative anaerobe* can grow in the presence or absence of oxygen.

Anaphylaxis: a hypersensitivity reaction.

Antagonism: one antimicrobial drug interferes with another so that the sum of the effect is less than if either were given alone, e.g. penicillin and tetracycline.

Antibiotic: a substance which is toxic to microorganisms; the first antibiotics to be used were derived from other microorganisms but many are now partly or wholly synthesised = antimicrobial agent.

Antibody: a protein produced by B lymphocytes which appears in the body fluids after contact with a foreign molecule, 'antigen', and which combines specifically with that antigen.

Antimicrobial agent: see antibiotic.

Antiseptic: a chemical used to kill microbes on body surfaces.

Antiserum: a serum that contains antibodies to a particular antigen.

Antitoxin: a serum containing antibodies to a toxin, either as a result of natural infection or, more often, in response to injection of toxoid.

Arthropod: an animal which has a hard outer 'skeleton' and jointed legs; examples are insects, ticks and lice.

Aseptic: free of microorganisms.

Attenuated: a microbe that is *attenuated* has lost its virulence and can be safely used as a vaccine.

Autoclave: a machine in which materials can be exposed to steam under pressure and therefore at a temperature higher than that of boiling water.

Autogenous: arising within the individual.

Bacillus: any rod-shaped bacterium; also the name of a genus of Gram-positive bacteria, often found in soil and dust.

Bacteraemia: the presence of bacteria in the blood without clinical signs or symptoms of infection.

Bactericidal: capable of killing bacteria, e.g. penicillins.

Bacteriophage: a virus which infects bacterial cells.

Bacteriuria: colonisation of the bladder by microorganisms without causing signs or symtoms of infection.

Bacteriostatic: a drug which prevents bacteria from replicating; if the drug is withdrawn, bacteria can multiply again, e.g. tetracycline. (A drug that is bacteriostatic may in high concentration or in certain circumstances become bactericidal, e.g. fusidic acid.)

Basophil: a white cell of the blood which attracts lymphocytes to the site of an infection by release of vasoactive chemicals that increase blood flow to the area.

B-cell: one of the two main cell types of the immune system, chiefly involved in the production of antibodies.

BCG strain of tubercle bacili: an attenuated strain that is used as a vaccine against tuberculosis.

Binary fission: division of one cell into two daughter cells, the usual method of reproduction in bacteria.

Broad-spectrum: agents which work against many types of bacteria. Often used for treatment initially when the cause of an infection is unknown.

Capsid: protein coat of a virus, which is made up of polypeptide sub-units.

Carrier: an individual who has a body surface colonised by a pathogen, but without being affected by disease.

Cell-mediated immunity: the part of the immune response medicated by T-Lymphocytes and directed against intracellular pathogens, e.g. viruses, malignant cells.

Cell wall: the rigid outer layer of most prokaryotic cells and of some eukaryotic cells.

Centrifuge: an instrument which can spin liquids in containers at high speed, thus depositing particles on the bottom of the tube. It is often used to concentrate bacteria from body fluids for examination.

Cercaria: the final larval stage of a fluke (trematode).

Chemotaxis: movement of a cell in response to the presence of a chemical.

Chemotherapy: treatment of disease with chemicals; with reference to infection, this means antibiotics.

Clone: a group of organisms descended from a single parent by asexual reproduction and therefore exact copies of it.

Coccobacillus: a short oval rod, i.e. between a coccus and a bacillus in shape.

Coccus: a spherical bacterium.

Colonisation: a microbe that establishes itself in a particular environment such as a body surface without producing disease is said to 'colonise' the site.

Colony: when a bacterial cell (or a few cells) multiplies on a solid medium until the group is visible to the naked eye, the group is called a colony. A typical colony contains 10-100 million cells.

Commensal: a commensal organism lives in association with another, without benefiting or harming it. Many members of the gut flora appear to be commensals. Commensals may be pathogenic if the host is immunocompromised.

Communicable: a disease that can be transmitted from one person to another is communicable (= contagious, = infectious).

Complement: a complex of proteins in the blood; sequential reactions between the component proteins triggered by micro-organisms or an antigen-antibody complex) promote the activity of phagocytic cells.

Conjugation: the transfer of genetic material from one bacterial cell to another by means of a small tube (sex pili) which forms between them.

Conjugative plasmid: a plasmid which causes the genes necessary to form a sex pili and transfer plasmid DNA into another cell.

Contagious: *see* communicable.

Counterstain: a stain used to enhance contrast in a differential stain.

Culture: a culture of microbes is the result of inoculating a medium with them and incubating it until large numbers are present.

Cutaneous: relating to the skin.

Cyst: (a) a sac or closed cavity in the (human or animal) body, filled with fluid or other material; (b) a stage in the lifecycle of some protozoan parasites, in which the organism is encased in a tough outer wall.

Cysticercus: a larval stage of some tapeworms, in which a fluid-filled cyst is formed.

Cystitis: infection of the bladder.

Cytoplasm: in a prokaryote, everything inside the cytoplasmic membrane; in a eukaryote, everything inside the cytoplasmic membrane, except the nucleus.

Cytoplasmic membrane: the membrane which surrounds the cell and retains the cytoplasm.

Cytotoxic: toxic to cells.

Dane particle: a complete and infectious hepatitis B virion; it consists of DNA enclosed in a protein capsid.

Definitive host: the host organism in which the adult form of a parasite lives.

Delayed(-type) hypersensitivity: a hypersensitivity reaction which develops 24 or more hours after exposure to an antigen.

Denaturation: (a) of proteins, the loss of folding brought about by heat or chemicals; associated with the loss of normal biological activity. (b) of DNA, breaking the hydrogen bonds that hold two DNA strands together, resulting in their separation.

Deoxyribonucleic acid (DNA): the large molecule in which genetic information is encoded, the genetic material. The component nucleotides contain the sugar deoxyribose.

Dermatophyte: a fungus that infects the skin, hair and nails without invading the deeper tissues.

Differential stain: a staining procedure that can dye some objects in the preparation but not others.

Diffusion: the process whereby random movement of molecules tends to equalize their concentration across areas of higher and lower concentration.

Diploid: a diploid cell contains two copies of each chromosome. The body cells of most eukaryotic organisms are diploid.

DNA: see deoxyribonucleic acid.

Dysentery: a severe form of infectious diarrhoea, characterised by blood and mucus in the stools.

Enctoparasite: a parasite that lives on the outer surface of the host, e.g. a tick or louse.

Electron: a negatively charged particle.

Electron microscope: a microscope in which a beam of electrons is used instead of light rays to produce an image.

Electrophoresis: the separation of molecules by subjecting them to an electric field in which they move at different rates.

ELISA (enzyme-linked immunosorbent assay): a technique for detecting antigens and antibodies, in which a coloured compound is formed by an enzyme linked to the detector antibody.

Encephalitis: inflammation of the brain.

Endemic: if a disease is endemic, cases regularly occur in the population with little variation in incidence. See epidemic.

Endocarditis: an inflammation, especially one due to infection, of the lining of the heart, including its valves.

Endogenous: arising within the body; an endogenous infection is caused by microorganisms which form part of the normal floral.

Endoplasmic reticulum: a complicated membrane system extending throughout the cytoplasm of the eukaryotic cell.

Endotoxin: lipopolysaccharides in outer membrane of Gram-negative cells. When cells are lysed these are released and can cause severe systemic symptoms (endotoxic shock).

Envelope: an outer membrane that surrounds the capsid of some viruses and may be derived partly or wholly from the host cell.

Enzyme: a protein which catalyses a biochemical reaction.

Eosinophil: a white cell of the blood whose main role is to attack large microorganisms, e.g. protozoa.

Epidemic: when the incidence of an endemic infection increases to an unusually high level or infections not usually seen in that population occur.

Epidemiology: the study of the occurrence of diseases, how and when they occur, how and why they are transmitted.

Eukaryotic cell: one of two types of living cells, in which the nucleus is delimited from the cytoplasm by a membrane.

Exogenous: derived from outside the body; compare 'endogenous'. Exogenous infections are caused by microorganisms acquired from another person, animal or the environment.

Extracellular: outside the cell.

Exotoxin: proteins secreted by bacteria which damage host tissues.

Facultative: an organism which can adapt its metabolism; thus a facultative anaerobe can live in the absence or presence of oxygen.

Fermentation: production of energy from carbohydrates in the absence of oxygen. The electrons generated are passed to organic molecules.

Fibrin: The final product of blood coagulation, formed by the action of the enzyme thrombin on the precursor fibrinogen. Makes a meshwork which seals off damaged blood vessels, i.e. a clot.

Fix: to prepare a specimen for staining; heating causes most bacterial specimens to adhere to the glass slide and is an adequate preparation for staining, other specimens need to be soaked in liquids such as formalin.

Flagellum: a hair-like appendage on the surface of the cell and used for locomotion.

Flatworm: any of the flat-bodied worms, especially the flukes and tapeworms, which are important parasites.

Flora: originally the plant life of an area or period (Flora was the Roman goddess of flowers); bacteria were originally considered to be plants, hence the term is still applied in microbiology to the community of microbes colonising a body region.

Fluke: a parasitic flatworm (= trematode). Adult flukes are important parasites of man, e.g. Fasciola, the liver fluke.

Fluorescent antibody technique: a technique for detecting microbes in which the antibody is tagged with fluorescent dyes and thus rendered visible when viewed with a special microscope (fluorescence microscope) in which ultraviolet light is used.

Fomites: inanimate objects or material on which disease-producing agents may be conveyed, e.g. patients' personal possessions such as bedding, clothes.

Gangrene: Death of tissue or part of the body due to deficiency or cessation of the blood supply.

Gas gangrene: Death of tissue or part of the body due to infection by *Clostridium perfringens*.

Gene: a 'unit of heredity', a segment of DNA that encodes the structure of a protein.

Generation time: the time required for a microbe to undergo division, producing two individuals.

Genetics: the science of heredity.

Genome: the complete set of hereditary genes contained in the chromosomes.

Genus: in biological nomenclature the *genus* is the larger grouping and is written with a capital; the species is the smaller grouping. Both words are modern Latin and are printed in italics.

Glycocalyx: a more or less diffuse layer outside the cell wall of prokaryotes; it consists of polysaccharide, polypeptide or both.

Glycogen: a polysaccharide stored by animals and some bacteria.

Golgi complex: an organelle present in the cytoplasm of eucaryotic cells; it is involved in the secretion of proteins from the cell.

Gram stain: a staining procedure that distinguishes two types of prokaryotes: Gram-positive and Gram-negative.

Habitat: the part of an ecosystem (environment) in which a creature lives.

Haemolysin: an enzyme that lyses red cells. Many bacteria produce haemolysins.

Haploid: a haploid cell contains only one copy of each chromosome. The cells of prokaryotic organisms are haploid. Compare *'diploid'*.

Heat-labile: easily destroyed by heat.

Helix, helical: spiral.

Herd immunity: protection of an entire population against a particular infection, through induction of immunity in at least 60% of individuals.

Hermaphrodite: possessing both male and female sex organs.

Histamine: a molecule released by mast cells; it causes increased permeability of blood vessels, and is responsible for the signs of inflammation; excess is associated with hay fever, asthma, etc.

Histocompatibility antigens: cell-surface antigens involved in many aspects of immunological recognition; they are the main antigens recognised in the rejection of grafts. In humans the chief group of such antigens is called the *HLA antigens*.

HLA antigens: See histocompatibility antigens.

Hypersensitivity: an exaggerated or inappropriate immune response, leading to inflammation or tissue damage.

Icosahedron: a solid figure with 12 (vertices) corners and 20 triangular faces.

Immunity: protection against infection by a particular microbe. Results from infection by or immunisation against that microbe.

Immunisation: the process of artificially inducing immunity to infection by a microbe.

Immunoglobulin: an antibody.

Incubation period: the interval between contact with the microbe and the development of the symptoms and signs of infection.

Infection: entry of a harmful microbe into the body and its multiplication in the tissues.

Inflammation: a response to infection or other injury characterised by swelling, heat, redness and pain.

Inoculum: material (containing bacteria) added to a growth medium to initiate a culture; hence 'inoculate'.

Interferons: a group of immunological proteins which carry signals between cells.

Interleukins: immunological proteins, messenger molecules released by cells of the immune system.

Intermediate host: a host organism in which the larval form of a parasite lives.

In vitro: 'in glass', i.e. carried out in the test-tube, in the laboratory.

In vivo: 'in the living', i.e. in the animal (or patient).

Intracellular: inside cells.

Latent infection: a condition in which the clinical signs of infection are absent and the causative organism may be temporarily undetectable; under certain conditions the infection may again become obvious.

Leucocyte: phagocytic white blood cell, e.g. neutrophil, eosinophils, basophils.

Lipid: a fat, a molecule made up of glycerol and fatty acids.

Lipopolysaccharide: a constituent of the Gram-negative bacterial cell wall, in which chains of various sugars are linked to lipid A.

Lymphocyte: cells involved in the specific immune response. B-lymphocytes produce antibodies, T-lymphocytes attack intracellular pathogens and malignant cells and co-ordinate the activity of other immune system cells.

Lyse: to cause or produce disintegration of a compound, susbtance or cell, to undergo lysis.

Lysis: destruction or decomposition of a cell under the influence of a specific agent.

Lysosome: an intracellular organelle, contains enzymes that digest unwanted molecules.

Lysozyme: an enzyme that can dissolve the cell walls of certain bacteria.

Malaise: a general feeling of being unwell.

Macrophage: a type of phagocyte mainly found in the tissues.

Mantoux test: a tuberculin skin test.

Mast cell: mediator cells in the tissues which influence the response of the immune system by releasing vasoactive chemicals, e.g. histamine. Responsible for the inflammatory response and hypersensitivity reactions.

Meiosis: a form of cell division, characteristic of eukaryotic cells; it results in haploid progeny cells (male and female gametes).

Membrane filter: a filter, usually made from a cellulose derivative, which contains large numbers of pores of a specified size.

Messenger RNA: the transcript of the DNA from which a polypeptide is synthesised by the ribosome.

Metabolism: a general term for all the biochemical process that occur in a living cell.

Metabolite: break-down products of the process of metabolism. This may pertain to bacterial or human cell metabolism.

Micrometre (μm): a unit of length, $= 10^{-6}$ metres.

Microorganism: a creature too small to be seen with the naked eye (or only just visible); the term includes bacteria, fungi, protozoa, some of the algae and the viruses.

Minimal inhibitory concentration (MIC): the lowest concentration of an antibiotic or other agent that will inhibit the growth of a microorganism.

Mitochondrion: an intracellular organelle that contains the energy-generating systems of eukaryotic cells.

Mitosis: division of a eukaryotic cell into two diploid daughter cells.

Monocyte: a white cell of the blood, which develops into the tissue macrophage.

Monolayer: a single layer of tissue cells used to culture viruses.

Mutation: a change in the sequence of the bases in the DNA strand.

Myalgia: pain in the muscles, a feature of many viral infections.

Mycelium: an intertwined mass of filaments (hyphae), typical of the growth of fungi.

Mycoses: infections caused by fungi; can be superficial, e.g. affecting the skin, or deep, invading tissue causing systemic infection.

Nanometer: a unit of length, $= 10^{-9}$ m (10^{-3} micrometer).

Narrow-spectrum: an antibiotic with activity against only one, or a limited range of bacteria.

Natural killer cells: large lymphoid cells capable of killing cells with the appropriate receptors on the surface.

Neutrophil: a phagocytic white cell of the blood. Accounts for most white cells circulating in the blood.

Nitrogen cycle: the series of reactions whereby nitrogen is converted from atmospheric nitrogen gas to organic compounds and back to gas again.

Normal flora: the community of microbes that colonises a body surface.

Nosocomial: acquired or occurring in a hospital; e.g. a nosocomial infection. = a hospital-acquired infection.

Nucleolus: an area in the nucleus of a eukaryotic cell where RNA is synthesised.

Nucleotide: a constituent of DNA or RNA, made up of a sugar, an organic base and a phosphate group.

Nucleus: (a) the central part of an atom, made up of protons and neutrons. Or (b) the part of the eukaryotic cell that contains the genetic material.

Objective lens: the lens of a microscope which forms the primary image of the specimen.

Obligate: an obligate organism is restricted to a particular way of life; e.g. an obligate parasite cannot live free without a host.

Obligate aerobe/anaerobe: see aerobe, anaerobe.

Ocular lens: the lens of a microscope which further magnifies the primary image formed by the objective lens.

Opportunistics organism: one capable of causing infection when the immune system of the host is impaired.

Organelle: a distinct structure within the cytoplasm of a eukaryotic cell that possesses a separate function; e.g. the mitochondria, Golgi complex.

Organic: an organic compound is one that contains carbon.

Oxidation: the addition of oxygen to, or the removal of electrons from, a substance.

Pandemic: a worldwide outbreak of an infectious disease.

Parasite: an organism that lives in or on another creature and obtains food and shelter without benefitting the host. Hence 'parasitism'. See commensal, symbiosis.

Parenteral: administered by injection directly into the tissues, e.g. subcutaneously, intramusculary, intravenously.

Passive immunity: immunity conferred on the host animal by antibodies made in another host.

Pathogen: a microbe capable of causing disease.

Pathogenicity: the ability of a microbe to invade and cause disease.

Peptide: a chain of amino acids.

Peptidoglycan: a major structural component of bacterial cell walls, consisting of chains of sugars cross-linked by peptides.

Peptones: short chains of amino acids derived from the breakdown of proteins.

pH: the symbol denoting hydrogen ion concentration; the pH ranges between 0 and 14 and its value indicates the relative acidity or alkalinity of a solution.

Phagocyte: a cell capable of phagocytosis.

Phagocytosis: the ingestion of material by a cell either in order to destroy foreign matter or for its own nutrition.

Phase-contrast microscope: a microscope which is fitted with a special illumination system that reveals the structure of living cells without the need for staining.

Photosynthesis: the use of solar energy by green plants and some bacteria to synthesise carbon compounds from CO_2 and water.

Plasma: the fluid in which blood cells are suspended. It contains a high concentration of protein, and inorganic salts, e.g. sodium, potassium, calcium.

Plasma cell: a cell that develops from a B-lymphocyte and that manufactures a specific antibody.

Plasmid: a small circle of DNA which may be present in the cytoplasm of a microbial cell. Plasmids often carry genes for antibiotic resistance.

Pleomorphic: varied in shape.

Polymer: a molecule made up of similar subunits.

Polymorphonuclear leucocyte: the blood contains three polymorphonuclear leucocytes, the neutrophil, the eosinophil and the basophil.

Polypeptide: a chain of amino acids, containing at least four and usually more.

Precipitate: the result of a reaction between two soluble substances to form an insoluble material that 'falls' out of solution.

Precipitin reaction: a reaction between antigen and antibody which results in a visible precipitate.

Primary response: the production of antibody in response to the first contact with the antigen.

Probe: a short single-stranded segment of DNA or RNA which is identical in base sequence to a part of a gene, plasmid, ribosome, etc., and which can be used to detect the presence of the gene or plasmid, and hence to identify the microbe of which it is a part, or to detect a hereditary defect.

Prokaryotic cell: one of two chief types of living cells, in which the nucleus is not delimited from the cytoplasm by a membrane. In general prokaryotic cells are smaller and of less complex structure than eukaroyotic cells.

Prophylaxis: treatment which is intended to prevent disease rather than cure it after it has developed; e.g. prophylactic antibiotic therapy.

Protein: a large molecule, one of the main constituents of living matter; it consists of one or more polypeptide chains.

Protozoa: microscopic single-celled eukaryotic microbes; some are free-living, others are important parasites.

Pseudopod: an extension of the cytoplasm of a cell; pseudopods are formed for the purposes of feeding and locomotion.

Pus: an accumulation of fluid due to infection; it consists of living and dead microbes, phagocytes and tissue cells, together with the fluid that has accumulated in the tissue because of inflammation.

Reservoir (of infection): the site where a microorganism normally lives and the permanent source of infection; e.g. foxes are a reservoir of rabies in Western Europe.

Respiration: the generation of energy by the conversion of organic compounds to carbon dioxide and water.

Reverse transcriptase: an enzyme that synthesises DNA from an RNA template. The human immunodeficiency virus contains a reverse transcriptase.

Ribonucleic acid (RNA): a nucleic acid in which the component nucleotides contain the sugar ribose. The ribonucleic acids of cells are messenger RNA, transfer RNA and ribosomal RNA; in addition the genome of some viruses consists of RNA.

Ribosome: the protein-synthesising 'factory' of the cytoplasm.

Saprophyte: an organism that lives on dead organic matter.

Scolex: the head of a tapeworm, armed with suckers and often with hooks.

Sensitivity: the susceptibility of certain organisms to specific agents.

Septicaemia: bacteraemia accompanied by symptoms and signs of infection and illness with no other recognised cause.

Serotype: a strain of a bacterial species which can be differentiated by the antigens present on its surface; these are detected by antibodies (serological methods).

Serum: the liquid that separates from clotted blood. Similar composition to plasma but without substances used in coagulation, e.g. fibrinogen.

Species: *see* genus.

Subclinical infection: an infection which produces no symptoms or signs of disease; said of the early stages or a very mild form of the disease.

Subcutaneous: beneath the skin.

Superinfection: acquisition of a more resistant strain of the organism already causing infection, or replacement of normal flora by antibiotic-resistant organisms because of antibiotic use.

Symbiosis: an association between two species in which there is mutual benefit.

Symptoms and signs: symptoms are the patient's complaints; signs are the physical evidence of disease.

Syndrome: a set of symptoms and signs that forms a distinctive clinical picture suggesting a particular disease.

Synergy: when the effect of two antiboitics (or other drugs) given together is greater than can be accounted for by the effect of each acting alone, this is said to be due to synergy.

Systemic: involving the whole body.

Teichoic acid: a polymer of an alcohol, phosphate and other molecules found in Gram-positive cell walls.

Titre (titer): a measure of the concentration of an antibody in serum.

Topical: a drug that is applied directly to the affected part (e.g. skin or eye) is applied *topically*.

Toxin: any poisonous substance produced by a living organism, especially a microbe.

Toxoid: a microbial toxin treated (usually with dilute formaldehyde) so that its toxic activity is destroyed, but it is still capable of stimulating the production of antibodies which recognise the microbial toxin.

Trace element: a chemical element required for growth, but only needed in very small amounts.

Transcription: copying the sense strand of the DNA into messenger RNA.

Transduction: the introduction of new genes into a bacterial cell, by a bacteriophage. The new genes are derived from the bacterium in which the phage previously replicated.

Transfer RNA: small RNA molecules which carry individual amino acids to the ribosome.

Transformation: the introduction of new genes into a cell by the uptake of fragments of DNA from solution.

Translation: synthesising a polypeptide chain from the messenger RNA template.

Tuberculin test: a skin test used to detect infection by mycobacteria.

Ultraviolet light: invisible light of wavelength shorter than the light at the violet end of the visible spectrum.

Uracil: an organic base found in RNA.

Vaccination: the process of inducing immunity by administering a vaccine.

Vaccine: a preparation of killed or inactivated microbes, inactivated microbial toxins or microbial antigens used to induce immunity.

Vector: an animal, usually an arthropod (insect or tick) that transfers an infectious microbe from one host to another.

Virulence: the ability of an organism to cause disease.

Zoonosis: an infectious disease of animals that may be transmitted to man. Brucellosis, rabies and toxoplasmosis are examples.

Index